Color Atlas of

VETERINARY CARDIOLOGY

Peter GG Darke
BVSc, PhD, DVR, DVC, MRCVS
Department of Veterinary Clinical Studies
Royal (Dick) School of Veterinary Studies
University of Edinburgh, UK

John D Bonagura
DVM. DACVIM (Cardiology, Internal Medicine)
Gilbreath-McLorn Professor of Veterinary Cardiology
University of Missouri–Columbia College of Veterinary Medicine
USA
Formerly
Professor of Veterinary Clinical Sciences
The Ohio State University College of Veterinary Medicine
USA

Donald F Kelly
MA, PhD, BVSc, MRCVS, FRCPath
Professor of Veterinary Pathology
University of Liverpool, UK

Mosby-Wolfe

London Baltimore Barcelona Bogotá Boston Buenos Aires Caracas Carlsbad, CA Chicago Madrid Mexico City Milan Naples, FL New York
Philadelphia St. Louis Seoul Singapore Sydney Taipei Tokyo Toronto Wiesbaden

Acknowledgements
The following illustrations have been reproduced with the permission of the publishers:
13.1, 13.4b and c, 14.2, 15.1b and 15.7c from Ettinger, Textbook of Veterinary Internal Medicine, W.B.Saunders, 1995.
1.10, 5.6, 9.15, 15.15, 17.4, 18.1, 19.6 and 20.2 from Sherding, The Cat, Diseases and Clinical Management. W.B.Saunders, 1995.
7.1, 7.2a, 7.3, 7.18, 9.20a, 9.22b, 11.9a, 21.7a–c from Darke PGG. Doppler Echocardiography. *J Small Anim Pract* 1992; **33**: 104–12.

Published in 1996 by Mosby-Wolfe, an imprint of Times Mirror International Publishers Limited

Printed by G. Canale & C.S.p.A. – Borgaro T.se – TURIN

ISBN 0 7234 1907 8

For full details of all Times Mirror International Publishers Limited titles, please write to Times Mirror International Publishers Limited, Lynton House, 7–12 Tavistock Square, London WC1H 9LB, England.

A CIP catalogue record for this book is available from the British Library.

Library of Congress Cataloging-in-Publication Data applied for.

Project Manager: Deborah Russell

Layout Artist: Jonathan Brenchley

Cover Design: Paul Phillips

Illustration: Lee Smith

Production: Siobhan Egan

Index: Angela Cottingham

Publisher: Jane Hunter

Contents

Preface

To many practitioners, cardiac diseases retain an unjustified mystique. Cardiac disorders can be overlooked easily or blamed unjustly for many ills. However, the correlations between cardiovascular pathology and pathophysiology and the resultant clinical signs are both logical and increasingly understood. The sophistication of cardiac diagnosis has improved remarkably in the last decade. Although a thorough clinical examination remains the cornerstone of accurate diagnosis and clinical assessment, the appropriate selection of noninvasive cardiac examinations is increasingly important. These studies, which include radiography, electrocardiography and echocardiography, can provide accurate insight into the anatomic and functional nature of most circulatory disturbances, even if the precise aetiology remains obscure. Our greater understanding of pathophysiology also has important implications for therapy, which can increasingly be directed at reversing dysfunction, in addition to symptomatic treatment. Likewise, the range of drugs with proven efficacy available to the clinician is at last expanding.

This Atlas aims to illustrate and summarize the most common cardiac disorders in dogs, cats, horses and cattle. The practice of clinical cardiology is largely visual: we inspect animals, anatomic lesions, radiographs, electrocardiograms and echocardiographic studies. There are, of course, restrictions to this approach. A thorough clinical examination cannot readily be portrayed in this format, nor can we adequately portray the physical characteristics of heart sounds and murmurs in a Colour Atlas! Despite these limitations, we hope that students and veterinary practitioners will find the figures, accompanying text, and the tables educational and useful for managing patients with cardiac disease. We believe that this Atlas will find a place between more extensive textbooks of cardiovascular pathology, medicine and surgery.

The authors have divided this Atlas into 23 chapters. Chapters 1 and 2 offer a general discussion of cardiac failure and its therapy as well as a description of proper techniques for the post mortem cardiac examination. Chapters 3 to 8 consider the principal diagnostic studies used in clinical cardiology. The relative merits of the main clinical diagnostic techniques, with normals, variations of normal, and some classic disturbances are illustrated. The bulk of this Atlas, Chapters 9 to 23, uses case materials to review the most important congenital and acquired heart diseases. Included are summaries of: valvular heart disease, myocardial diseases, pericardial diseases and cardiac tumours, vascular diseases, and cardiac dysrhythmias. These chapters use optimal illustrations, obtained from different animals, to represent the typical clinical features of important disorders. While we aim to emphasize the usual, the reader should bear in mind that the next case of any encountered disorder may not be a 'typical' representation. Since the clinical presentation of most cardiac disorders differs little among species, we have elected to include dogs, cats, horses and cattle in our discussions – emphasizing commonality while identifying differences when clinically important.

Each of the authors has been privileged to work with many talented clinical colleagues. A number of the cases illustrated in this Atlas are derived from examinations and studies performed in collaboration with these outstanding individuals, including: Drs Jim Buchanan, Helio DeMorais, Virginia Luis Fuentes, Bruce Keene, Linda Lehmkuhl, Karen Long, Matt Miller, Mike O'Grady, Don Patterson, Rebecca Stepien and Wendy Ware.

This work is not intended to be comprehensive or to replace detailed textbooks of internal medicine or pathology. Nevertheless, we have tried to fill the text with the concepts, facts and experiences we believe are most useful for clinical practice. We have endeavoured to give the reader important clinical information in tabular form. It is our hope that this information will be concise and practical. Finally, we hope to emphasize throughout that optimal management of cardiac disease requires a veterinarian with these qualities: a knowledge of relevant pathology and pathophysiology; an ability to conduct a careful clinical examination; the willingness to investigate clinical signs by choosing appropriate diagnostic tests; and a logical approach to the diagnosis and treatment of defined disorders.

Peter Darke
John Bonagura
Donald Kelly

1. Heart Failure

CONCEPTS OF CARDIAC FAILURE

The circulation has an enormous reserve capacity, and a fit animal's cardiac output can increase severalfold during vigorous exercise. The circulation can, therefore, accommodate considerable cardiac disease in a sedentary animal before signs of cardiac failure are noticed. However, a performance animal, such as a racehorse, a racing greyhound or a working collie, may demonstrate a lack of circulatory reserves when affected by relatively minor disease. In fact, one definition of cardiac failure is the failure to perform exercise owing to cardiac limitations and the inadequate perfusion of skeletal muscle.

Insufficient cardiac output, and hence low arterial blood pressure, may develop from disorders of the heart that lead to either systolic dysfunction or diastolic dysfunction, or both. Arrhythmias further reduce cardiac output because electrical activity dictates mechanical activity. Regardless of the underlying cause, compensation for insufficient cardiac output can include any or all of the following: activation of the sympathetic nervous system, systemic arterial vasoconstriction, redirection of cardiac output among the various regional circulations, renal retention of sodium and water, and cardiac dilatation and hypertrophy. Each of these mechanisms is a useful short-term adaptation to a decline in cardiac output; however, chronic activation of these systems can injure the animal and lead to clinical signs that we associate with heart failure.

Sympathetically mediated tachycardia, myocardial stimulation, and vasoconstriction are effective methods for maintaining blood pressure; however, these adaptations may limit the diastolic interval for ventricular filling, increase myocardial oxygen demand, precipitate arrhythmias and injure the myocardium. In myocardial failure, chronic sympathetic activation actually shortens the life span.

Systemic vasoconstriction develops through one or more mechanisms, including sympathetic alpha-adrenergic mediated vasoconstriction, the renin–angiotensin system, release of arginine vasopressin (ADH), and inhibition of various vasodilator mechanisms. Vasoconstriction can impose an afterload 'mismatch' on a failing ventricle and further reduce stroke volume; mitral regurgitation is also exacerbated. These concepts form the basis for using vasodilators to increase stroke volume in dilated cardiomyopathy and mitral regurgitation.

Peripheral vasoconstriction leads to increased systolic tension (afterload) in the ventricular myocardium (which increases the myocardial demand for oxygen and may impede its coronary supply), and it may reduce the blood supply to regional tissues such as skeletal muscle, prompting loss of condition of muscle cells. Moreover, the renin–angiotensin–aldosterone system has been shown to be directly injurious to the myocardium, and angiotensin-converting enzyme (ACE) inhibitors prolong life and decrease clinical signs of congestive heart failure in chronic myocardial failure.

The renal retention of sodium and water characterizes all forms of heart failure, particularly those that involve a component of right-sided failure. Expanding the plasma volume leads to an increase in preload via improved venous return and ventricular filling. Sodium and water retention is mediated partly by aldosterone and ADH secretion, and also by intrinsic changes in renal blood flow that develop in heart failure. Sodium and water retention, when severe, leads to volume overload and tissue oedema in the syndrome known as congestive heart failure (CHF).

The failing heart may be stimulated to contract more vigorously through increased sympathetic drive and cardiac dilatation (Frank–Starling effect), but this response is optimal only if the myocardium is healthy. Sympathetic stimulation and cardiac dilatation lead to increased oxygen consumption and predispose to numerous arrhythmias. Furthermore, extreme dilatation or hypertrophy impair the diastolic properties of the ventricle and reduce ventricular filling (or require it to occur at higher than normal venous pressures).

Failure to respond to a sudden drop in arterial pressure will cause signs of *low cardiac output*: acutely, this may cause weakness, syncope or death; chronically, it may cause weakness or exercise intolerance. Low output is typically caused by myocardial disease with loss of systolic function, cardiac dysrhythmias (bradycardias or tachycardias) or ventricular outflow obstruction, but it is also encountered with mitral regurgitation and pulmonary hypertension.

CLINICAL SIGNS OF CARDIAC FAILURE

Cardiac failure is manifested in many ways. Few clinical signs are unique to cardiac failure, and a clinician can easily be confused by the coincidental detection of insignificant cardiac disease in one animal with clinical signs that might represent cardiac failure in another. For example, an ageing pet dog with a systolic murmur of mild mitral regurgitation may develop a cough. This cough may be secondary to the mitral regurgitation (especially due to the compressive effect of the dilated left atrium on the left mainstem bronchus), or it may be due to some other disease (such as pulmonary neoplasia or chronic bronchitis), with the mitral regurgitation being a confusing irrelevance. Similarly, a dog with clinical bradycardia and poor exercise tolerance may have a bradycardia sufficient to limit cardiac output at exercise. Alternatively, the bradycardia and muscle weakness might be caused by some metabolic disturbance (e.g. hypothyroidism or hyperkalaemia), and the bradycardia be a minor factor in the exercise intolerance.

Thorough cardiopulmonary assessment is vital for correct treatment, and careful evaluation of the entire animal is imperative. Most cardiac diseases are easily detected by any clinician reasonably proficient with a stethoscope. The important question is whether this disturbance is the cause of clinical signs, or whether these signs perhaps result from another disease process, elsewhere in the body.

The *breed*, *age* and *sex* of the animal can often guide the clinician to a possible diagnosis. For example, murmurs in young animals are likely to be associated with congenital heart disease, although innocent murmurs are often also found in young dogs; however, it should always be borne in mind that a murmur from a congenital lesion may still be identified when the animal is ageing. Conversely, in ageing animals, neoplasia must be an increasing possibility and, in dogs and horses, degenerative heart-valve disease becomes increasingly prevalent with age. Furthermore, chronic respiratory and endocrine diseases, and renal failure, occur more frequently in ageing animals, and may compromise cardiac function.

Many breeds of animal are predisposed to particular diseases. For example, congenital aortic stenosis is seen most frequently in certain larger breeds of dog such as golden retrievers, boxer dogs, German shepherd dogs and Newfoundlands; Arabian horses are predisposed to ventricular septal defects and other complex malformations; dilated cardiomyopathy is prevalent in large and giant breeds of dog, together with cocker and springer spaniels; while mitral valve disease is found in certain ageing smaller breeds (e.g. Pekinese and cavalier King Charles spaniels).

Many cardiac diseases are found more frequently in males than females (e.g. cardiomyopathies). However, a few (e.g. patent ductus arteriosus) occur more frequently in females.

CARDIAC OUTPUT FAILURE

Signs of low cardiac output include depression, exercise intolerance, weakness or collapse. Collapse may be solitary, recurrent and episodic, or terminal (cardiac arrest). Objective assessment of exercise tolerance is not easily achieved in animals: of the domestic species, only horses readily cooperate with exercise testing. Furthermore, exercise intolerance can be due to disorders of other body systems (e.g. respiratory or musculoskeletal), or to some psychological, metabolic or neurological disturbance.

Collapse associated with low cardiac output is often provoked by excitement or exercise, and it tends to be syncopal in nature: the animal shows sudden weakness, and then falls down unconscious, often with brief vocalization and opisthotonos, but otherwise with little muscular movement. Urination may occur, but other signs of autonomic release are uncommon. The mucous membranes are initially likely to be pale rather than cyanosed; recovery may be swift, and complete within seconds or minutes.

In contrast to this, epileptiform seizures occur most often when the animal is at rest or waking, and although the animal may be unconscious, muscle tremor or tonic/clonic spasm is often seen. Many activities are stimulated – the eyes may move rapidly, there may be tachypnoea, salivation, vocalization, and urination or defecation. Another type of collapse is tussive syncope. This resembles a cardiac event but invariably follows an episode of coughing.

Not all animals that collapse follow one of these patterns slavishly, but careful history-taking is vital in trying to classify the disorder.

CONGESTIVE CARDIAC FAILURE

The development of congestive cardiac failure is often relatively slow, especially with diseases such as mitral regurgitation. However, acute failure can be seen with pericardial haemorrhage, for example, or with rupture of chordae tendineae. In most cases, congestive failure is a debilitating state, with cachexia, fluid accumulation in vital tissues such as the liver and lungs and pooling in body cavities, and there are often concurrent signs of insufficient cardiac output, with tissue hypoxia, lethargy, exercise intolerance and weakness.

Congestive failure is often primarily right- or left-sided in the early stages. For example, left-sided failure is typically associated with mitral regurgitation and some cases of cardiomyopathy, while signs of right-sided failure are encountered with pericardial effusions, cor pulmonale, tricuspid or pulmonic valve diseases, and many chronic cardiomyopathies. Left-sided failure typically leads to respiratory signs and loss of cardiac output, while right-sided failure is seen as accumulation of fluid in body cavities and peripheral oedema.

The classic signs of congestive failure may include tachypnoea and respiratory distress (due to pulmonary oedema or hydrothorax) and abdominal enlargement (due to ascites and hepatomegaly). Right-sided failure frequently causes subcutaneous oedema in large animals, but this sign is seen less often in small animals.

Coughing is a prominent sign of left-sided failure in dogs, but this may be due to the gross enlargement of the left atrium that is especially characteristic of the slow development of mitral valve regurgitation in this species. This large left atrium can cause partial airway obstruction which may be the major contributor to coughing: some dogs cough prior to the development of overt pulmonary oedema. Many animals tolerate congestive cardiac failure reasonably for weeks or months, but are incapable of sustaining much physical activity. Nonetheless, congestive failure often responds very well to symptomatic therapy, which is optimized by an understanding of the pathophysiology of this type of cardiac failure.

THERAPY FOR CARDIAC FAILURE

Careful management of an animal with cardiac failure can be as important as specific therapy. Few cardiac disorders can be cured, and although animals can compensate reasonably for severe cardiac disease if they are adequately rested, many show gross exacerbation of signs of cardiac failure with any activity. Sedentary domestic cats and housed pigs often show few signs of cardiac failure until the disease is well advanced. Any animal with cardiac failure may benefit from moderate-to-severe exercise restriction. In severe cardiac failure, sedation may be required; opiates such as morphine may be indicated, as may careful use of phenothiazine derivatives such as acepromazine, or benzodiazepines such as diazepam.

Plans for urgent treatment should be separated from chronic heart failure therapy. Often the goals and type of therapy will differ. Chronic therapy for syndromes involving systolic dysfunction (e.g. dilated cardiomyopathy or chronic mitral valvular insufficiency) usually involves the administration of diuretics, ACE inhibitors, and digoxin. Diastolic dysfunction (e.g. hypertrophic cardiomyopathy or pericardial diseases) may require a different approach (see specific chapters for details).

Diuresis is of paramount importance in congestive failure. Diuretics are needed to reduce oedema rapidly in severe CHF and are also important for preventing the chronic retention of sodium and water in chronic heart failure. Furosemide (frusemide) is generally the agent of first choice in all species, but other drugs such as thiazides and amiloride (which act at other sites in the kidney) may also be indicated in resistant fluid retention.

In mitral regurgitation or dilated cardiomyopathy, vasodilators have proven value through alterations in haemodynamics or neurohormonal activity. Arteriolar dilators should increase cardiac output, reduce mitral regurgitation, and reduce left ventricular myocardial tension (afterload). Venodilators should reduce venous congestion, particularly in the lungs, by pooling blood in systemic veins. The first choice for *chronic therapy* is an ACE inhibitor such as enalapril. This should also decrease plasma aldosterone, and may suppress other inappropriate sympathetic activity. Hydralazine, entirely an arteriolar dilator, has been used widely in dogs, and has its greatest value in the management of severe life-threatening pulmonary oedema caused by mitral regurgitation or in the 'last-ditch' therapy for chronic heart failure that has not responded to other therapy. Very potent agents such as sodium nitroprusside are used at centres with intensive monitoring, in animals with severe life-threatening cardiac failure, but this drug cannot be safely used without strict supervision. Venodilators such as nitroglycerine (glyceryl trinitrate), available as a cream for percutaneous absorption, have been widely used in small animal centres to reduce pulmonary overload, particularly in pulmonary oedema.

Cardiac glycosides have been used in veterinary medicine for over a century. The rationale for their use is usually two-fold: as positive inotropes, and to sensitize baroreceptors which withdraws sympathetic tone and increases vagal activity. Digitalis exerts a favourable effect on the resting heart rate and may improve haemodynamics in some patients. Digoxin is the glycoside favoured by most cardiologists, but it must always be used with great care, as the therapeutic margin for this drug is very narrow. The prime indications for glycosides in dogs are dilated cardiomyopathy (in which the loss of contractility calls for inotropic support) and atrial fibrillation (which often calls for control of the ventricular rate response). However, the inotropic support provided by glycosides is mild and, in severe cases of low cardiac output due to dilated cardiomyopathy, a 24–72 hour intravenous infusion of dobutamine or dopamine is often more effective. The use of glycosides in cardiac failure due to other disorders such as primary mitral regurgitation is more controversial, though the tendency is to prescribe digoxin when signs are related to CHF rather than a cough from a compressed bronchus. Digitalis glycosides may still help by improving autonomic balance and either suppress or help to control supraventricular tachyarrhythmias, especially atrial fibrillation. Glycoside toxicity takes the form of an ill-defined poisoning: acute lethargy and anorexia, often with vomiting or diarrhoea. Administration of the drug should always be stopped, at least temporarily, if these signs are seen. The best way to monitor digoxin therapy is to measure blood concentrations of the drug on a regular basis, using the laboratory's guidelines for therapeutic concentrations. The dose of digoxin can be calculated on the basis of body surface area, but probably the best guideline is to start with a conservative dose (see Appendix) and then adjust the dose according to serum concentrations. The dosage should be reduced in azotaemia, hypokalaemia, hypothyroidism, or in aged or obese animals.

According to the animal's status, there may be a need for other symptomatic therapy for heart failure. In dogs, coughing is frequently encountered in advanced mitral regurgitation, due partly to mechanical compression of the left mainstem bronchus by the dilated left atrium. Treatment of chronic airway disease may be required with bronchodilators such as aminophylline, cough suppressants such as butorphanol or hydrocodone, and even a brief course of glucocorticoids to reduce the cough. In small animals, pleural effusion can be life-threatening, and thoracocentesis may be essential. It is generally undesirable to drain retained fluids such as ascites repeatedly, as this will cause severe protein loss and the loss of plasma volume will simply trigger further sodium and water retention. Adequate diuresis is preferable, and may be best performed in the hospital.

Although few cardiac disorders can be cured, specific therapies have been developed for a number of lesions, including congenital heart disease, pericardial effusions, dirofilariasis, some cardiomyopathies and many cardiac dysrhythmias. Of the congenital malformations, patent ductus arteriosus can be occluded by careful surgery in all species. In dogs, pulmonic stenosis can be effectively relieved in most cases by transvenous balloon valvuloplasty, and palliative surgery can be undertaken to reduce the adverse effects of tetralogy of Fallot and septal defects. For pericardial effusions in any species, pericardiocentesis should help in diagnosis, as well as therapeutically. If pericardial effusions are persistent or recurrent, thoracotomy may be indicated to try to identify a source of the effusion, or to provide permanent relief of tamponade, either by pericardiectomy or by marsupialization. In cardiomyopathies (notably in cats, in which the precise type of dysfunction should be identified), the animal may require therapy with a calcium antagonist such as diltiazem or a beta blocker such as propranolol or atenolol to prevent further bouts of congestive cardiac failure (see Chapter 17). Therapy for cardiac dysrhythmias can be life-saving (e.g. with cardiac pacemakers in heart block), or in the suppression of tachycardias with appropriate drugs. These are addressed in Chapter 23. Some specific treatment plans for common conditions are summarized below.

TREATMENT PLANS FOR COMMON CONDITIONS

CHRONIC MITRAL VALVE REGURGITATION

- The clinician must distinguish between true congestive heart failure (pulmonary oedema) and clinical signs that result from bronchial compression. Any drug that decreases heart size (e.g. furosemide plus an angiotensin inhibitor, or furosemide plus digoxin) may relieve the mechanical cough.
- Acute life-threatening pulmonary oedema is treated with intravenous furosemide, oxygen, oral hydralazine, and percutaneous nitroglycerine (see Appendix for dosages). Less severe cases usually respond to cage rest and one or two doses of furosemide. Longer-term therapy can then begin.
- Prolonged therapy for congestive heart failure may include dietary sodium restriction, digoxin, furosemide, and an ACE inhibitor (e.g. enalapril).
- In advanced cases that are becoming refractory to increasing diuretic doses, both enalapril (decreased to once daily) and hydralazine (twice daily) can be prescribed, as well as a maintenance dose of digoxin. Arterial blood pressure and renal function should be monitored when using such therapy.
- Cough suppressants (e.g. butorphanol or hydrocodone) may be beneficial for coughing secondary to bronchial compression, but the clinician should first ensure that pulmonary oedema has been effectively treated.

DILATED CARDIOMYOPATHY WITH LEFT-SIDED OR BIVENTRICULAR HEART FAILURE

- Digoxin, furosemide, enalapril, and dietary sodium restriction are prescribed.
- Some dogs with substantial mitral regurgitation (and marked left atrial dilatation) respond better

to enalapril or lisinopril (0.25–0.5 mg/kg) plus hydralazine twice daily. Blood pressure must be monitored.
- Antiarrhythmic drugs are often necessary for control of heart rate in atrial fibrillation (add diltiazem or a beta blocker) or for control of recurrent or complex ventricular tachycardia (procainamide, tocainide, quinidine or mexiletine).
- A few animals respond to supplementation with taurine or L-carnitine (see Chapter 16).

FELINE HYPERTROPHIC CARDIOMYOPATHY

- Emergency therapy for dyspnoea includes furosemide, oxygen, cage confinement and nitroglycerine ointment. Thoracocentesis is required if there is a large pleural effusion.
- Prolonged therapy includes furosemide if needed, dietary sodium restriction, and either a beta blocker (propranolol, atenolol) or a calcium-channel blocker (diltiazem), or both (see Chapter 17).
- In cats without signs, or in those with trivial left ventricular hypertrophy diagnosed by echocardiography, a long-acting beta blocker (atenolol – 1/4 of a 50 mg tablet once daily) is more easily administered by clients.
- If CHF has already developed or echocardiography shows moderate to severe left ventricular hypertrophy (e.g. wall thickness > 7 mm), diltiazem is often preferred.
- If CHF advances (progressive pulmonary oedema or pleural effusion), enalapril is added once daily and twice daily after 2 weeks.
- Aspirin is given empirically as an anti-platelet drug to prevent systemic embolization if the left atrium is > 1.8 cm in diameter. Warfarin (0.5 mg daily) has been used in place of aspirin, but this requires *strict* evaluation of the prothrombin times to avoid haemorrhage. If renal failure or chronic vomiting occurs, consider discontinuing aspirin.

ADVANCED HEARTWORM DISEASE THAT IS COMPLICATED BY RIGHT-SIDED CHF

- The patient is first stabilized with strict cage rest, furosemide, aspirin (4–5 mg/kg q12h) to reduce pulmonary vascular reaction, and dietary sodium restriction.
- Oxygen therapy (for 24–48 hours) may also reduce pulmonary artery pressures by raising the alveolar pO_2, causing arterial vasodilatation. A short, anti-inflammatory dose of prednisolone may be helpful if there is active pulmonary parenchymal disease (this can be evaluated by X-ray), since reduction of infiltrate may improve ventilation–perfusion inequalities.
- When these treatments (including parenteral furosemide) fail to control ascites, hydrochlorothiazide plus spironolactone is added once daily and a cautious maintenance dose of digoxin is administered.
- Should this therapy fail, a cautious dose of enalapril (0.25 mg/kg daily or less) can be tried. A cardiologist should be consulted if this fails.
- After 2–4 weeks of stabilization, adulticide therapy is instituted.

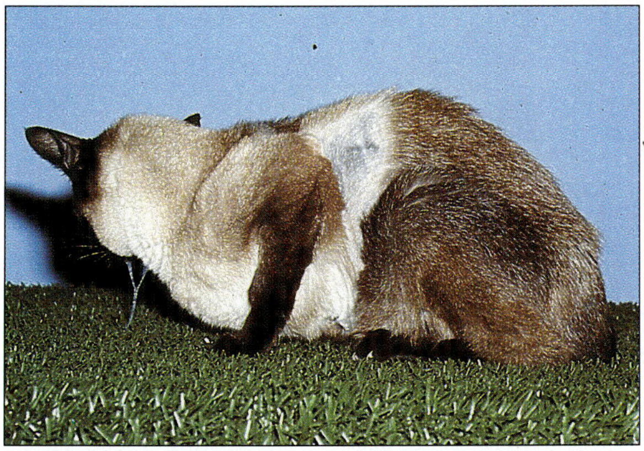

1.1 Cat with dyspnoea due to pleural effusion adopting a position of relief in sternal recumbency and with abducted elbows.

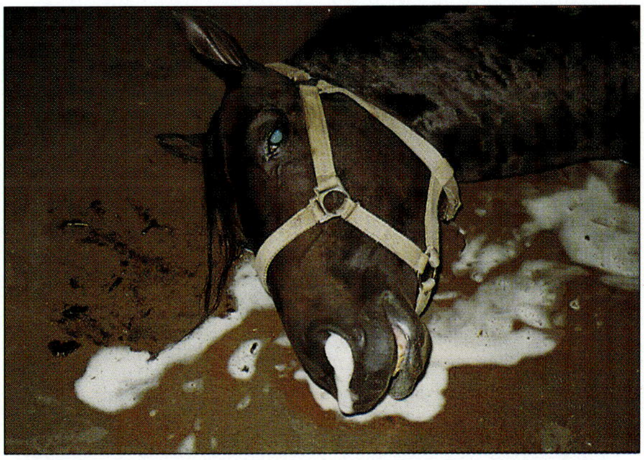

1.2 Severe pulmonary oedema in a horse presented with dyspnoea and heart failure due to ruptured mitral valve chordae tendineae. Large quantities of frothy oedema are observed exiting the nostrils. This finding can also be an agonal artifact of death caused by leakage of plasma into the alveoli.

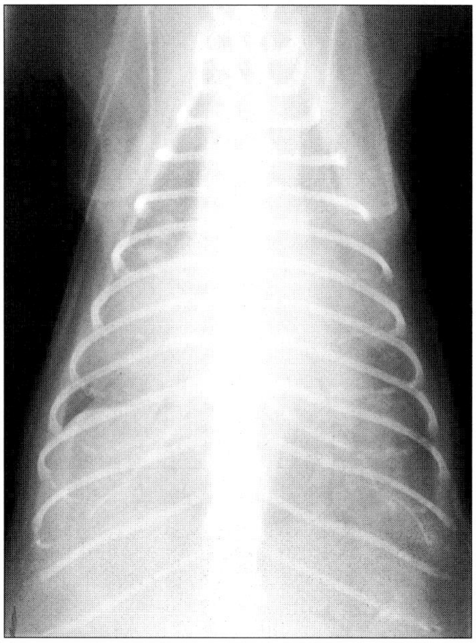

1.3 Dorsoventral radiograph of a cat with hypertrophic cardiomyopathy and pleural effusion. The cardiac outline cannot be identified, but caudal lobe pulmonary vessels are much enlarged.

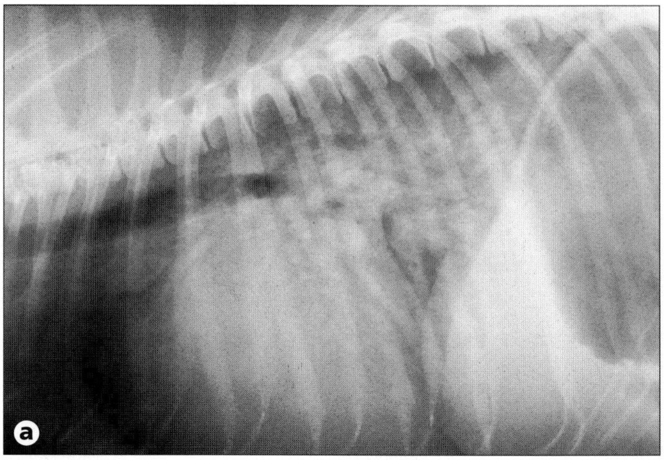

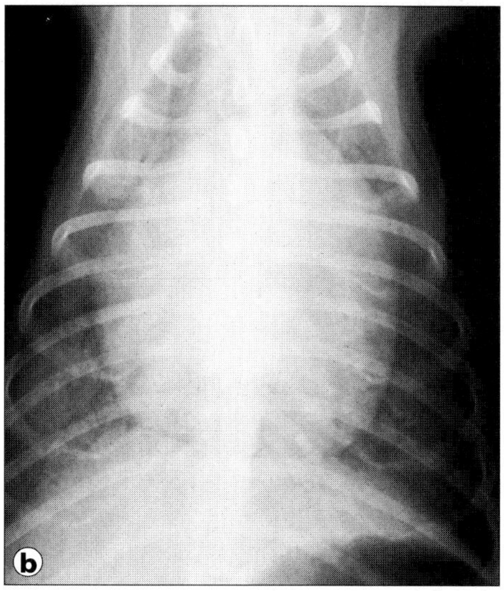

1.4 a, b Radiographs of a cocker spaniel with dilated cardiomyopathy. There is generalized cardiomegaly and a diffuse alveolar pattern representing pulmonary oedema. This affects the right caudal lobe more than the left – a common finding in cardiac failure.

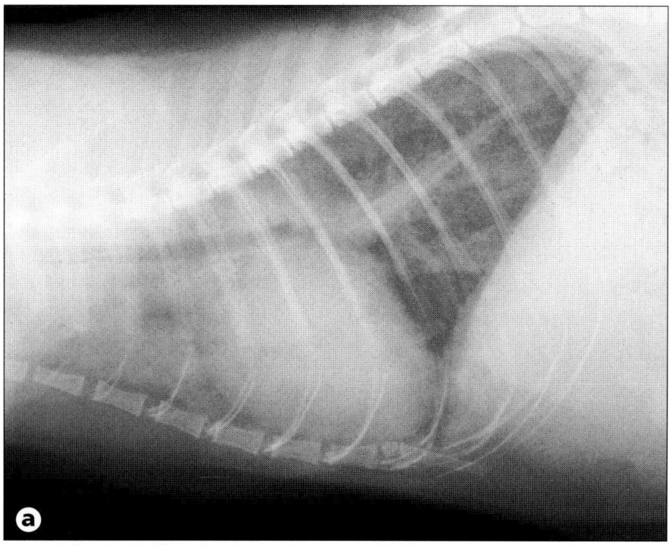

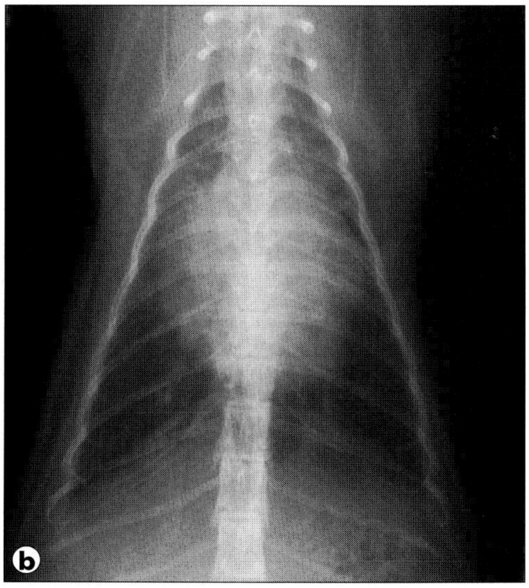

1.5 a, b Radiographs of a cat with hypertrophic cardiomyopathy and cardiac dilatation, showing generalized cardiomegaly and pulmonary oedema, which is diffuse, but which affects the cranioventral lobes.

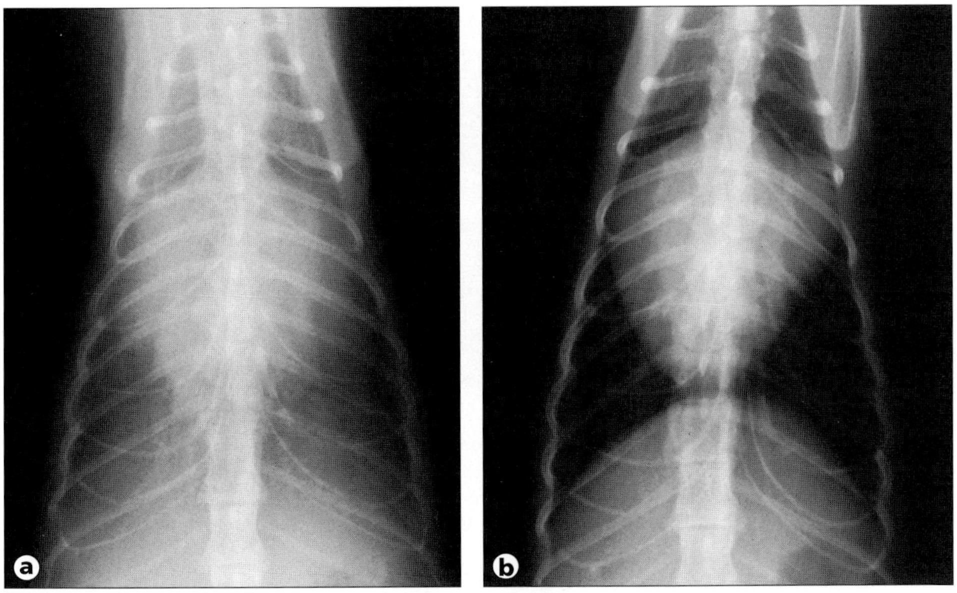

1.6 Dorsoventral radiographs before and after therapy for cardiac failure from a cat with hypertrophic cardiomyopathy. (**a**) Initially there is pulmonary oedema and pleural effusion partly obscuring an enlarged cardiac silhouette. (**b**) After therapy, bi-atrial enlargement is obvious.

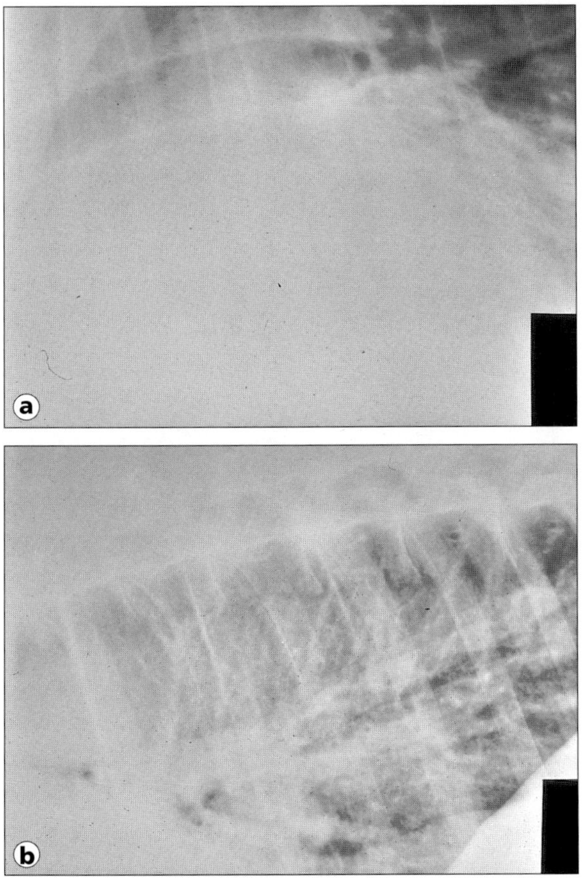

1.7 Thoracic radiographs showing cardiomegaly and pulmonary oedema in a horse with cardiac failure. (**a**) Rounding of the cardiac borders and tracheal elevation are evident, indicating cardiomegaly. (**b**) A marked increase in caudal lobe pulmonary densities and prominent vascular pattern are suggestive of cardiac failure.

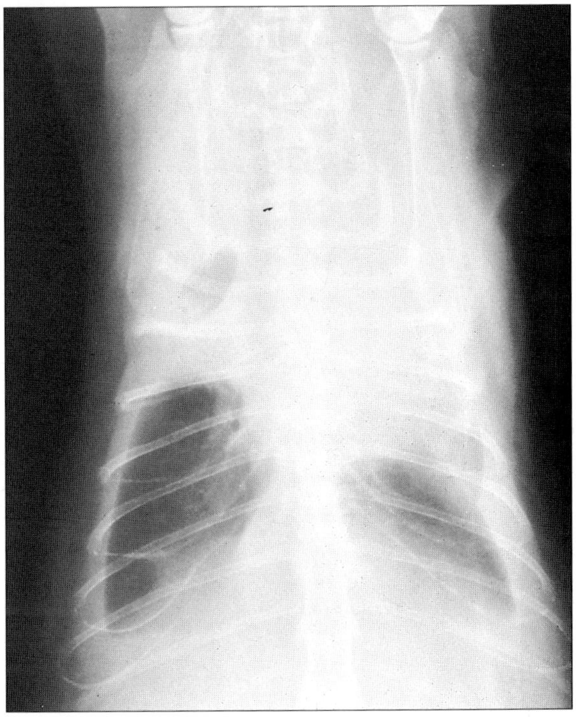

1.8 Ventrodorsal radiograph showing pleural effusion in a cat with dilated cardiomyopathy. There is blunting of the costophrenic angles and obscuring of the diaphragm and cardiac borders by free pleural fluid.

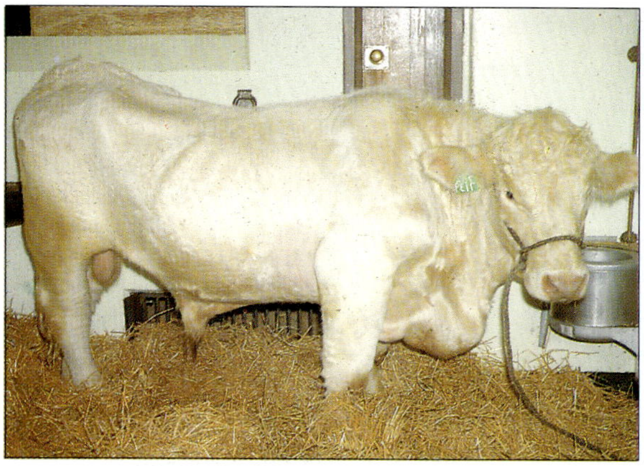

1.9 Subcutaneous oedema ventral to the sternum ('brisket oedema') in a bull with right-sided heart failure caused by bacterial endocarditis of the pulmonary valve.

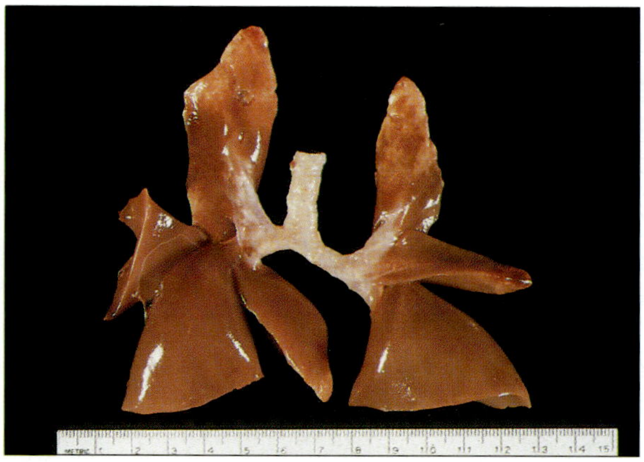

1.10 Lungs from a cat that died of pulmonary oedema viewed from the dorsal perspective. Diffuse oedema is evident, especially in the caudal lung lobes. The most cranial portions of the lung (top of picture) are unaffected.

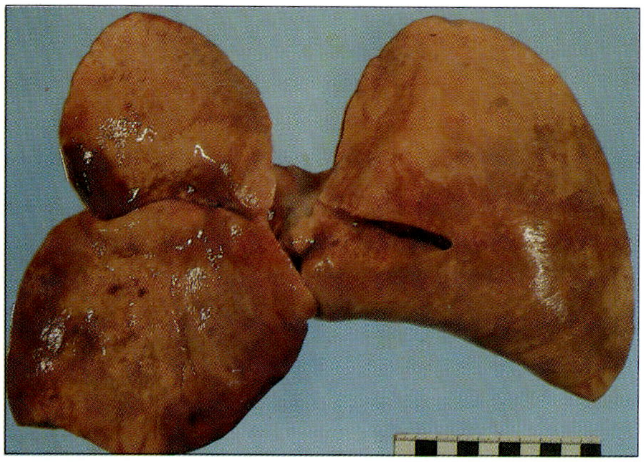

1.11 Pulmonary infarction in a Great Dane with congestive heart failure.

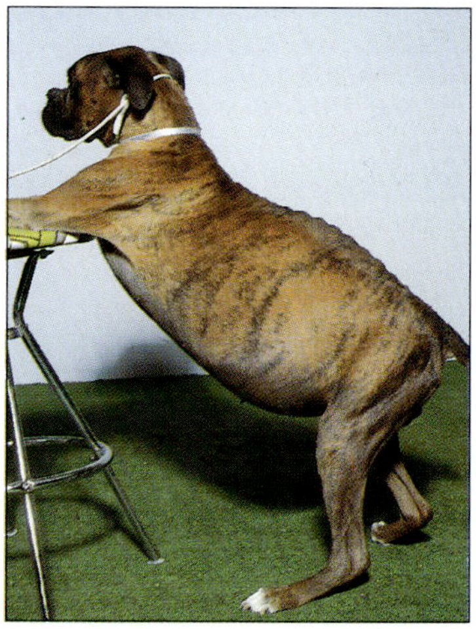

1.12 Severe ascites in a boxer dog with right-sided congestive heart failure. The abdominal distension partially masks the cardiac cachexia, which is evident as loss of muscle mass along the spine.

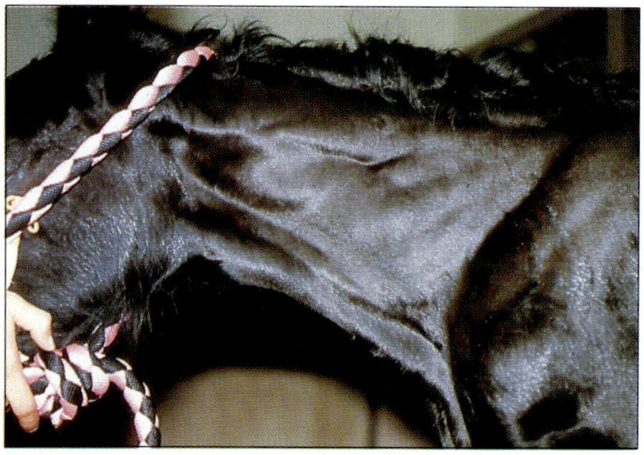

1.13 Elevated jugular venous pressure as a sign of right-sided heart failure in a shire foal.

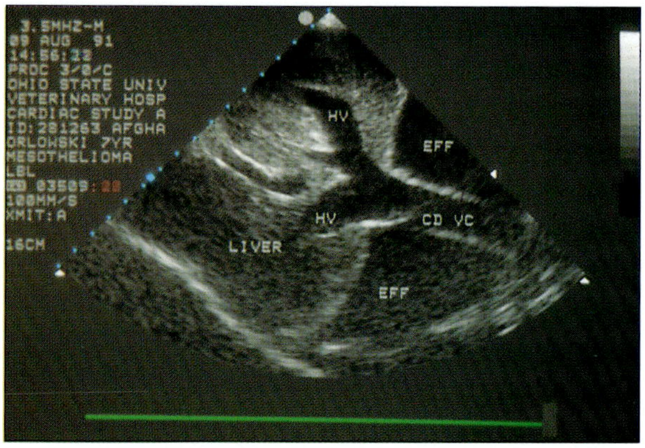

1.14 Ultrasound image demonstrating distended caudal vena cava (CD VC) and hepatic veins (HV) in a dog with pericardial disease and heart failure. Pleural effusion is evident (EFF) cranial to the diaphragm and liver.

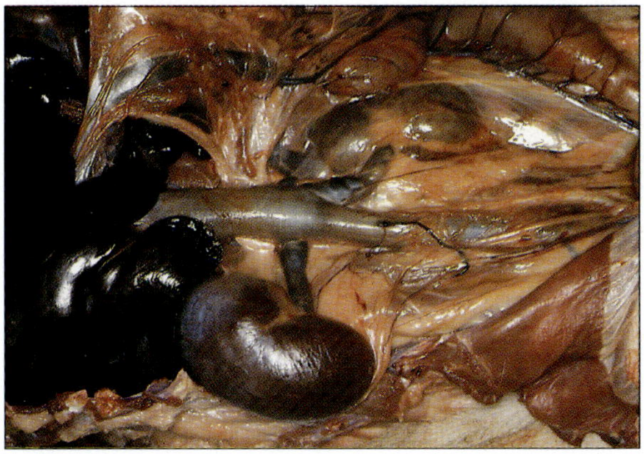

1.15 Splanchnic venous bed in a 3-year-old Great Dane with venous obstruction. There is marked distension and engorgement of the caudal vena cava and renal and mesenteric veins. Similar findings can be made in chronic congestive heart failure.

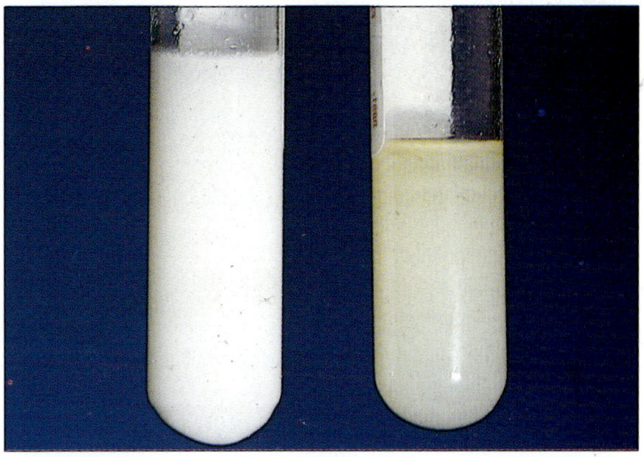

1.16 Chylothorax in a cat with severe heart failure. A sample of the aspirated effusion is shown (left). The effusate becomes more translucent following addition of anhydrous ether (right).

2. Post Mortem Examination of the Cardiovascular System

GENERAL INTRODUCTION

Post mortem examination of the cardiovascular system is directed at answering two questions:

1. Is there a demonstrable organic basis, at gross and/or microscopic levels, for clinical cardiovascular dysfunction recognized in a live animal?
2. Is it possible to demonstrate or exclude the presence of organic heart lesions in animals that have died suddenly, and in which there may be clinical suspicion of heart disease?

In the past, post mortem examination of the heart has been of major importance in recognizing and describing congenital and acquired forms of heart disease in domesticated and wild animals. Thus, much veterinary cardiology has depended on post mortem confirmation of the basis for valvular murmurs, acute and chronic congestive cardiac failure, congenital shunting defects, syncope and exercise-related unexpected death. Hence, pathology has a valuable role in complementing the observations derived from clinical investigations such as percussion, auscultation, radiography, electrocardiography and cannulation studies. The increasing use of more sophisticated, discriminating and quantitative investigations (such as Doppler echocardiography) has now provided much more secure ante mortem backgrounds of functional heart disease against which necropsy investigation can take place. In spite of the recent development of such non-invasive diagnostic techniques, there remains an important role for necropsy pathology in evaluating and recording the morphological basis for cardiovascular disease.

This chapter summarizes the important principles of these morphological investigations.

POST MORTEM EXAMINATION OF THE HEART AND BLOOD VESSELS

Important general principles underlie examination of the cardiovascular system:

- Be thorough
- Use a consistent technique
- Open all hollow structures
- Examine all solid structures by careful systematic incisions to expose small and deeply situated lesions.

Examination of the cardiovascular system is undertaken during the course of systematic post mortem examination of the whole body. Detailed guidance on necropsy techniques is readily found in published sources (Kelly, 1982; Strafuss, 1988).

Instruments suitable for use in necropsy are illustrated in **2.1**.

In the context of investigating cardiovascular disease, general examination of the body should look for abnormalities that might indicate cardiovascular disease; these can include subcutaneous and pulmonary oedema, venous congestion of liver, lungs and mesentery, and excess fluid accumulation in serosal cavities (e.g. hydropericardium, pleural effusion and ascites). Excess serosal fluids should be collected and their volumes measured and recorded. Animals that die suddenly from putative cardiac dysrhythmia may, however, have no organic sign of heart failure (Kelly and Newsholme, 1993).

The lungs, heart, trachea, oesophagus, tongue and pharynx are removed together, and are dissected systematically. The heart can be separated from the lungs and then examined, or it can be dissected while still attached to the lungs and great vessels; the latter may be preferable when dealing with complex congenital cardiac malformations.

Examination of the heart should be systematic and complete, but should be conducted so that anatomical relationships can be satisfactorily demonstrated and photographed (McGavin and Thompson, 1988) at the conclusion of the prosection. The following sequence is based on following the circulation of blood returning to the right atrium: the anterior and posterior vena cavae are opened longitudinally and post mortem blood clot removed; the right atrium is opened along its length (blood clot is common in the atrium and should be removed gently so the endocardium can be examined); the tricuspid valve orifice is inspected for patency and the atrial aspect of the valve examined for the presence of endocarditis or thickening; the right ventricle is next opened with a knife or scissors, cutting through the tricuspid valve and continuing towards the apex, keeping close to the interventricular septum; from the apex, the incision is continued towards the base of the heart so that the lateral wall of the right ventricle is reflected, followed by incision through the pulmonary valve; the tricuspid and pulmonary valves, cusps and chordae tendineae are now fully exposed for careful examination. An alternative approach to the right side of the heart starts by opening the pulmonary artery and exposing the ventricle and atrium in the reverse order; in this approach, the cranial vena cava is not incised, so the sinus node is left intact for histological examination (Bishop, 1988).

The left side of the heart is opened in a similar systematic manner, beginning with the pulmonary veins and finishing by opening the aortic valve, aortic trunk and extramural coronary arteries. The valves and chordae tendineae are examined systematically after any post mortem blood clot is removed from the space between the endocardium and the chordae. In opening the ventricles, the prosector should avoid cutting through moderator bands that cross the lumen of the chamber. These are normal features in the feline right ventricle and in both ventricles of the dog and horse, but can also occur in excessive numbers or thickness in cats with heart failure (Liu, 1988). The endocardium of the left atrium is normally slightly thicker and hence more opaque than on the right side (see **2.13** and **2.14**). The myocardium is examined by making multiple, serial, transverse incisions of the ventricular free walls and interventricular septum. Myocardial infarcts (see Chapter 19) can easily be missed if the myocardium is not examined in this systematic manner. Assessment of atria is best done histologically, using serial transverse blocks; this can reveal small mural thrombi, providing inferential evidence of atrial fibrillation (Kelly, Gaskell, Lee, 1992) in animals that have congestive heart failure.

Subjective assessment of cardiac chamber dilatation or myocardial hypertrophy is relatively easy when examining hearts from animals with marked adaptive changes, such as those that occur in animals that live for some months with congenital heart disease. Objective quantitation of equivocal dilatation and hypertrophy can be made by measuring body weight, total heart weight, chamber weights and valve circumferences (Bishop, 1988; Turk, Turk and Root, 1983) and relating these parameters to reference values from normal animals. These reference values are shown in **2.2** and **2.3**.

Histological examination of the heart is best carried out after the heart is first hardened by fixation *in toto*. This allows the trimming of symmetrical blocks of tissue. The heart is wiped free of major blood clots and then immersed (or suspended by the great vessels) in a large volume (at least ten times greater than that of the heart) of buffered 10% formalin. The heart should not be packed into a small container with other tissue samples, since this inhibits good fixation. After hardening by fixation for at least a week, the heart is washed and tissue blocks trimmed and further fixed for several days. Tissue blocks should not exceed 3 mm in thickness if good fixation is to be achieved. Ten percent buffered formalin is a suitable fixative for most routine examinations of cardiovascular tissue (Luna, 1992).

Selection of heart tissue samples for histological examination will often be based on the clinical and gross necropsy findings. In investigation of sudden cardiac death, where no gross organic lesion is found at necropsy, it is important to sample the heart in a systematic way so as to include all the major anatomical regions of the conducting tissue, myocardium and valves. Such a sampling protocol is illustrated in **2.4**.

Post mortem examination of the vascular system involves systematic opening of the main arteries and veins throughout their length, noting patency, the presence of smooth or rough intima, the presence of valves in veins, the presence of post mortem blood clot or ante mortem thrombi. The former have glistening smooth surfaces and can be easily removed from the vessel lumen or heart chamber (**2.5**); they have a soft, gelatinous consistency and are usually dark red but, in anaemic animals, may be pale and resemble chicken fat. By contrast, thrombi have a rough surface and have dull, often lamellated, cut surfaces (**2.6**). Older thrombi may be firmly adherent to the vessel intima, but recent thrombi may be only loosely attached. Such recent lesions should be fixed, without tissue disturbance, so they can be evaluated histologically for evidence of organization and recanalization. Patency of the ductus arteriosus should be assessed by gentle probing and the dimensions of the vessel recorded by accurate measurement.

Post mortem examination of the cardiovascular system is incomplete without a full report of the observations. This should include a complete, concise account of the size and shape of the chambers, and a record of measurements of weights and valve dimensions, together with comments on the naked-eye appearance of the pericardium, epicardium, myocardium, endocardium, valves and great vessels. The report (Prichard, 1966) is best supplemented by photographic records of gross abnormalities (McGavin and Thompson, 1988).

NORMAL ANATOMICAL AND HISTOLOGICAL FEATURES

The heart and blood vessels vary considerably in size between different animal species, but basic anatomical and histological features have more in common than they have differences.

The major anatomical features of the heart, and the principal histological features of the heart and blood vessels, are shown in **2.7–2.16**.

AGONAL CHANGE

This term refers to those changes that occur immediately prior to death. They result largely from terminal vascular congestion and bleeding from small blood vessels.

Terminal petechial and ecchymotic haemorrhage is a common finding in the hearts of large animals, such as cattle and horses. These agonal haemorrhages are most common on the epicardium and endocardium and are very common in animals that die in convulsions (e.g. in hypomagnesaemia in cattle), or following painful illness (e.g. colic in horses). These agonal changes are seen in **2.17** and **2.18**.

ARTIFACTS OF EUTHANASIA

These are commonly encountered in domestic animals and can produce striking changes in the heart and blood vessels. If the prosector is the person who euthanased the animal, then these artifacts are unlikely to cause confusion, but if this is not the case, the prosector should always be aware of the method used to produce euthanasia.

Euthanasia artifacts can result from agonal cardiac puncture for blood sampling or intracardiac injection, shooting and pithing, or injection of barbiturate solutions into solid tissues. These common artifacts are illustrated in **2.19–2.26**.

ARTIFACTS PRODUCED BY INJECTION OF BARBITURATE EUTHANASIA SOLUTIONS

These concentrated euthanasia solutions can produce darkening of endocardium and intima because of the imbibition of haemoglobin liberated by haemolysis (**2.22**), crystalline deposits in endocardium (**2.22**) and epicardium (**2.24**), and localized alterations in colour and texture of solid tissues (such as myocardium) into which barbiturate solution is injected (**2.23**, **2.25** and **2.26**).

These artifacts associated with barbiturate euthanasia can become accentuated after fixation of the tissues in formalin (**2.25** and **2.26**).

INCIDENTAL LESIONS OF NO CLINICAL SIGNIFICANCE

Post mortem examination of the cardiovascular system is directed primarily at the identification and evaluation of lesions that relate to heart disease.

There are a small number of lesions that are common incidental post mortem findings and that may be found in normal healthy animals. It is important to recognize these as incidental findings so that they are not erroneously given clinical significance. Some of these incidental findings may result from disease elsewhere in the body, but may not, of themselves, be of clinical significance. These incidental lesions are illustrated below (**2.27–2.40**).

ACKNOWLEDGEMENTS

Figures **2.2–2.4** are republished, with the author's permission, from: Bishop SP. Necropsy Techniques for the Heart and Great Vessels, Chapter 31; in *Canine and Feline Cardiology*. 1988. Ed. Fox PR. Churchill Livingstone, New York .

REFERENCES

Bishop SP. Chapter 31: Necropsy Techniques for the Heart and Great Vessels in *Canine and Feline Cardiology*. Ed. Fox PR. Churchill Livingstone, New York 1988.

Kelly DF, Gaskell CJ, Lee MA. Arteriosclerosis of extramural coronary arteries in Labradors with congestive heart failure. *Journal of Small Animal Practice* 1992; **33**: 437–42.

Kelly DF. Chapter 4: Necropsy Procedures in D F Kelly, V M Lucke, C J Gaskell. *Notes on Pathology for Small Animal Clinicians*. Wright P S G, Bristol, 1982.

Kelly DF, Newsholme SJ. Sudden death in related bloodhounds. *Journal of Small Animal Practice* 1993; **34**: 390–392.

Liu S-K. Chapter 32: Cardiovascular Pathology in *Canine and Feline Cardiology*. Ed. P R Fox. Churchill Livingstone, New York 1988.

Luna LG. *Histopathologic Methods and Color Atlas of Special Stains and Tissue Artifacts*. American Histolabs. Gathersburg, 1992.

McGavin MD, Thompson SW. *Specimen Dissection and Photography for the Pathologist, Anatomist and Biologist*. Charles C Thomas, Springfield, 1988.

Prichard RW. Descriptions in Pathology, Avoiding Pathological Descriptions. *Pathologia veterinaria* 1966; **3**: 169–77.

Strafuss AC. *Necropsy Procedures and Basic Diagnostic Methods for Practicing Veterinarians*. Charles C Thomas, Springfield, 1988.

Turk JR, Turk MAM, Root CR. Necropsy of the Canine Heart: A Simple Technique for Quantifying Ventricular Hypertrophy and Valvular Alterations. *Compendium on Continuing Education for the Practicing Veterinarian* 1983; **5**: 905–10.

For further references on cardiovascular pathology, see References and Further Reading, pp 177–179.

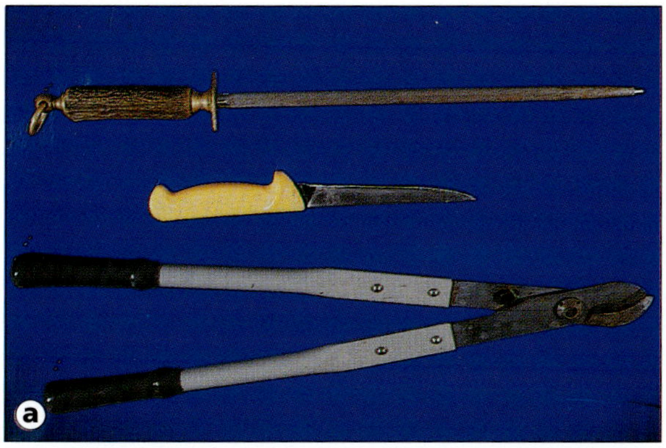

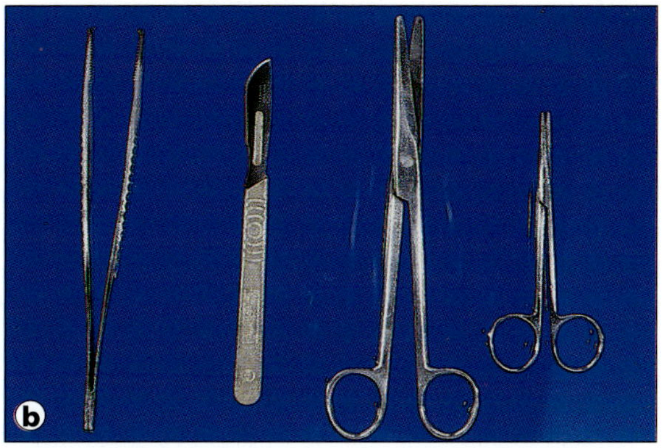

2.1 (**a**) Instruments suitable for post mortem examination of the heart and great vessels: rib shears for opening the thorax and a sharp knife for excision of soft tissues and examination of the myocardium. (**b**) Smaller instruments suitable for finer prosection of the heart and great vessels: large and small dissecting scissors, tissue forceps, surgical scalpel.

Heart Weight, Body Weight, and Associated Ratios in Normal Dogs and Cats

		BW (kg)	HW/BW (g/kg)	RV/BW (g/kg)	(LV+S)/BW (g/kg)	RV/HW	(LV+S)/HW	(LV+S)/RV
Normal beagles	Mean	10.22	6.69	1.37	4.25	0.207	0.650	3.13
(N=26)	SD	1.23	0.68	0.17	0.42	0.014	0.034	0.23
Normal mixed-	Mean	13.49	7.41	1.67	4.71	0.225	0.635	2.82
breed dogs (N=47)	SD	5.18	1.02	0.26	0.67	0.020	0.028	0.23
Normal cats	Mean	3.08	3.68	0.67	2.41	0.184	0.659	3.56
(N=33)	SD	0.57	0.60	0.15	0.37	0.025	0.025	0.23

BW = body weight, HW = heart weight, LV+S = left ventricle plus septum, RV = right ventricular free wall, SD = standard deviation.

2.2 Heart weight, body weight, and associated ratios in normal dogs and cats.

Heart Weight, Body Weight, and Associated Ratios in Normal and Cardiomyopathic Cats

Myocardial disease	**Number of cats**	**BW** (kg)	**HW** (g)	**HW/BW** (g/kg)
Hyperthyroid related	23	3.3±0.3	22.6±2.1	7.0±0.3
Restrictive	15	4.6±0.2	30.6±1.7	6.4±0.3
Symmetric hypertrophic	35	4.5±0.2	27.5±0.8	6.3±0.1
Asymmetric hypertrophic	16	4.4±0.1	27.5±0.8	6.3±0.3
Dilated (congestive)	21	4.5±0.1	24.1±0.9	5.4±0.3
Excessive moderator bands	21	4.5±0.2	21.6±0.8	4.5±0.2
Control (normal)	36	4.8±0.2	18.4±0.6	3.83±0.2

BW = body weight, HW = heart weight.
(Liu SK, Peterson ME, Fox PR: Hypertrophic cardiomyopathy amd hyperthyroidism in the cat. *J Am Vet Med Assoc* 1984; **185**:52.)

2.3 Heart weight, body weight, and associated ratios in normal and cardiomyopathic cats (Mean ± SEM)

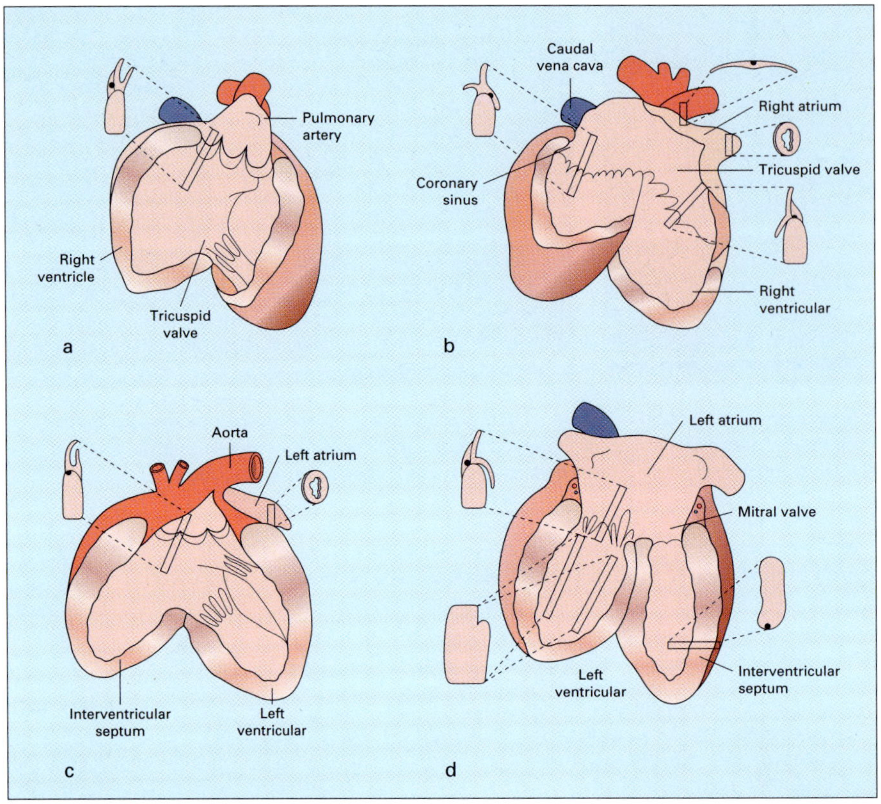

2.4 Diagram of the heart opened along the lines of blood flow. Numbered drawings illustrate the shape of the tissues as removed for histologic section. (**a**) Right ventricular cavity and pulmonary outflow tract. (**b**) Right ventricle and right atrium. (**c**) Left ventricle and aortic outflow tract. (**d**) Left ventricle and left atrium.

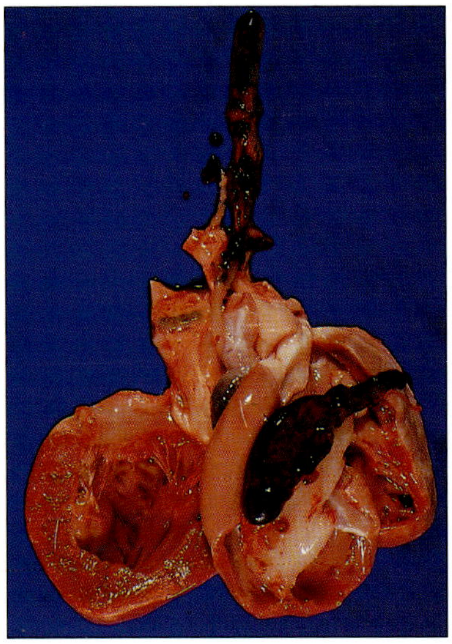

2.5 Post mortem blood clots. In the right ventricular lumen there are distinct, separate, dark red and pale post mortem clots. These have glistening surfaces and are easily removed because they do not adhere to the endocardium. (From a 4-year-old Jack Russell terrier.)

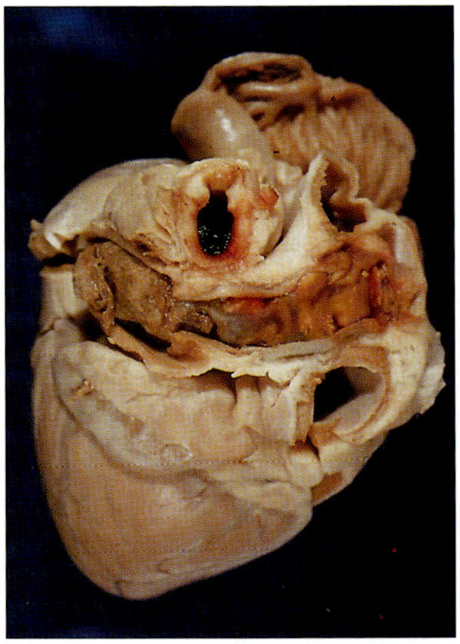

2.6 Thrombosis of pulmonary artery. The outflow tract from the right ventricle is completely occluded by a dull, rough thrombus. (From a 6-year-old dachshund bitch that was found dead without previous illness.)

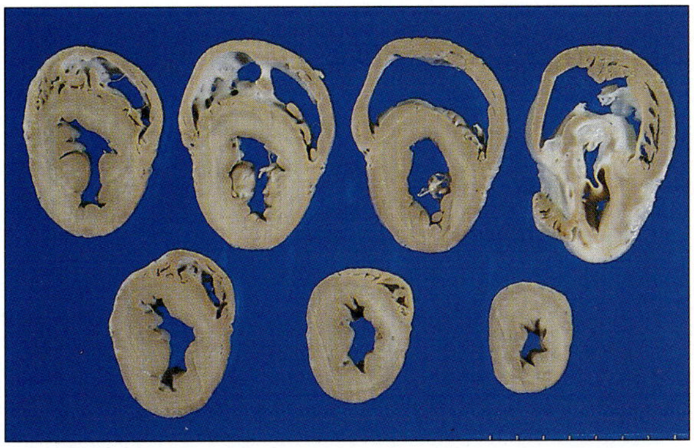

2.7 Normal heart. Coronal sections of fixed heart from a 7-month-old Akita puppy. The sections are mounted from the dorsal part of the heart to the apex, showing the normal relative thickness of left and right ventricles and the positions of the atrioventricular valves.

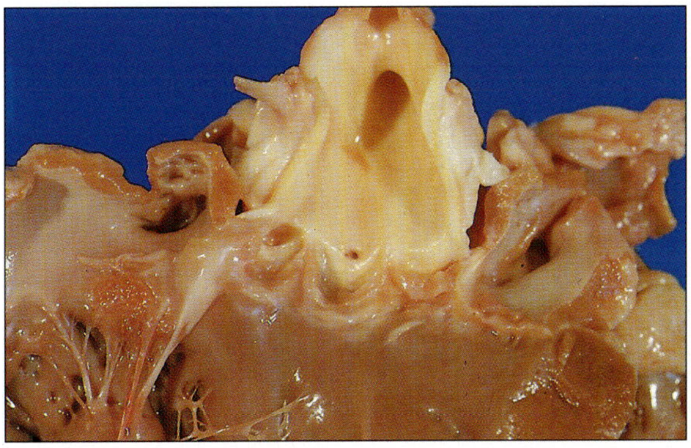

2.8 Normal aortic valve, showing the three separate valve cusps and the origin of a coronary artery. (From a 2-year-old boxer dog.)

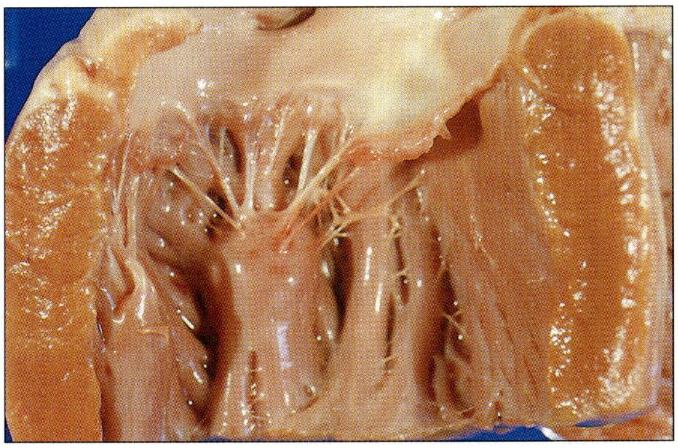

2.9 Normal mitral valve, papillary muscles and chordae tendineae. The cusp margins are transparently thin and without nodularity. Chordae tendineae are uniformly slender. (From a 2-year-old boxer dog.)

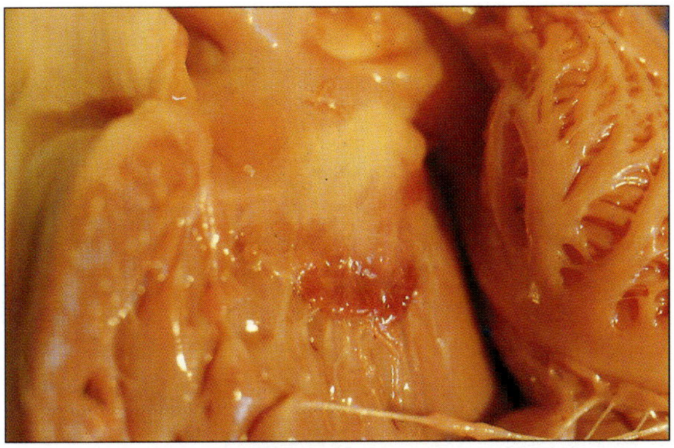

2.10 Normal tricuspid valve. In the dog, the septal cusps of the right atrioventricular (triscuspid) valve are anatomically slightly thicker than those on the left side, and chordae tendinae are shorter. This normal feature should not be mistaken for early endocardiosis. (From a 2-year-old boxer dog.)

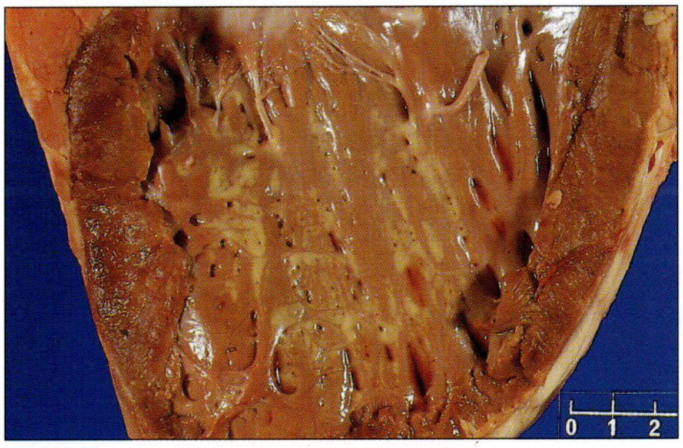

2.11 Subendocardial adiposity. Patchy pallor of subendocardial myocardium is a common finding in dairy cows. It is associated with increased deposition of adipose tissue between myocardial fibres and often results from overfeeding during late pregnancy. Similar adiposity is also conspicuous in the epicardial coronary grooves. (From a 3-year-old Friesian cow.)

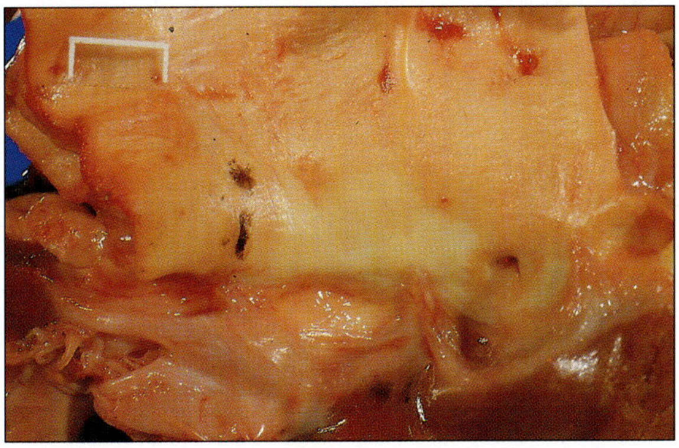

2.12 Melanosis of the aorta. Grey-black discoloration of the intima of large blood vessels is a common, but variable, normal anatomical feature of some species, especially in ruminants. (From a 5-year-old ewe.)

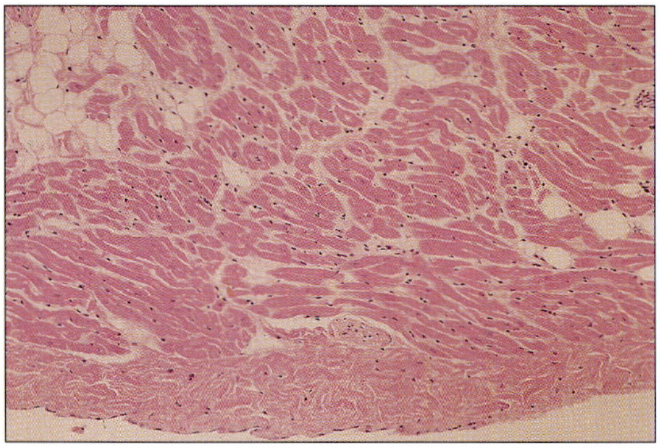

2.13 Normal histology. The section illustrates the relatively compact appearance of normal left atrial myocardium (above) and the fibroelastic tissue of the endocardium. There are regional variations in the relative thickness of the atrial endocardium: it is normally thicker in the left than in the right (see **2.14**). (From a 2-year-old boxer dog.)

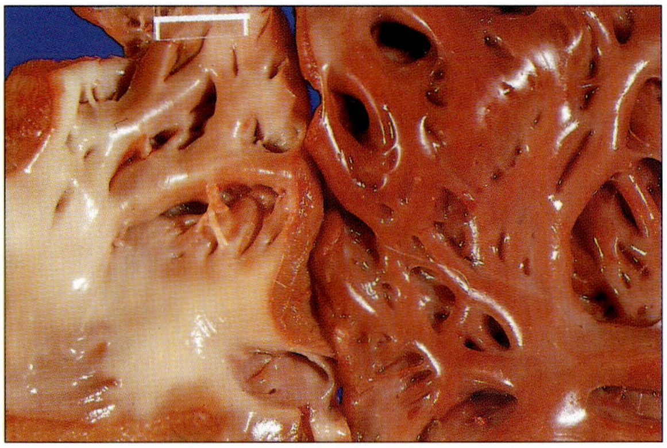

2.14 The left and right atrial endocardium are compared in this photograph. On the left, the endocardium is pale and opaque; on the right, the thinner endocardium reveals the underlying dark atrial myocardium. (From a 5-year-old pony gelding.)

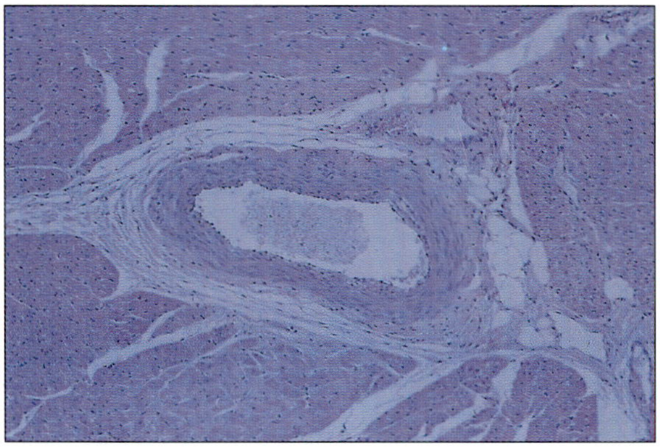

2.15 Normal intramural coronary artery. Photomicrograph showing the normal thickness of the tunica media, and the normal proportions of wall thickness/luminal diameter. (From a 4-month-old German shepherd bitch.)

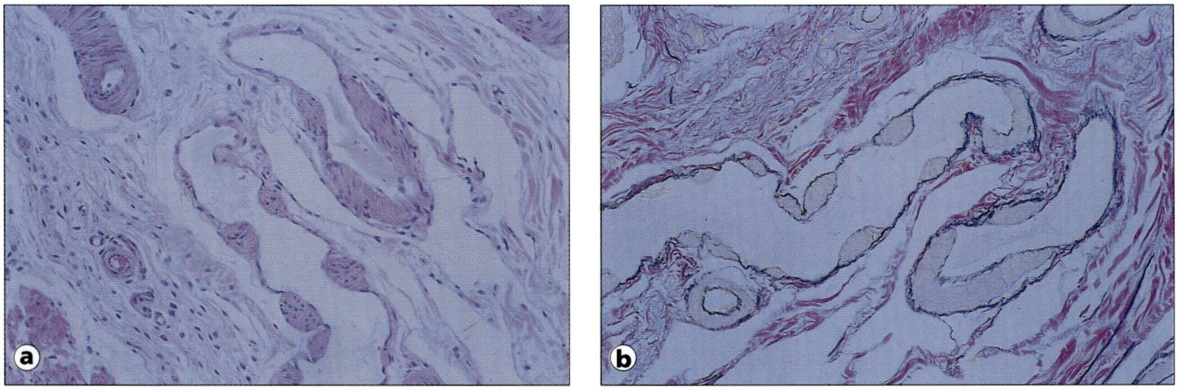

2.16 Photomicrograph of normal blood vessels in equine intestinal submucosa. (**a**) These annular cushions of smooth muscle are a normal histological feature of these arteriovenous vessels. (H&E stain). (**b**) Smooth muscle cushions closely apposed to adjacent elastic fibres. (Elastic – van Gieson stain)

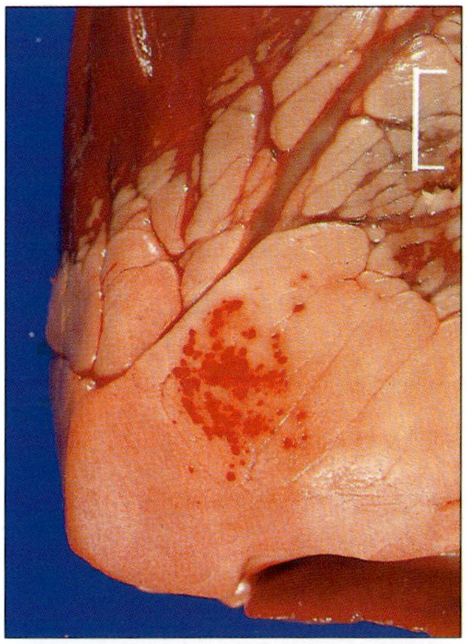

2.17 There is a cluster of agonal haemorrhages that contrast sharply with the underlying pale apical epicardial adipose tissue. (From a Friesian bullock.)

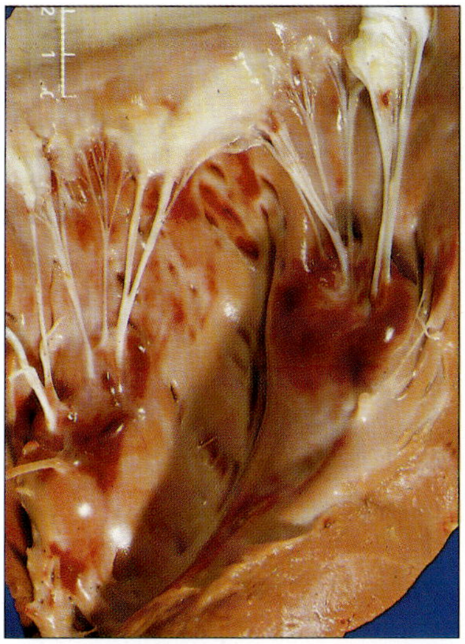

2.18 There is extensive subendocardial agonal haemorrhage. The bleeding extends no more than a millimetre into adjacent myocardium. (From an 18-month-old Dutch warmblood mare that died after splenic rupture.)

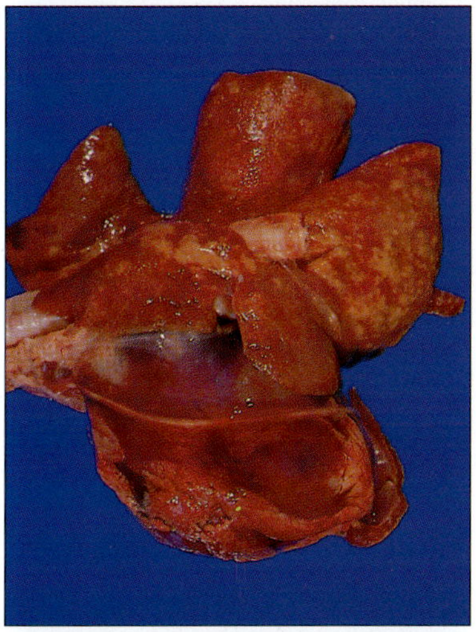

2.19 Euthanasia haemorrhage. There is haemorrhage into lung overlying the heart following attempts at terminal exsanguination. (From an 18-month-old Cairn terrier.)

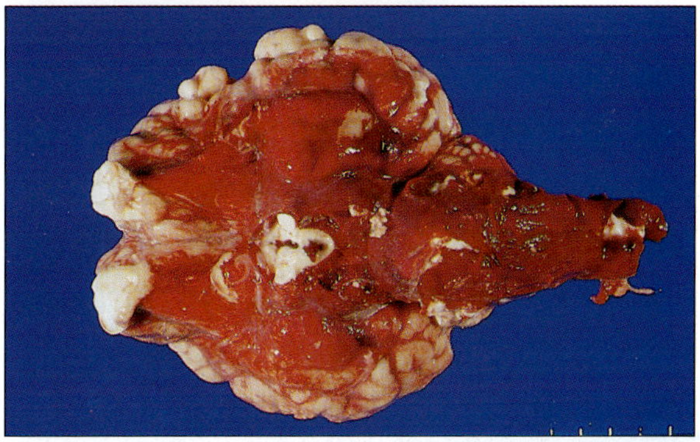

2.20 Euthanasia haemorrhage. There is extensive haemorrhage over the ventral surface of the brain and upper cervical spinal cord. (From a 7-year-old Holstein cow.)

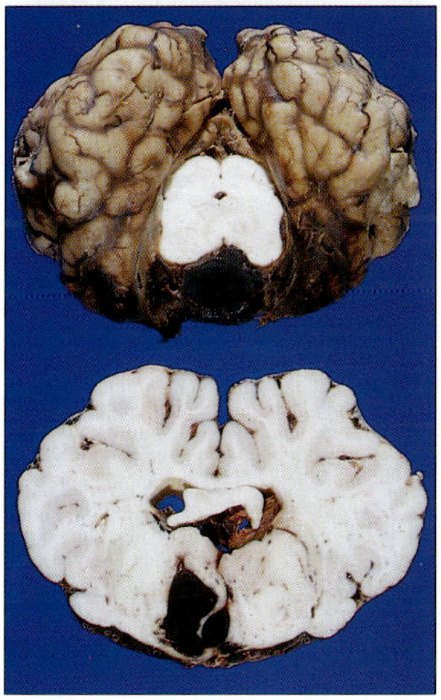

2.21 Euthanasia haemorrhage. There is extensive haemorrhage within the lateral ventricles and in the thalamus as a result of trauma produced by pithing. (From a 4-year-old Friesian cow.)

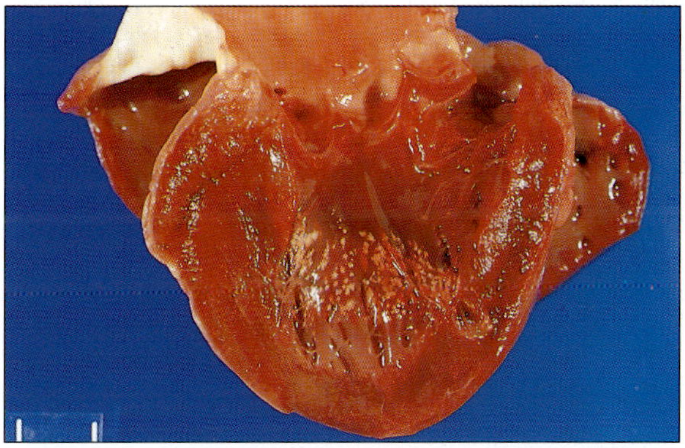

2.22 Euthanasia artifact. The left ventricular endocardium is discoloured by injection of barbiturate into the underlying myocardium and bears a 'snowflake' pattern of crystal deposition. Note the normal, pale-cream appearance of the pulmonary arterial intima, and the dark haemoglobin-stained aorta. Barbiturate solutions are haemolytic, so released haemoglobin discolours adjacent tissues. (From a 4-year-old Jack Russell terrier.)

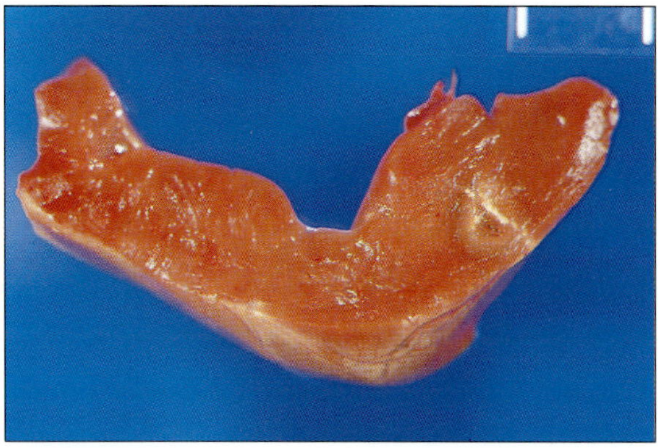

2.23 Euthanasia artifact. In the apical myocardium, there is a linear artefact produced by injection of barbiturate into the heart. (From a 4-year-old Jack Russell terrier.)

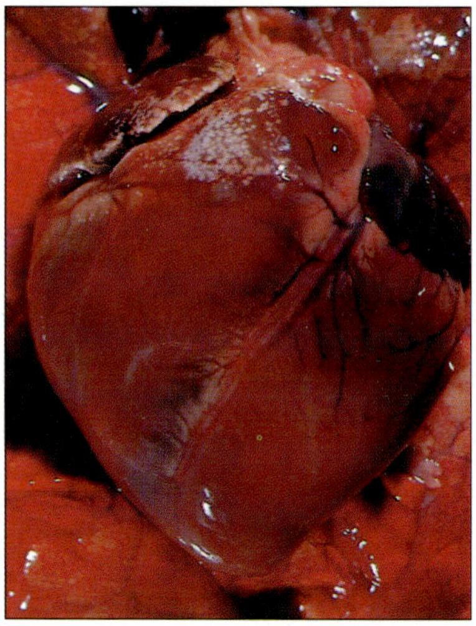

2.24 Euthanasia artifact. There are numerous 'snowflake' crystals on the right atrial and ventricular epicardium, following intracardiac injection of barbiturate.

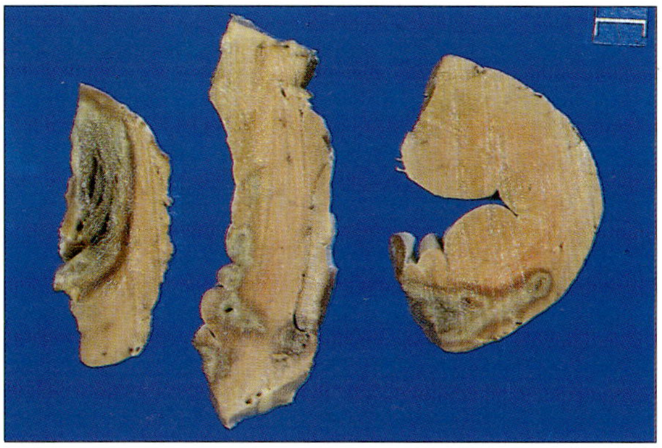

2.25 Coronal slices of interventricular septum and left ventricular free wall after formalin fixation. There is artifactual darkening of myocardium caused by intramyocardial injection of barbiturate.

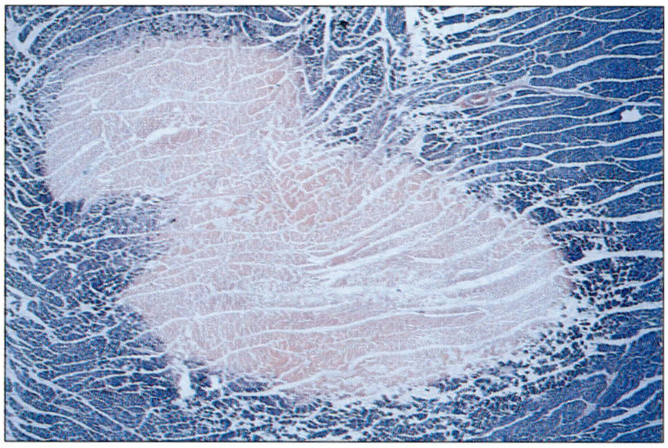

2.26 A section of myocardium showing the artifact illustrated in **2.25**. There is a large, well-demarcated area of myocardium that is unstained by the dye (PTAH) that stains the surrounding unaffected normal fibres.

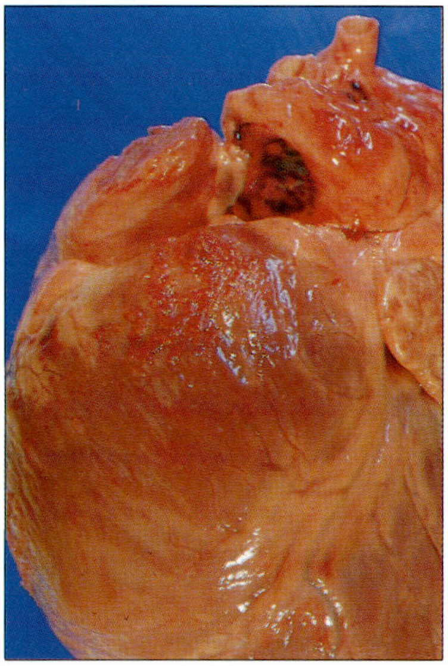

2.27 Epicardial fronds. The epicardium is patchily roughened by filiform projections of fibrovascular connective tissue covered by mesothelium. Occasionally, these fronds contain minimal foci of haemosiderin, suggesting that there has been past bleeding into the epicardium or into the pericardial sac. (From a 2-year-old bloodhound.)

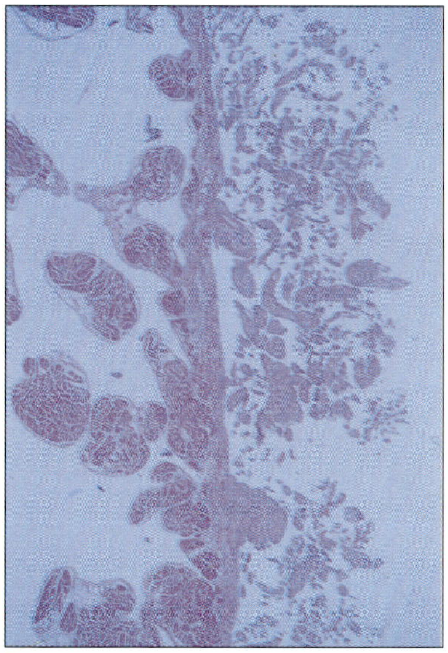

2.28 Photomicrograph of atrial epicardium showing diffuse proliferation of arborizing fibromesothelial fronds. (From a 2-year-old bloodhound.)

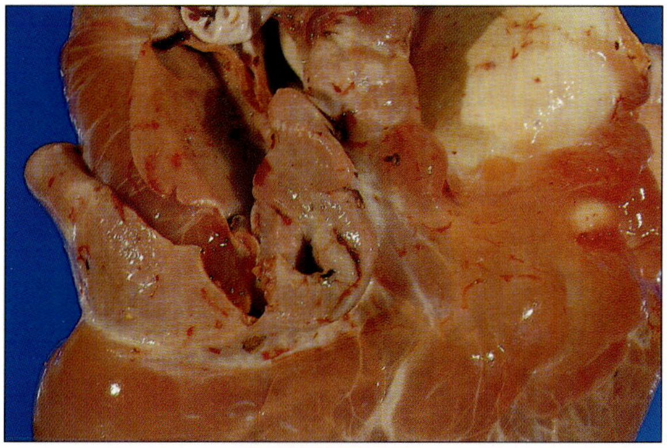

2.29 Serous atrophy of epicardial fat. Normal coronary-groove fat is firm and pale-cream or yellow. In this animal, the epicardial fat is pale and gelatinous. This change results from mobilization of body-fat reserves, so this is a common feature in cachectic animals that have chronic wasting diseases such as parasitism, mycobacterial infections, chronic renal or liver disease. Histological examination of this softened adipose tissue often shows focal necrosis of fat cells and associated steatitis (see **2.30**). Similar changes are common in other body-fat depots. (From an emaciated 10-year-old female giraffe.)

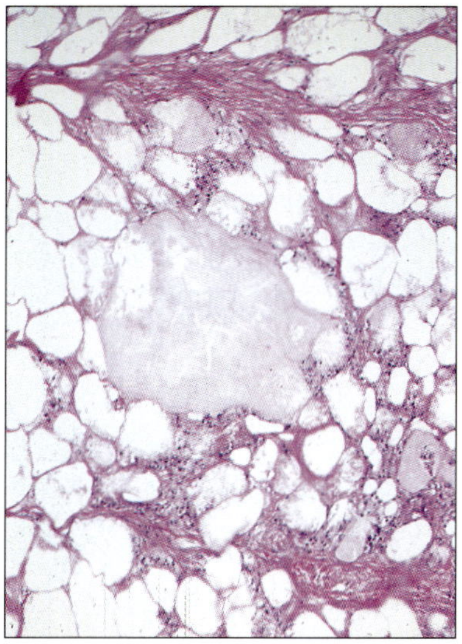

2.30 Photomicrograph of adipose tissue showing necrosis of fat and chronic inflammatory cell reaction. (From a 9-year-old Ayrshire cow.)

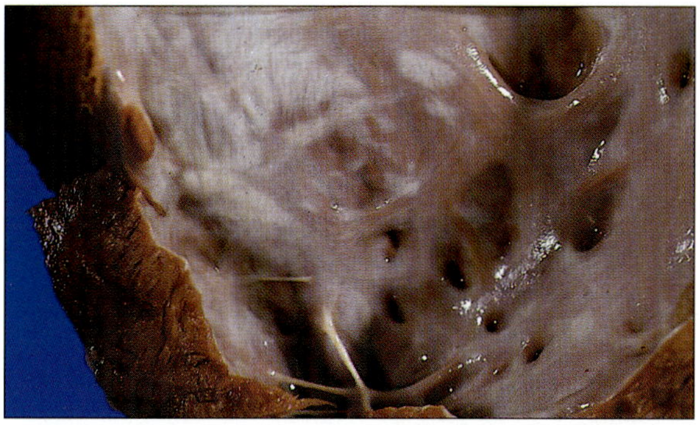

2.31 Endocardial elastosis in a 9-year-old thoroughbred mare. There is patchy opacity and wrinkling of the endocardium of the left ventricular free wall. This is a common age-related change in the horse; it is of no clinical significance.

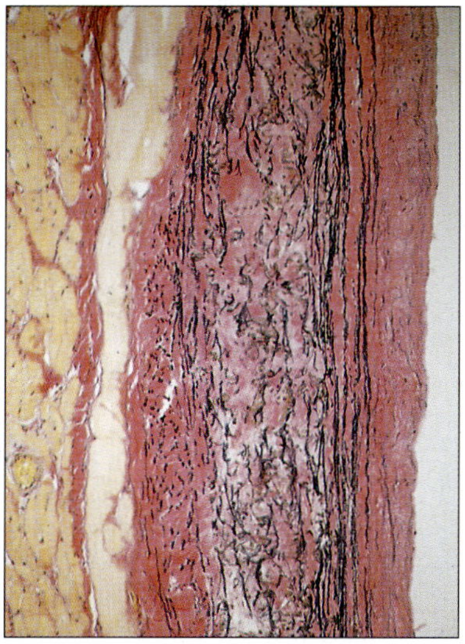

2.32 Photomicrograph of left ventricular endocardium from a 9-year-old mare. There is thickening of the endocardium by collagen fibres; elastic fibres are thickened, fragmented and calcified. (Elastic–Van Gieson stain)

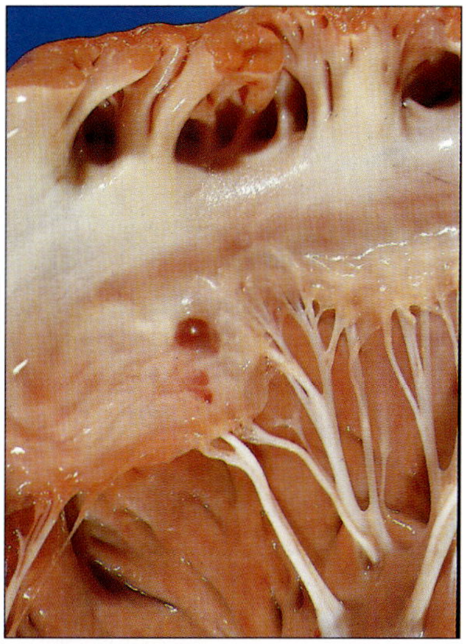

2.33 Telangiectasia in the mitral valve of a Friesian bullock. These well-circumscribed intravalvular cysts are common incidental findings in the atrioventricular valves of cattle. They are also known as haematocysts.

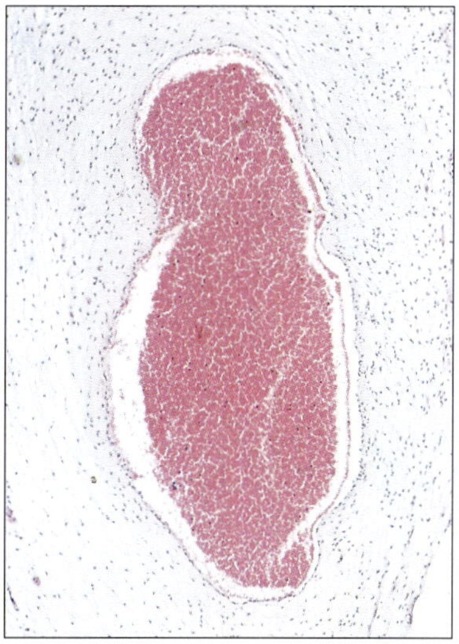

2.34 Photomicrograph of mitral valve telangiectasia from a calf, showing the endothelial lining and erythrocytes in the cyst lumen. (H&E stain)

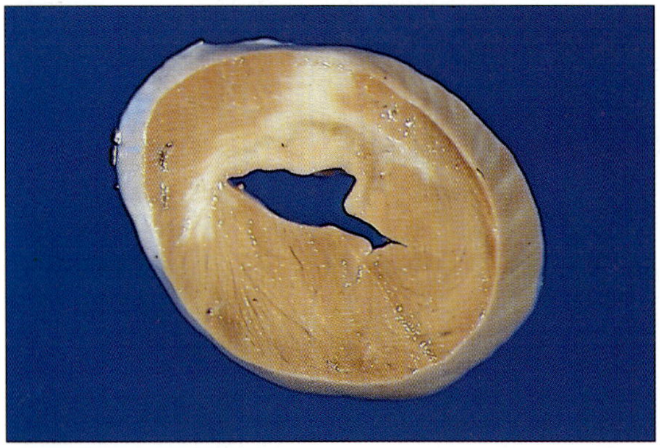

2.35 Myocardial scarring. The coronal cut surface of the apex shows tough patchy myocardial scarring. Such lesions are common incidental findings in elderly horses in which there is no clinical evidence of cardiac dysfunction. (From an 18-year-old thoroughbred mare.)

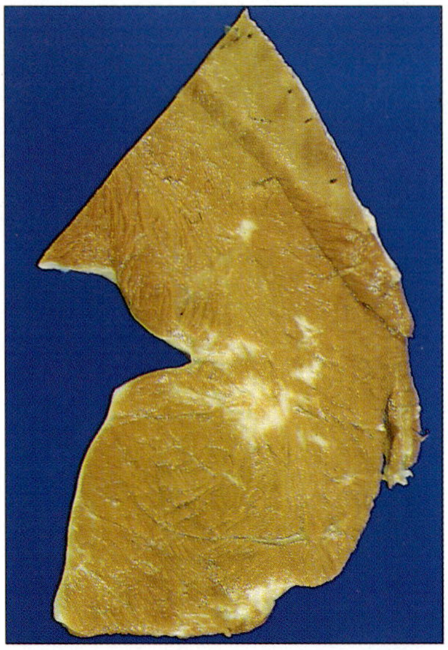

2.36 Incidental myocardial scarring in the subendocardial left ventricular free wall of a 20-year-old Suffolk punch mare.

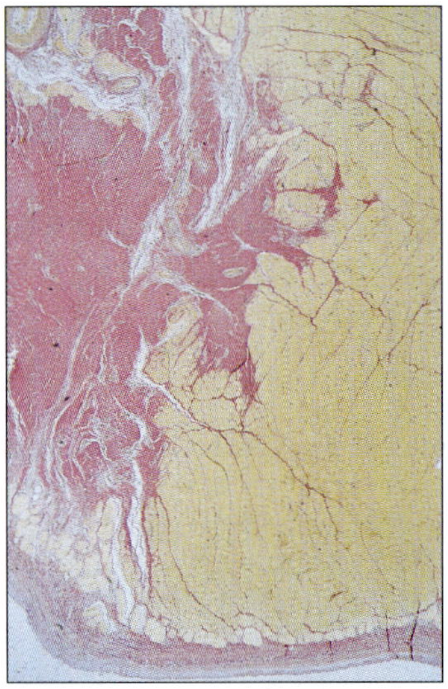

2.37 Photomicrograph of the left ventricular free wall showing the contrast between myocardium (yellow) and scar tissue (red). (From a 5-year-old hunter gelding.)

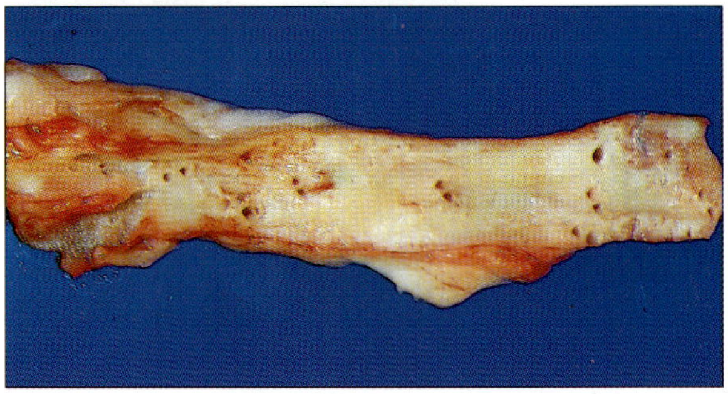

2.38 Aortic intimal fibrosis. The intima is patchily rough and opaque because of focal thickening of intimal fibroelastic tissue. These lesions are common incidental findings in older dogs: they usually contain only minimal amounts of lipid. (From an 11-year-old cocker spaniel bitch.)

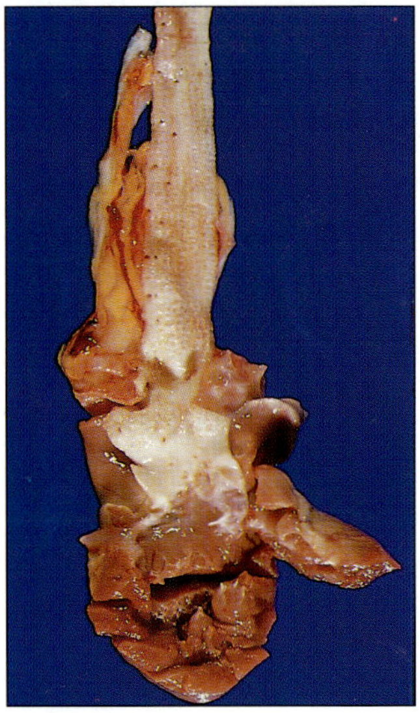

2.39 Aortic calcification. The tunica intima is rough and wrinkled because of extensive soft tissue calcification. (From a 10-year-old male cat with hypercalcaemia caused by chronic renal failure and secondary hyperparathyroidism.)

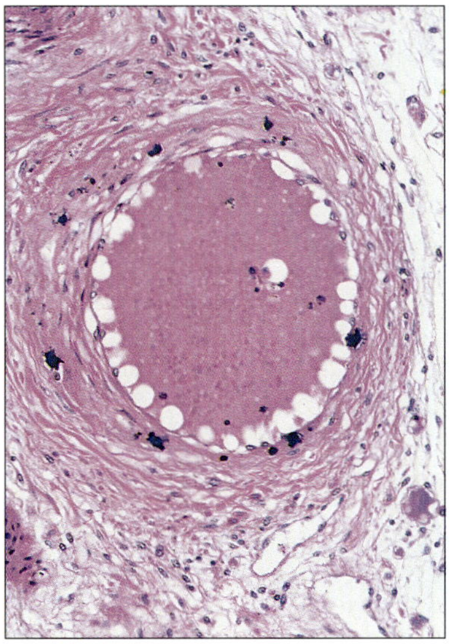

2.40 Basophilic bodies. In the horse, intestinal submucosal arteries invariably contain intimal asteroid basophilic bodies. These are derived from degeneration and calcification of subendothelial smooth muscle cells. These bodies exert no harmful effect on the arterial intima. (From a 14-year-old pony mare.)

3. The Clinical Examination

Thorough clinical examination is of paramount importance in even the most sophisticated investigation of the heart. It can provide valuable information about cardiac functional status, circulatory physiology, and the likely cause of heart disease. This complete cardiovascular (CV) examination includes many elements (**3.1**), but should always begin with a conversation with the owner, and a complete physical examination of the patient. Pertinent aspects include an overall inspection and assessment of the heart and circulation, particularly the identification of heart murmurs, gallop sounds, arrhythmias or congestive heart failure (CHF). The most important aspect of physical examination is careful cardiac auscultation, which remains one of the most sensitive and cost-effective techniques for cardiac diagnosis. The establishment of anatomic, aetiologic and physiologic diagnoses (**3.2**) facilitates an accurate prognosis and appropriate therapy.

GENERAL CONSIDERATIONS

The *species, age, breed and sex* should be considered, as certain disorders are associated with particular signalments. For example, virtually all cases of right-sided CHF in cattle would be due to ventricular septal defect, tricuspid or pulmonic valve endocarditis, septic pericarditis, right atrial lymphosarcoma, or severe, diffuse pulmonary disease (cor pulmonale). A left-sided systolic heart murmur in a golden retriever puppy is most likely to be caused by either subvalvular aortic stenosis or mitral valve dysplasia. The most important cardiac arrhythmia leading to exercise intolerance in a performance horse is atrial fibrillation. Almost all cases of aortic thromboembolism in cats can be attributed to a form of cardiomyopathy or (rarely) bacterial endocarditis. Heart failure in a 3-year-old male Doberman pinscher is almost certainly caused by dilated cardiomyopathy. An older, small breed of dog, with a loud systolic murmur of mitral regurgitation is assumed to be affected with degenerative mitral valve disease (endocardiosis) until proven otherwise. Experienced clinicians recognize well these predispositions to cardiac disease.

No complaints are specific for cardiovascular disease. A systematic clinical evaluation includes a client interview, complete physical examination of the patient, and selection and interpretation of appropriate laboratory studies. Nevertheless, the clinician should be attuned to potential cardiovascular disease whenever certain clinical signs are evident, including exercise intolerance, sudden weakness or collapse, syncope (**3.3**), fatigue or poor performance, difficult

Diagnostic Studies in Cardiovascular Disease

- Signalment (age, breed, sex) and the animal's use
- Client complaint and patient history (anamnesis)
- Physical evaluation of the arterial pulses
- Inspection of the venous pressure and pulses
- Palpation of the precordium
- Measurement of arterial blood pressure
- Auscultation of heart and lungs
- Percussion of thorax
- Radiographic examination
- Electrocardiography
- Echocardiography, ultrasound imaging of blood vessels, and Doppler studies
- Ultrasound examination of noncardiac structures, including liver and hepatic veins, spleen, peritoneal and pleural cavities and mediastinum
- Appropriate clinical laboratory tests, including: tests for microfilaria or heartworm antigens (heartworm enzootic areas), blood cultures (for endocarditis), haemoglobin, serum chemistries including electrolytes, serum myocardial enzymes, serum thyroxin concentration, plasma taurine or plasma carnitine, titres (e.g. Chagas' disease or parvovirus)
- Cytologic evaluation and culture of peritoneal, pleural or pericardial effusions
- Noninvasive graphic studies – phonocardiography, measurement of systolic time intervals
- Cardiac catheterization – for determination of intravascular pressures, cardiac output, oxygen saturation and intracardiac electrocardiography
- Angiocardiography and angiography
- Radioangiocardiography (nuclear cardiology)
- Myocardial biopsy

3.1 Diagnostic studies in cardiovascular disease.

Cardiac Diagnoses		
Anatomic diagnoses – morphologic diagnosis/area of injury • Cardiac valves • Endocardium • Myocardium (including cardiac septa) • Pericardium and pericardial space • Specialized impulse forming and conduction system • Arteries Pulmonary Coronary Systemic • Veins	**Aetiologic diagnoses –** the cause of cardiovascular injury • Anomalous • Degenerative • Endocrine • Genetic • Metabolic • Nutritional • Neoplastic • Iatrogenic • Idiopathic • Immune-mediated • Infectious • Inflammatory • Ischaemic • Space occupying (e.g. pericardial effusion, intracardiac tumour) • Toxic • Traumatic • Other (e.g.foreign body)	**Physiologic diagnoses –** the functional consequence • Valvular regurgitation • Valvular stenosis • Intracardiac obstruction • Intracardiac shunting • Cardiac arrhythmia • Shock • Syncope • Systolic heart (cardiac) failure • Diastolic heart (cardiac) failure • Congestive heart (cardiac) failure • Vascular obstruction • Vascular shunting • Hypotension • Hypertension • Sudden cardiac death

3.2 Cardiac diagnoses.

breathing, coughing, cyanosis, acute limb paresis, regurgitation of food in neonates (vascular ring anomaly) and abnormal fluid accumulation.

The *general inspection and physical examination* of an animal may indicate whether clinical signs are likely to be of cardiac origin, although there are few totally reliable indicators of heart disease. Certain clinical findings, however, should influence the differential diagnosis. Two simple examples are body weight and heart rate in dogs: loss of body condition is typical of advanced heart failure in dogs and, conversely, dogs with chronic airway diseases (e.g. bronchitis, fibrosis or tracheal collapse) are more often overweight or obese. The finding of resting bradycardia associated with exertional weakness or collapse in a dog may suggest reduced cardiac output caused by a primary bradyarrhythmia, such as in sick sinus syndrome or atrioventricular (AV) block. However, sinus bradycardia also can result from noncardiac disorders (see Chapter 23). Further observation may be helpful: a dog with chronic bradycardia associated with sinus node or AV nodal disease is usually alert at rest, whereas marked depression or subdued mentation would suggest that bradycardia might be secondary to a metabolic disturbance (e.g. hypothyroidism or hyperkalaemia) or abnormally high vagal tone (e.g. elevated cerebrospinal fluid pressure or chemical/plant intoxication).

Vital signs, heart and respiratory rate, and rectal temperature should be recorded. Persistent fever is typical of infective endocarditis or pericarditis. Hypothermia can be an ominous sign of cardiogenic shock and low cardiac output. It is important to monitor hydration status, especially in animals receiving diuretic therapy. Mucous membranes should be examined for cyanosis, which is a sign of systemic arterial hypoxemia (right-to-left shunt or pulmonary dysfunction), low cardiac output, or both. Pallor of the mucous membranes typically indicates either anaemia or intense peripheral vasoconstriction related to low cardiac output. Bodyweight should be monitored in all cardiac patients.

Respiratory signs are commonly observed in animals with heart disease. High pitched respiratory noise (wheezing or stridor) tends to indicate airway obstruction. This may be due to laryngeal paralysis, collapsed or obstructed trachea or bronchus, bronchial asthma, or compression of the left bronchus by an enlarged left atrium. Differential diagnosis of cough, tachypnoea and dyspnoea must include each of these conditions as well as infectious, oedematous, neoplastic, parasitic and inflammatory bronchopulmonary disorders. Pleural effusion is a common cause of tachypnoea and respiratory distress. Most respiratory signs related to CV disease stem from either pulmonary oedema or pleural effusion (signs of CHF), bronchial compression, or pulmonary thromboembolism.

The numerous interactions between the CV and other organ systems must be considered. For example, older cats should be examined for palpable thyroid tumours, and the ocular fundus should be examined for retinal lesions of taurine deficiency or hypertension. Heart failure can disrupt normal neurohormonal balance (see Chapter 1), decrease renal perfusion, disrupt normal pulmonary function and

Cardiovascular Causes of Syncope	
Cardiac arrhythmias – particularly sinus arrest, complete AV block, and paroxysmal tachycardias **Congenital heart diseases** – particularly cyanotic heart disease (e.g., tetralogy of Fallot), pulmonic valve stenosis, and aortic stenosis **Acquired heart disease** – any condition serious enough to limit cardiac output such as mitral or tricuspid valve regurgitation, dilated cardiomyopathy **Pulmonary hypertension** – animals with pulmonary hypertension (e.g. heartworm disease; acute pulmonary thromboembolism) seem at risk for exertional syncope **Cough (tussive) syncope** – a syndrome that may be caused by abrupt reductions in venous return and/or increases in cerebrospinal fluid pressure **Cerebral vascular haemorrhage**	**Dysautonomia (vagal-induced syncope)** – a syndrome of inappropriate sinus bradycardia and peripheral vasodilation; possible causes include hyperactive baroreceptors (e.g. brachycephalic breeds), cervical tumours, and chronic heart failure (desensitization). **Plasma volume contraction** – as with Addison's disease (hypoadrenocorticism), administration of diuretic drugs, severe diarrhoea **Obstruction to venous return** – related to vascular tumours (e.g. obstructing the caudal vena cava) or intracardiac masses (e.g. right atrial haemangiosarcoma) or pericardial effusion **Vasodilator drugs** – administration of prazosin, hydralazine, angiotensin-converting enzyme (ACE) inhibitors, calcium channel antagonists
Cardiovascular syncope is usually caused by arterial hypotension, therefore *excessive arteriolar vasodilatation, reduced cardiac output*, or *excessive plasma volume contraction* will be the underlying mechanism for syncope. Other mechanisms of importance include moderate-to-severe (often acute) anaemia which limits oxygen delivery, microvascular sludging of RBC in severe polycythaemia and shock, arterial hypoxaemia from severe pulmonary dysfunction and hypoglycaemia.	

3.3 Cardiovascular causes of syncope.

even lead to colic or vomiting (horses with low output or cats with heartworm disease). Similarly, diseases of the respiratory system (e.g. diffuse pulmonary fibrosis), endocrine system (e.g. Addison's disease and thyroid disorders), kidneys (e.g. hypertension, or potassium depletion in cats), brain (e.g. dysautonomia), and gastrointestinal system can lead to secondary cardiac effects.

PERIPHERAL INDICATORS OF CIRCULATION

The *arterial pulse* rate, character and rhythm should be evaluated. The pulse and heart rates are slowed by vagal activity and increased by sympathetic stimulation, as found in overt cardiac failure. The pulse strength is related to myocardial contractility, stroke volume, aortic compliance, peripheral vascular resistance, and diastolic 'run off' of blood.

For example, the pulse tends to be notably weak in systolic failure, as with dilated cardiomyopathy, or in aortic outflow obstruction (aortic stenosis). Conversely, the pulse is accentuated but 'falls away' quickly in many cases of patent ductus arteriosus or aortic regurgitation. Particularly strong or hyperkinetic pulses may also be evident in hyperthyroidism, moderate-to-severe anaemia, and fever.

With many cardiac dysrhythmias (e.g. atrial fibrillation or ventricular premature beats) the pulse will have a variable intensity, related to variations in the left ventricular preload, arterial blood pressure (afterload), and cardiac cycle length; this can be accentuated by an absence or lack of coordination of the ventricular beats with the atrial contractions. Furthermore, with dysrhythmias, the pulse may be imperceptible or absent for some audible beats ('pulse deficit'). Absence of a pulse may indicate thrombosis or thromboembolism of a vessel. This situation is most often observed in cats with cardiomyopathy and thromboembolism of the terminal aorta. Finally, the clinician can measure arterial blood pressure indirectly using one of several devices. For example, a Doppler flow meter with a cuff and hand-held manometer is an effective and practical method. Blood pressure devices are invaluable in monitoring cardiac therapy and preventing untoward hypotension.

The *jugular veins* and peripheral veins should be scrutinized. The vein may be distended, or abnormal jugular pulsation may be appreciated in right-sided CHF or cardiac tamponade. To appreciate this fully, clipping the hair of the neck may be required (**3.7**). In normal animals, with the head in the normal position while standing, back-filling of the jugular vein may be seen about one-third of the distance up the neck, generally to the level of the point of the shoulder. The finding of jugular venous distension in the animal with ascites, pleural effusion, or subcutaneous oedema should lead the clinician to evaluate the heart carefully. However venepuncture, thrombosis, obesity and prior diuretic therapy may prevent adequate evaluation of the vein.

While abnormal fluid accumulation is an essential finding for a diagnosis of CHF, there are numerous noncardiac causes of fluid retention. *Subcutaneous oedema* of the ventral thorax and abdomen is a prominent sign of right-sided cardiac failure in horses and cattle (**3.11**), but not in small animals with CHF. When limb oedema develops in the absence of ventral oedema or ascites, heart failure is not usually the cause in any species. Most cases of generalized subcutaneous oedema in small animals are instead associated with hypoproteinemia (e.g. protein-losing enteropathy or nephropathy). Vasculitis can lead to subcutaneous oedema without jugular distension; this is most often observed in horses, but can be seen in other species as well. *Ascites* can be a sign of right-sided CHF. Even if ascites is not obvious, careful abdominal palpation may demonstrate hepatomegaly in right-sided congestive failure. *Hydrothorax* is also commonly found in left-sided or biventricular CHF, but this requires rather more careful clinical assessment. Tachypnoea is evident in moderate-to-severe pleural effusions, and there is accentuation of the contrast between dorsal resonance and ventral thoracic dullness on percussion. Airway sounds are often accentuated and displaced dorsally, and heart sounds are often muffled. Pleural effusions should be examined cytologically to assist in the differential diagnosis: a modified transudate is typical. *Pulmonary oedema*, a sign of left-sided CHF and some noncardiac pulmonary injuries, also often leads to tachypnoea and often respiratory distress. Surprisingly, coughing may be absent. In some cases, pulmonary oedema leads to audible 'crackles' – a sign of small airway dysfunction. Crackles are not pathognomonic for fluid accumulation, however, as bronchitis, fibrosis, and other bronchopulmonary disorders can produce crackles and lungs that 'sound wet' to the examiner.

The *cardiac impulse* should be palpated on both sides of the thorax (**3.10**). It becomes more prominent in cardiac enlargement, tends to be hyperkinetic with increased myocardial contractility (e.g. hyperthyroidism), but is usually weakened by severe myocardial failure, hypovolaemia or pericardial effusion. A precordial thrill is a palpable vibration indicating turbulence in blood flow. It is a reliable sign of significant cardiac disease. Many cardiac dysrhythmias can also be readily appreciated by palpation.

CARDIAC AUSCULTATION

Cardiac auscultation is essential to a thorough cardiac assessment, and it is vital that all areas of the thorax overlying the heart are examined thoroughly. Auscultation should be continued for at least two minutes in an attempt to detect transient cardiac dysrhythmias. Several phenomena can be evaluated:

The *audibility* of heart sounds: this is often accentuated by cardiac enlargement unless there is severe myocardial failure, in which case their audibility may be reduced. Sounds can be muffled by most pleural and pericardial effusions and evaluation may be difficult in dyspnoeic animals with pulmonary oedema, or in obese subjects.

The *area* over which cardiac sounds are heard: this is often increased, but may also be reduced in the presence of effusions. Heart sounds may be displaced by an abnormal mass or in cases of congenital peritoneopericardial diaphragmatic hernia.

The *heart rate*: this is usually, but not always, increased in cardiac failure, but it is also elevated by other states such as excitement, hyperthermia, fever and pain. In some dogs with significant heart disease and clinical signs (e.g. coughing from bronchial compression), but without CHF, the heart rate may be normal with prominent sinus arrhythmia. Finally, significant elevations or depressions in heart rate occur with many dysrhythmias.

The *cardiac rhythm*: regular sinus rhythm is normal in most species. However, at rest, most normal dogs and horses and some cattle exhibit 'sinus' arrhythmia – a phasic acceleration and deceleration of the heart rate which is often, but not always, synchronous with ventilation. The slowing is achieved through increased vagal tone, which tends to be abolished by sympathetic drive. In many normal horses (especially in fit animals) and in some dogs, 'missed beats' due to second degree AV block will be evident. This is also a vagally mediated rhythm and, like sinus arrhythmia, will abate if the animal is excited or exercised. Clinically significant dysrhythmias, such as ventricular tachycardia, tend to provoke a much more sudden change in heart rate, often accompanied by a change in intensity of heart sounds and of the pulse intensity, and any murmur may be modified. Bradydysrhythmias, such as complete (third degree) AV block, may often be manifest as unvarying bradycardia, and a notably strong pulse. Atrial fibrillation, an important and common arrhythmia in many species, gives a truly random arrhythmia, with variations in intensity of cardiac sounds and pulse. Furthermore, as with some premature beats, the second heart sound may be absent following particularly short cardiac cycles, adding to the chaos in the sounds. In large animal species, the normally present atrial (fourth) sound will be lost.

Cardiac murmurs: these are caused mainly by the vibrations associated with high velocity, disturbed and turbulent blood flow. These flow disturbances are most often related to valvular incompetence, valvular steno-

Clinical Features of Common Cardiac Murmurs

Auscultatory finding	Timing*	Point of maximal intensity [Valve area]
FUNCTIONAL MURMURS		
Systolic ejection	S	Lt base [Aortic/pulmonary valves] and craniodorsal to the semilunar valve (over the great vessels)
Early diastolic (protodiastolic) (horses, cattle)	D	Ventricular inlets (Lt/Rt)
Late diastolic (presystolic) (horses, cattle)	D	Ventricular inlets (Lt/Rt)
VALVULAR REGURGITATION		
Mitral regurgitation	S	Lt apex [mitral valve] – radiation to the right, cranial towards the aortic valve area and dorsally into the left atrium
Tricuspid regurgitation	S	Rt hemithorax [tricuspid valve] – radiation dorsad and to the left
Aortic regurgitation	D	Lt base [aortic valve] – radiates to the right and often caudad
Pulmonary insufficiency	D	Lt base [pulmonic valve] – usually very localized murmur, difficult to detect unless moderate to severe regurgitation or pulmonary hypertension
VALVULAR STENOSIS		
Pulmonic stenosis	S	Lt base [pulmonic valve] with dorsal radiation into main pulmonary artery [craniodorsal cardiac base]
(Subvalvular) aortic stenosis	S	Lt base [aortic valve] or immediately caudoventral to the aortic valve with radiation craniad, dextrad, up the carotids, and sometimes to the left apex
SHUNTS		
Atrial septal defect	S + D	Lt base [pulmonic valve] with radiation dorsad; the systolic murmur is due to relative pulmonic stenosis; a soft right-sided diastolic murmur of relative tricuspid stenosis might also be detected.
Ventricular septal defect	S	Right sternal border/left cardiac base [pulmonic valve]
Patent ductus arteriosus	S+D	Dorsal left base over pulmonary artery

*Systolic (S) or Diastolic (D)

- Only typical features are considered; 'apex' refers to the ventral part of the heart, at the point of the palpable cardiac impulse (apex beat); 'base' refers to the cranio-dorsal part of the heart over the outlet valves (aortic, pulmonic); the aortic valve area is that where the second heart sound is most intense.
- The exact causes of functional (flow) murmurs have not been determined.
- Ventricular inlets refer to the thorax overlying the ventricular inflow tracts. These include those regions just dorsal to the mitral and tricuspid valve areas and extend ventrally to the apical regions of the ventricles.
- Most cases of valve regurgitation are evident throughout systole or diastole and extend into the second heart sound (holo- or pansystolic) or first heart sound (holo- or pandiastolic); however, late systolic murmurs, which may be related to valve prolapse and minor chordal ruptures, have been identified with mitral or tricuspid valve insufficiency and the murmur of aortic insufficiency may not always be holodiastolic.
- Murmurs caused by septal defects in the right ventricular inlet septum are heard best below the tricuspid valve and above the right sternal border and generate a softer systolic ejection murmur of relative pulmonic stenosis over the left cardiac base; murmurs from defects in the RV outlet septum may be loudest on the left near the pulmonary valve; flow across very large nonrestrictive defects can be relatively soft.

3.4 Clinical features of common cardiac murmurs.

sis, or the presence of a shunt. Virtually all significant flow disturbances (e.g. those with valve regurgitation or stenosis, and shunts) can be detected by auscultation. However, disturbed flow that is trivial, or that is of low velocity flow (e.g. with pulmonic regurgitation) may not be heard; furthermore, murmurs can also be created by other physiological or pathological processes. For example, murmurs are often heard with changes in the viscosity of the blood (e.g. moderate-to-severe anaemia). Innocent 'flow' murmurs are found in many fit racehorses and in some normal young dogs (**3.4**). A few cardiac disorders are *not* associated with an audible murmur. For example, cardiomyopathies will be associated with a murmur only if there is concurrent valve regurgitation; pericardial effusions do not cause cardiac murmurs; cardiac dysrhythmias *per se* do not create murmurs, but valvular regurgitation or 'flow' murmurs may develop.

Cardiac murmurs may be classified in several ways:

Timing in the cardiac cycle – systolic, diastolic or continuous – and *duration* of the murmur, relative to the heart sounds: most murmurs are created by the pressures generated during ventricular systole, though there are some notable diastolic heart murmurs (e.g. aortic regurgitation). The duration of a murmur carries significance as well (**3.4**). The timing of some cardiac murmurs is notably characteristic of certain lesions. For example, murmurs of pulmonic or aortic stenosis begin after the first sound and always end by the second sound (ejection murmurs); mitral regurgitation typically is holosystolic, beginning with the first sound and ending after the second sound; the murmur of patent ductus arteriosus is usually prolonged, peaking at about the time of the second sound and waning at the end of diastole; the typical murmur of aortic regurgitation begins immediately with the second sound and is holodiastolic. In contrast, functional (innocent or physiological) murmurs are usually shorter in duration.

Intensity: cardiac murmurs are graded by intensity on a subjective scale (**3.5**). Generally, the more intense (and later peaking) the murmur, the more serious the lesion (e.g. aortic or pulmonic stenosis). However, loudness does not consistently correlate with murmurs of mitral or tricuspid regurgitation or ventricular septal defect, though there is usually a tendency for serious regurgitant lesions to cause very loud murmurs. Occasionally, severe lesions do not result in prominent murmurs; examples include tetralogy of Fallot with pulmonary atresia, unrestrictive ventricular septal defect, or severe tricuspid regurgitation.

Point of maximal intensity: this is the area of the thorax at which a murmur is most intense, and it generally relates closely to the underlying source of turbulent flow. For example, the murmur of patent ductus arteriosus is best heard over the dorsocranial heart base, essentially over the main pulmonary artery, at the left side of the thorax. Murmurs of mitral regurgitation project to the left apical impulse where they are particularly intense. The timing and point of maximal intensity are the best indicators of the haemodynamic basis of a cardiac murmur (**3.4**).

Radiation: murmurs may radiate widely from the point of maximal intensity. Generally, the wider the radiation, the more severe the lesion, while very localized murmurs often represent minimal disease. Some murmurs radiate in a fairly characteristic fashion. For example, the murmur of aortic stenosis may be heard radiating cranially and to the right, into the ascending aorta and then up the carotids; the murmur of pulmonary stenosis radiates dorsally from the pulmonary valve area into the main pulmonary artery, so this murmur tends to be quite loud over the left craniodorsal cardiac base.

Pitch and quality: these subjective descriptions are used to describe the character of a murmur. The terms are not precise and do not have the same objectivity as timing and point of maximal intensity. Most murmurs consist of mixed audible frequencies and sound 'harsh' – a very general term. The term 'ejection' refers to the murmurs generated when blood is ejected into a great vessel; on a phonocardiogram this is inscribed as a crescendo–decrescendo pattern that ends at the second heart sound. The term 'regurgitant' refers to holosystolic murmurs – usually those caused by mitral regurgitation, tricuspid regurgitation, or a ventricular septal defect; these murmurs are relatively plateau-shaped on a phonocardiogram recording. However, sometimes these lesions lead to a more decrescendo configuration on the phonocardiogram, and are characterized clinically as 'blowing'; aortic regurgitation produces a similar diastolic murmur. The term 'musical' indicates that the murmur has characteristics that result in phonocardiogram recordings of a fundamental frequency and harmonic; such sounds may be described as 'vibratory', 'cooing' or 'buzzing'. Musical murmurs are most often detected in aortic regurgitation in horses and in animals with ruptured mitral chordae tendineae.

Other abnormal cardiac sounds: in fibrinous pericarditis of large animals, friction sounds can be heard that are synchronous with the heart beat, usually evident in systole and in early and late diastole. However, this finding is rare in companion animal species. In pericarditis in cattle, splashing or tinkling sounds may be heard when gas-producing organisms are present within the pericardial space. Alternatively, as in any species, the heart sounds may be muffled by pericardial effusion.

The atrial (fourth) and ventricular (third) sounds are normal in horses and cattle, but indicate heart disease in small animals. When present in dogs and cats, the extra sounds cause a cadence similar to a galloping horse (*gallop sound*). Atrial and ventricular gallops indicate diastolic dysfunction, and are most often observed in dogs with volume overload (e.g. mitral regurgitation or dilated cardiomyopathy) and in cats with left ventricular hypertrophy. These sounds are often best heard with the bell of a stethoscope. The presence of the fourth (atrial contraction) sound in many normal horses can assist the clinician in assessing cardiac rhythm: it will be absent in atrial fibrillation, but it is often present in the pause of the missed beat of second degree AV block. A gallop sound should not be confused with a *systolic click* – a high-pitched, left apical, systolic sound indicative of mitral valve thickening or prolapse.

Splitting of the second heart sound can be heard in circumstances in which the closure of the pulmonic valve is delayed. This is a normal finding in some horses. When exaggerated, and especially when accompanied by a tympanic pulmonary component of the S2, pulmonary hypertension should be suspected. Causes include chronic respiratory disease, dirofilariasis in dogs, and left-sided CHF. Splitting of the first or second sound may become evident when there is abnormal ventricular activation as with bundle branch block or ventricular ectopic beats.

Grading of Cardiac Murmurs

Grade 1	A very soft, localized murmur detected only in a quiet room and after minutes of intense listening.
Grade 2	A soft murmur, heard immediately.
Grade 3	A low to moderate intensity murmur.
Grade 4	A moderate to loud intensity murmur; a consistent precordial thrill is not present.
Grade 5	A loud murmur accompanied by a palpable precordial thrill but cannot be detected when the stethoscope is removed from the thorax.
Grade 6	A loud murmur accompanied by a precordial thrill and audible when the stethoscope is removed from the thorax.

Intensity of the murmur is arbitrarily graded on a 1–6 scale (some use a 1–5 scale); this scale is adapted from that of Friedman; in some 1–6 systems, a grade 4 murmur is associated with a definite precordial thrill.

3.5 Grading of cardiac murmurs.

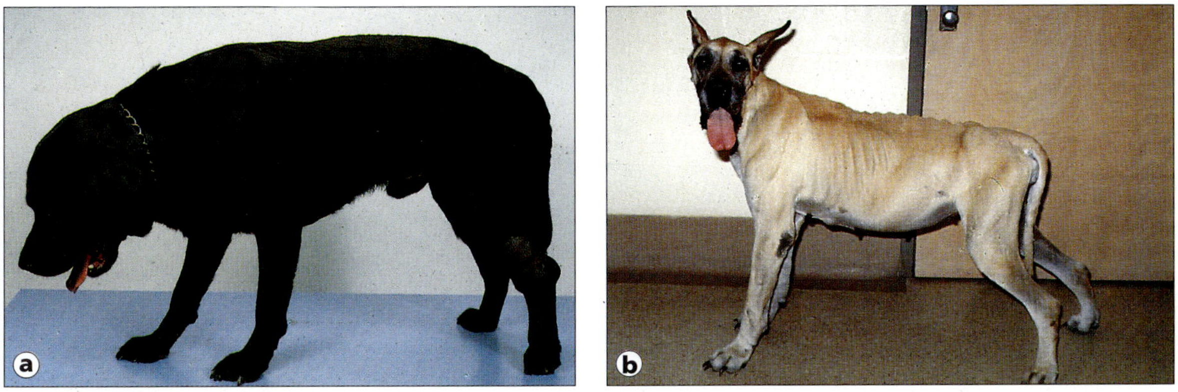

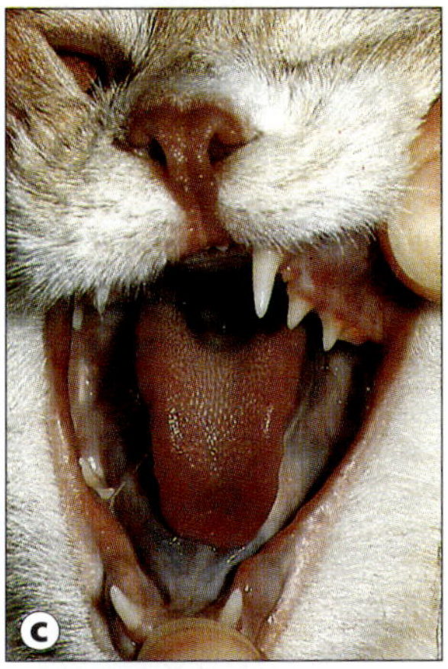

3.6 (**a**) The examination begins with a general inspection of the animal. This dog was exercise intolerant and had syncopal attacks related to heartworm disease. (**b**) Cardiac cachexia is evident in this Great Dane dog with chronic heart failure secondary to mitral malformation and atrial fibrillation. There is also a small degree of ascitic fluid accumulation that slightly distends the abdomen. (**c**) Cyanosis in a cat. This finding typically suggests either right-to-left shunting or severe pulmonary dysfunction, as might develop with pulmonary oedema or pleural effusion.

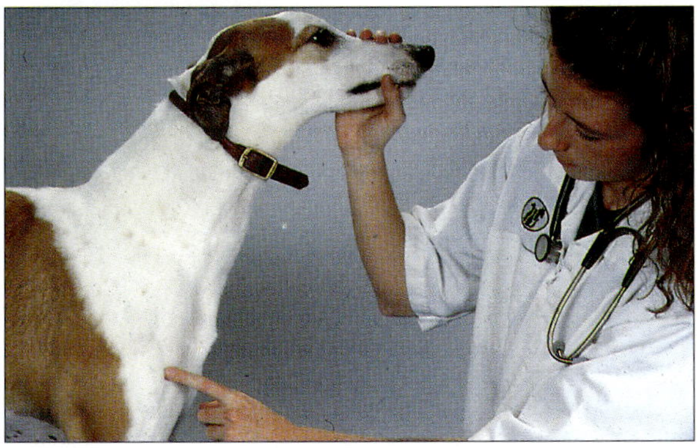

3.7 The jugular venous pressure and pulse are inspected. It is normal to observe transmission of right atrial pressure pulses to the level of the point of the shoulder.

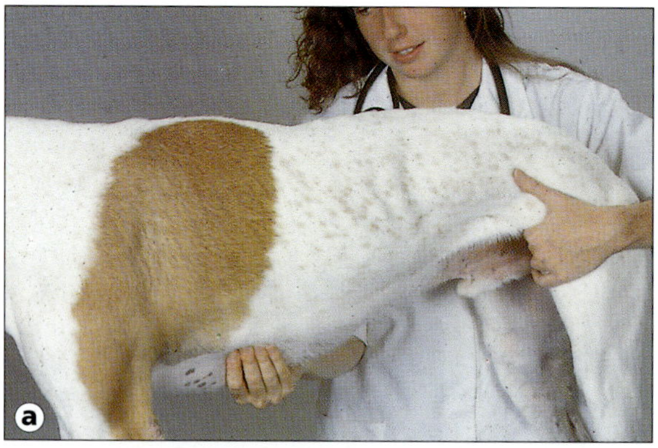

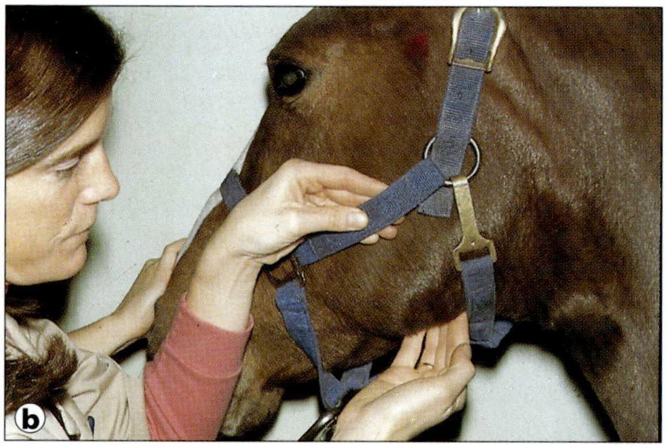

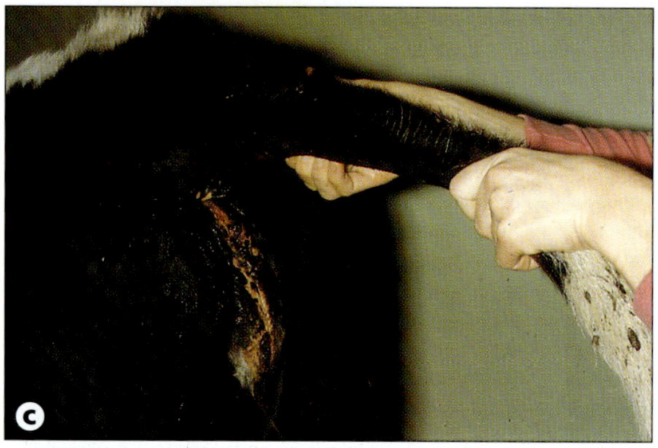

3.8 Palpation of the arterial pulse. (**a**) The femoral artery is used in the dog and cat. The cardiac impulse (apex beat) and pulse can be compared to detect pulse deficits. (**b**) The facial artery is typically palpated in the horse. (**c**) The coccygeal artery is examined in the cow.

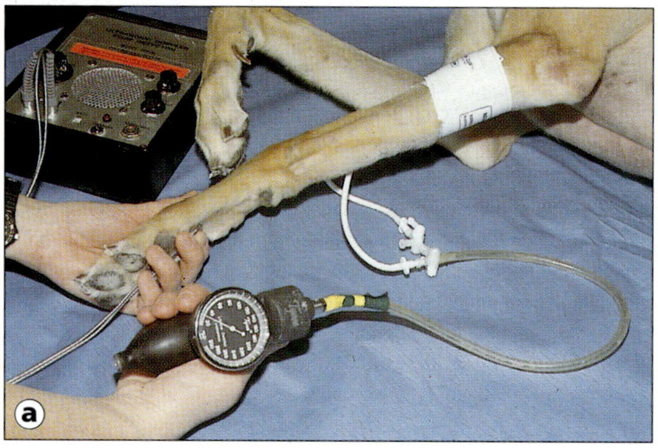

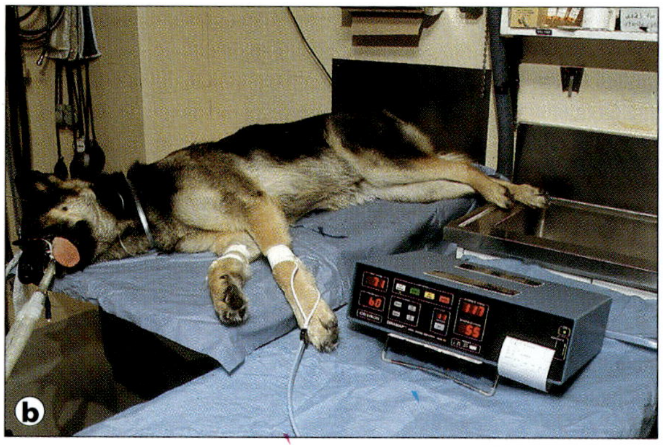

3.9 Measurement of the arterial blood pressure. (**a**) Using an ultrasound crystal to measure blood flow. The cuff inflation pressure is monitored as pressure is released to permit flow through the artery. (**b**) A fully automated device that measures blood pressure can be used to record blood vessel oscillations.

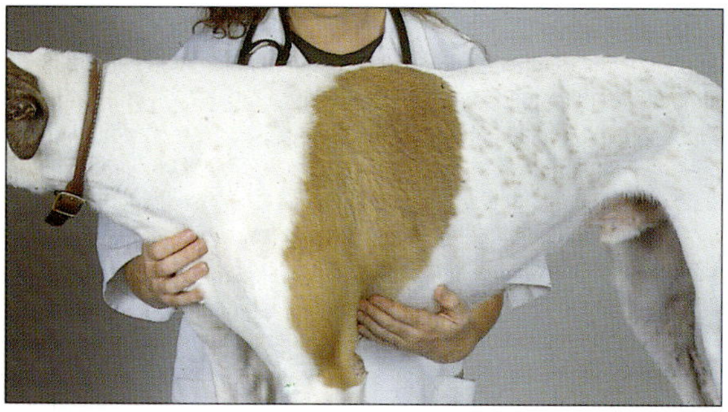

3.10 Palpation of the precordium to identify the apical impulse and precordial thrills.

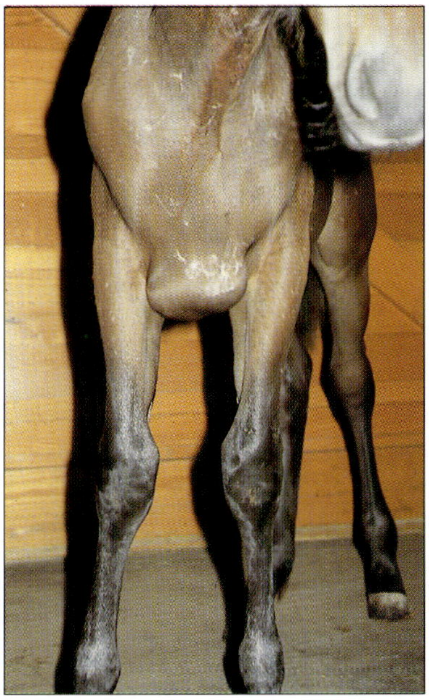

3.11 Ventral oedema caused by heart failure in a yearling with tricuspid valve endocarditis.

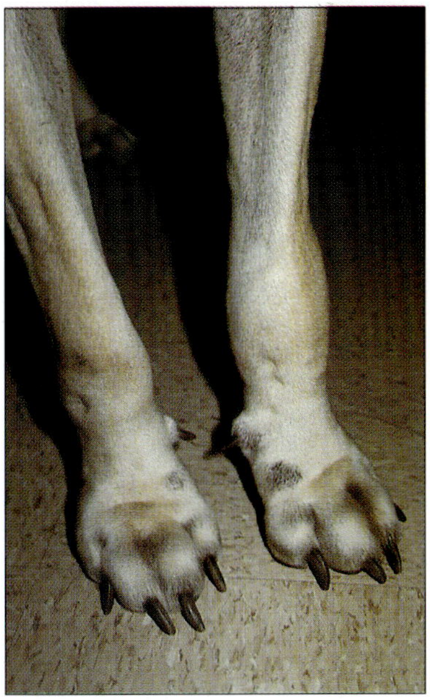

3.12 Distal limb oedema in a dog with severe right-sided heart failure. Limb oedema is more often a sign of non-cardiac diseases, such as hypoalbuminaemia.

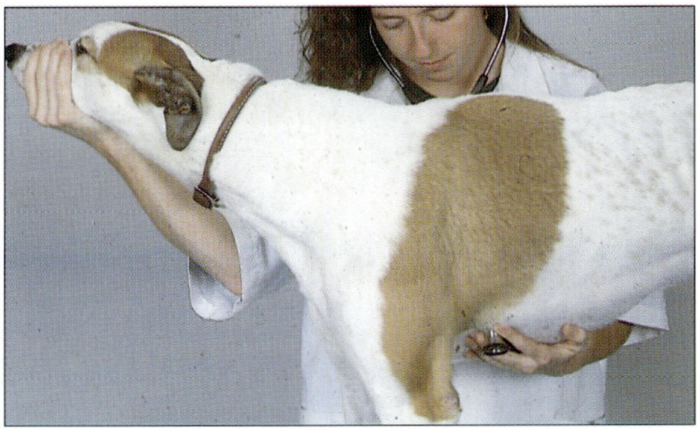

3.13 Auscultation of the heart. The stethoscope is placed over the cardiac apex in this picture.

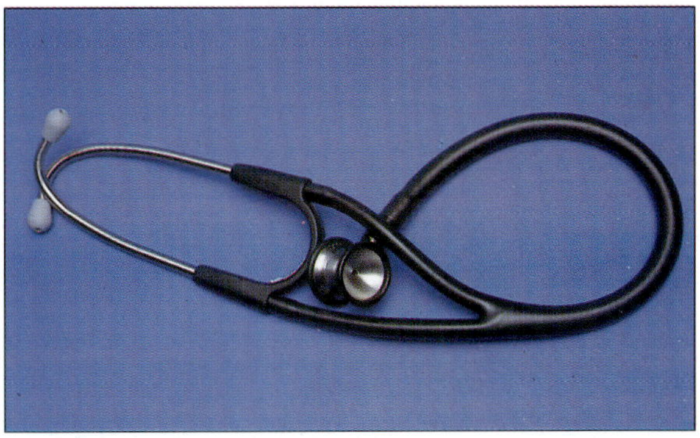

3.14 Parts of the stethoscope are evident, including the diaphragm and bell of the chest piece, tubes (double tubes eventually combined), biaurals and ear pieces, both of which are adjustable to the comfort of the examiner.

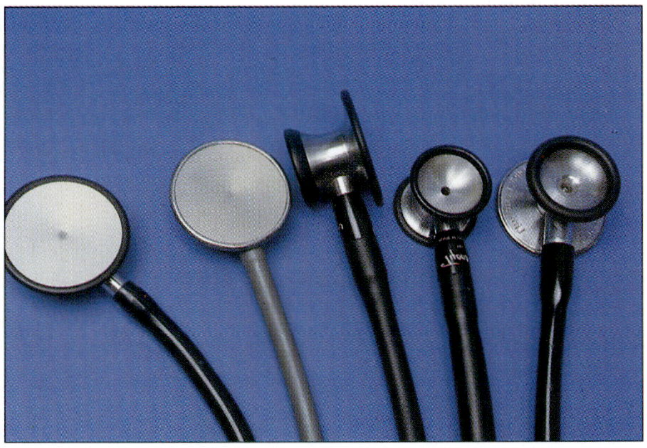

3.15 Various types of chest pieces. The small, paediatric-type diaphragms and bells are often more effective for auscultation of smaller animals. The bell is best used to detect low frequency sounds such as gallops and soft diastolic murmurs and should be applied with light pressure to the chest so as to create an air seal. Other models (not shown) include deep 'trumpet' bell chest pieces and single chest pieces in which the diaphragm and bell are combined and toggled by varying the pressure applied to the thorax.

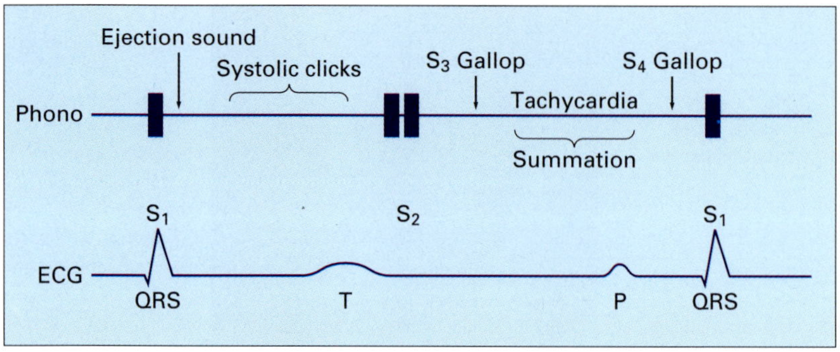

3.16 Timing of heart sounds. The relationship of the ECG to the heart sounds is demonstrated. The first sound indicates the onset of ventricular systole and coincides with closure of the mitral and tricuspid valves. The arterial pulse can be palpated following the first sound. The second sound indicates the end of systole and the closure of the aortic and pulmonic valves. The third sound, S_3, which occurs at the end of rapid ventricular filling and the fourth sound, S_4, which follows the atrial contraction are normally detected in horses and cattle. An S_3 or S_4 are considered signs of heart disease in the dog and the cat and when present often lead to a 'galloping' cadence. At rapid heart rates, an S_3 and S_4 may merge leading to a *summation gallop*. The timing of other transient sounds, such as the ejection or midsystolic click is shown. Often, a physiologic ejection murmur is heard in horses or cattle between the first and second sounds. In normal horses, one or two brief diastolic murmurs also may be detected; these occur between the second and third sounds (protodiastolic or rapid filling murmurs) and between the fourth and first sounds (presystolic murmur).

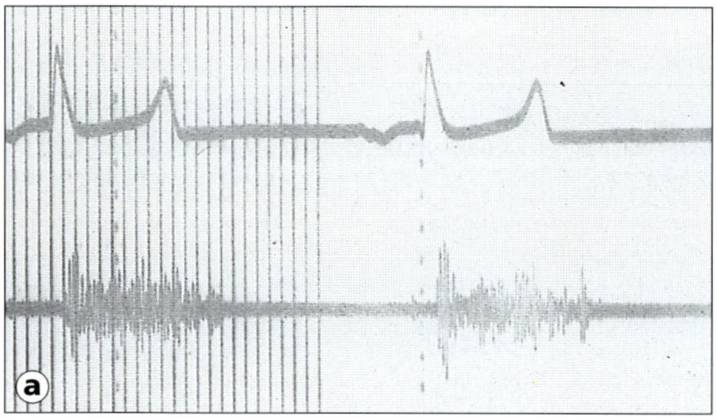

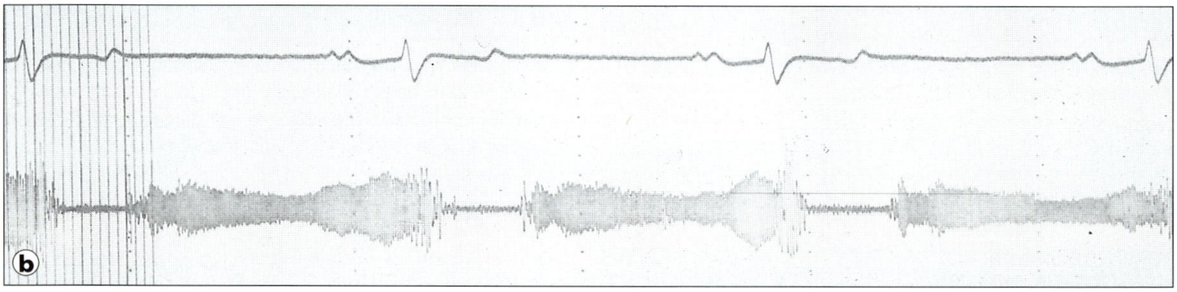

3.17 Cardiac murmurs. (**a**) ECG (top) and phonocardiogram demonstrating a systolic murmur in a foal with a ventricular septal defect. (**b**) ECG (top) and phonocardiogram demonstrating a holodiastolic murmur with presystolic accentuation recorded from a horse with aortic regurgitation.

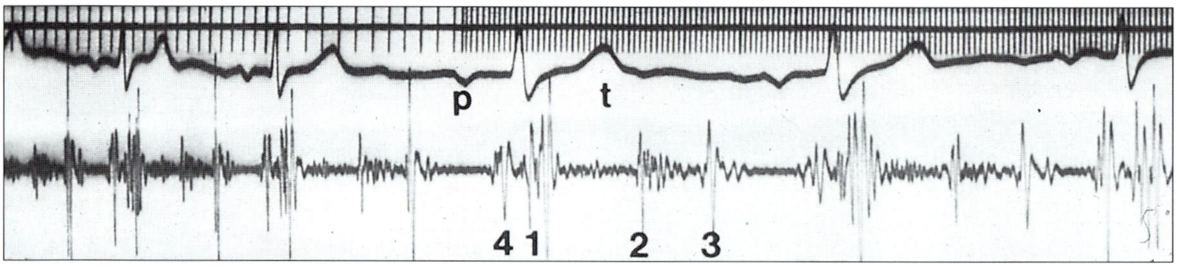

3.18 ECG (top) and phonocardiogram demonstrating both atrial (4) and ventricular (3) gallops in a Doberman pinscher with dilated cardiomyopathy. The first (1) and second (2) sounds also are demonstrated.

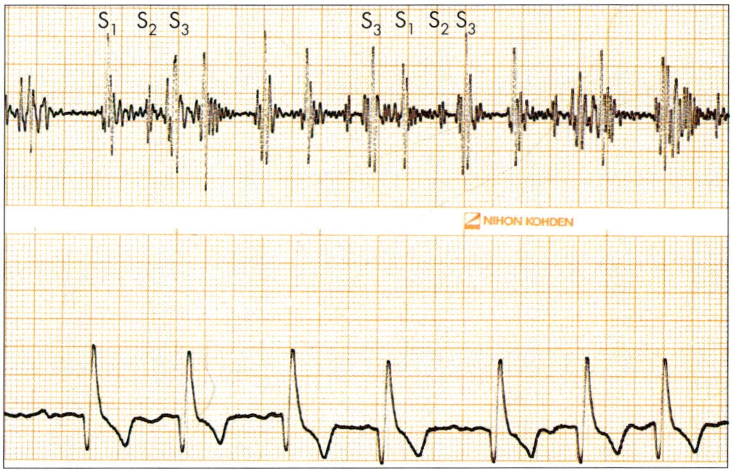

3.19 Phonocardiogram from a Doberman pinscher with dilated cardiomyopathy. There is atrial fibrillation, gallop sounds are shown to be due to a pronounced third heart sound (S_3), and the second heart sound (S_2) is variable – it disappears for some beats, in which ventricular filling has been inadequate to cause adequate stroke volume to open the aortic valve. This demonstrates the source of the pulse deficit in this case.

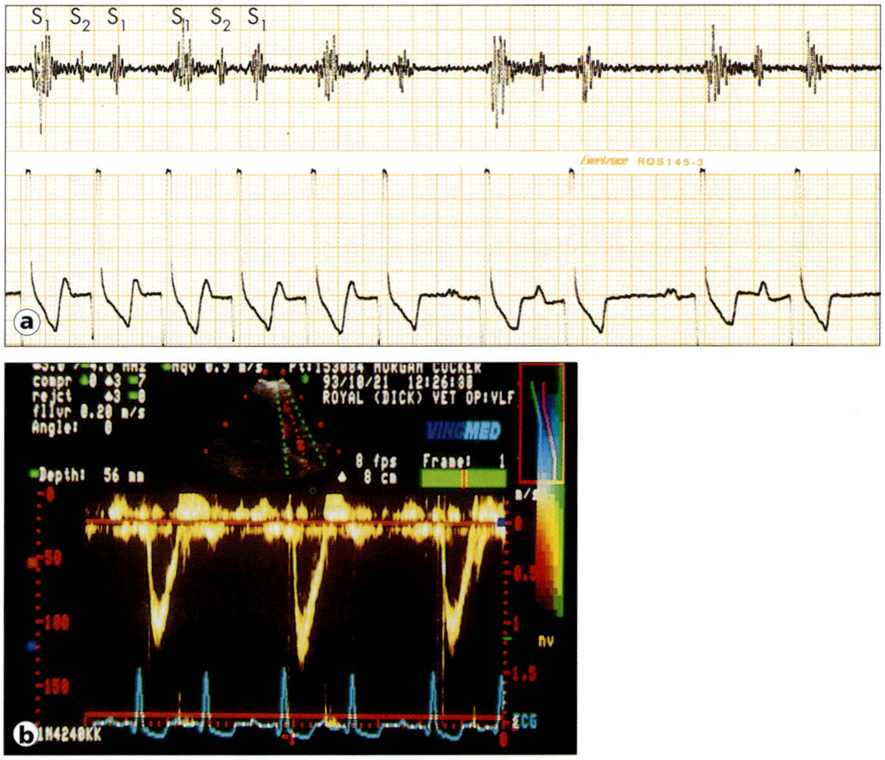

3.20 (**a**)Phonocardiogram from a cocker spaniel with dilated cardiomyopathy, showing alternans in the second heart sound (S_2), which is absent in every second beat, relating to the pulsus alternans in this case. (**b**) Pulsed-wave Doppler recording from the same cocker spaniel as in (**a**). Note the alternating stroke volume in the aortic outflow, which was associated with pulsus alternans. (Courtesy of Miss V Luis Fuentes)

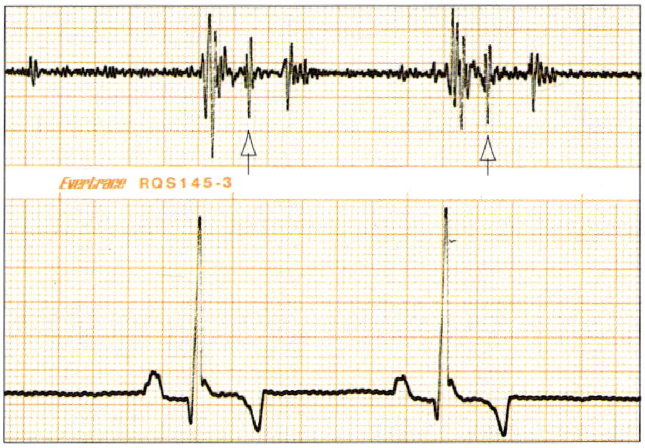

3.21 Phonocardiogram from a golden retriever with hypothyroidism. The systolic click (arrows) was an incidental finding of unknown aetiology in this case.

4.

Cardiac Radiography

Cardiac radiography is available to almost all small animal practitioners. However, radiography of the thorax presents the technical challenge of overcoming the effects of respiratory movement, especially in cardiac failure when dyspnoea may be present. This movement artifact may be reduced by the use of fast (e.g. rare earth) intensifying screens, and relatively high exposure voltages (e.g. 70–80 mV), which will minimize the current needed to achieve exposure, and therefore the exposure time. Good collimation will also help to improve the quality of films and minimize the effects of scattered radiation. Deep chests (> 12 cm) require the use of grids to minimize the effects of scattered radiation. Sedation may be needed for radiography, but heavy tranquillization is best avoided if the animal is dyspnoeic or showing other severe signs of cardiac failure. If the animal is relatively stable a mixture of acepromazine (0.03 mg/kg) with almost any opiate (e.g. buprenorphine 0.0075 mg/kg), given intravenously, will usually give sufficient sedation for an intractable dog to be positioned on a radiographic table without manual restraint being required. Cats may be sedated with a mixture of acepromazine (0.1 mg/kg) and butorphanol (0.2–0.3 mg/kg) administered intramuscularly. Low doses of ketamine (2–5 mg intravenously) can be used alone or with diazepam or midazdam for supplemental restraint.

Two views (lateral and dorsoventral or ventrodorsal) should be taken, and ideally the exposure should be made at peak inspiration. The animal should be carefully positioned to avoid rotation of the thorax, at this distorts the cardiac image. For detailed examination of the lung fields (e.g. for oedema), correct exposures, lack of movement and careful film processing are essential.

Thoracic radiographs indicate the volume load of the heart very well. Both congestive heart failure and the effects of hypovolaemia are well portrayed, and enlargement of specific cardiac chambers and great vessels may be demonstrated. Pulmonary overcirculation (as with left-to-right shunts), underperfusion (as with right-to-left shunts), pulmonary venous congestion (as with left-sided heart failure), and pulmonary hypertension (as with heartworm disease) may be suggested by inspection of lobar pulmonary arteries and veins. Left-sided congestive heart failure is best recognized by integration of clinical findings with thoracic radiographs. Typical features include left atrial enlargement, dilated pulmonary veins, and increased pulmonary interstitial and alveolar infiltrates. Right-sided heart failure may be suggested by distension of the caudal vena cava, hepatomegaly, ascites, and sometimes hydrothorax. In dogs with mitral regurgitation, left-mainstem bronchial compression by an enlarged left atrium can be demonstrated.

The detailed interpretation of thoracic radiographs demands considerable experience, however, and the technique is of less practical value in large animals. The large variation in shape and size of the thorax in dogs is challenging, especially when allied to variable exposure factors and stage of respiration. In the evaluation of thoracic films, the technical quality and artifacts should be assessed first, followed by systematic consideration of the following details:

1. The type of thorax: shallow-chested breeds of dog (e.g. bulldogs and some retrievers) have rounded cardiac outlines, while deep-chested breeds have more upright, triangulated hearts; and expiratory films tend to exaggerate the cardiac size.
2. Any evidence of cardiac enlargement – and which chambers may be involved.
3. The size of blood vessels (pulmonary arteries and veins; caudal vena cava).
4. The presence or absence, pattern, and distribution of abnormal pulmonary densities (which are exacerbated at expiration).
5. The presence of any pleural effusion or ascites.
6. The thoracic wall, mediastinum, diaphragm and abdominal contents.

A summary of radiographic findings is found in **4.1**. This chapter and others contain examples of various radiographic and angiographic patterns of cardiac disease. Angiography is discussed in Chapter 8.

Radiographic Features of Heart Disease								
DISORDER	**LV**	**LA**	**Ao**	**RV**	**RA**	**MPA**	**Pulmonary Circulation**	**Comments/ Additional findings**
Patent ductus arteriosus	+	+	+ Desc Ao.	0 [a]	0	+	+Artery +Vein	Left-sided CHF
Ventricular septal defect	+	+	0	+ [b]	0 [b]	+	+Artery +Vein	Left-sided CHF
Atrial septal defect	0	0 [c]	0	+	+	+	+Artery +Vein	Right-sided CHF
Mitral regurgitation	+	+	0	+ [b]	0	0	+Vein 0/+Artery	Left-sided CHF
Tricuspid regurgiatation	0	0	0	+	+	0	0	Dilated vena cava, right-sided CHF
Aortic stenosis	+	0/+	+ Asc.Ao	0	0	0	0/+Vein 0/+Artery	Left-sided CHF
Pulmonic stenosis	0	0	0	+	+	+	0/–Artery 0/–Vein	Right-sided CHF
Tetralogy of Fallot	0	0	+ [d]	+	+	[e]	–Artery –Vein	
Dilated cardiomyopathy	+	+	0	+	+	0	+Vein 0/+Artery	Biventricular CHF
Hypertrophic cardiomyopathy	+	+	0	0/+ [b]	0/+ [b]	0	+Vein 0/+Artery	Left-sided or biventricular CHF
Restrictive cardiomyopathy	+	+	0	+	+	-	+Vein 0/–Artery	Variable findings
Pericardial effusion	+	+	0	+	+	0	0/–Artery 0/–Vein	Possible mass lesion
Hyperthyroidism	+	+	+	+	+	0	0/+Artery 0/+Vein	Dilated or tortuous aorta
Pulmonary hypertension	0/+ [f]	0/+ [f]	0	+	+	+	–/0/+Artery –/0/+Vein [f,g]	Lungs may be abnormal or under-circulated
Heartworm disease	0	0	0	+	+	+	+Artery 0 Vein	Pulmonary infiltrate

Key: 0 (no change), + (enlarged or increased), – (decreased), Art (artery), Ao (aorta), MPA (main pulmonary artery)

Notes:

[a] While the RV may appear enlarged, echocardiographic studies demonstrate that left ventricular dilatation accounts for ventricular enlargement; in the rare case of reversed PDA the radiograph resembles that of pulmonary hypertension.

[b] Right-sided cardiomegaly will develop if there is pulmonary hypertension due to increased pulmonary flow, increased pulmonary vascular resistance, or right ventricular outflow obstruction.

[c] In the typical ostium secundum (high) ASD, blood flows immediately into the RA and the LA does not enlarge immediately. In cases of primum ASD with concurrent VSD or AV valve malformation (endocardial cushion defect), LA dilation also develops.

[d] The aorta is dextropositioned and receives most blood flow; this causes widening of the ventrocranial mediastinum on the lateral projection.

[e] The pulmonary artery is not dilated because blood preferentially shunts across the VSD into the aorta.

[f] In cases of pulmonary hypertension secondary to left-sided CHF, left heart structures will be enlarged.

[g] In cases of pulmonary hypertension secondary to left-sided CHF, pulmonary venous distension will also be present; in pulmonary hypertension caused by pulmonary vascular disease (e.g. reversed PDA, primary pulmonary hypertension), peripheral pulmonary vascularity will be decreased while central lobar vessels will be dilated from pressure.

From Myer CW and Bonagura JD: Cardiovascular Radiography; in *Manual of Small Animal Practice*. 1993. Eds: Birchard SJ and Sherding RG. WB Saunders Company, Philadelphia, with permission.

4.1 Radiographic features of heart disease.

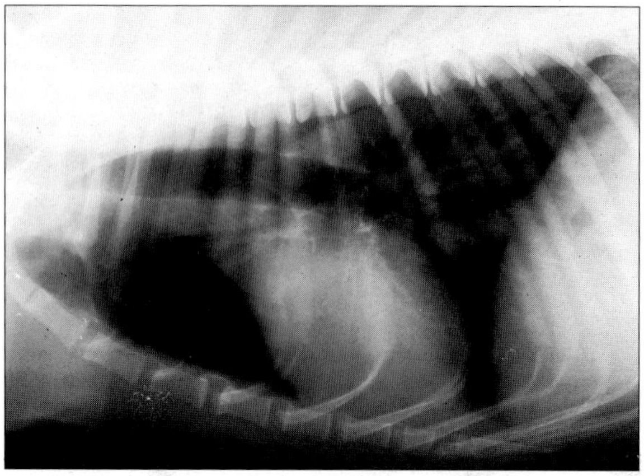

4.2 Thoracic radiograph from an Old English sheepdog with normal cardiac function showing clearly identifiable major peripheral and pulmonary vessels.

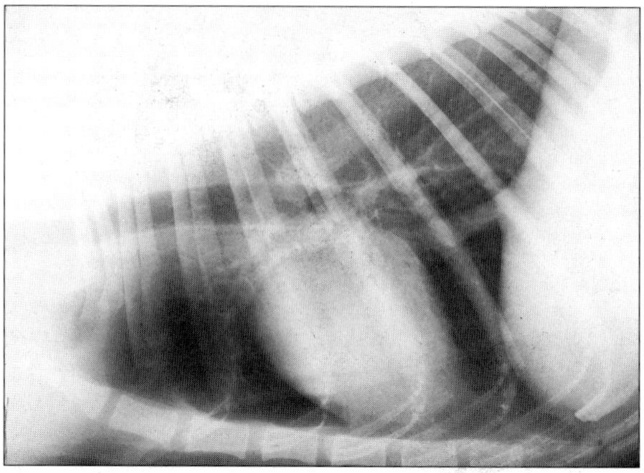

4.3 Radiograph from a cross-bred dog with hypovolaemia following emesis associated with a gastric foreign body. Although pulmonary vessels are easily seen, there is marked hypoperfusion and a small cardiac outline.

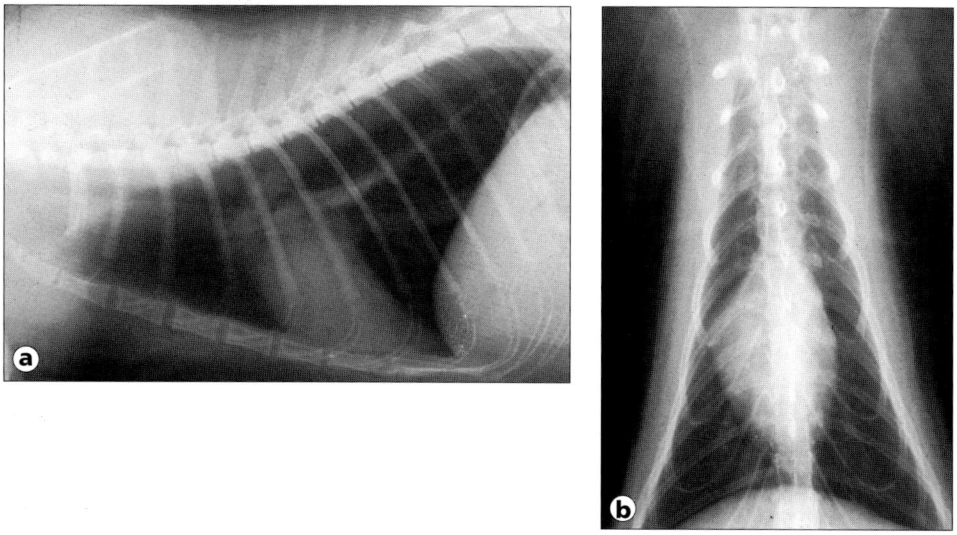

4.4 a, b Radiographs from a normal short-haired domestic cat.

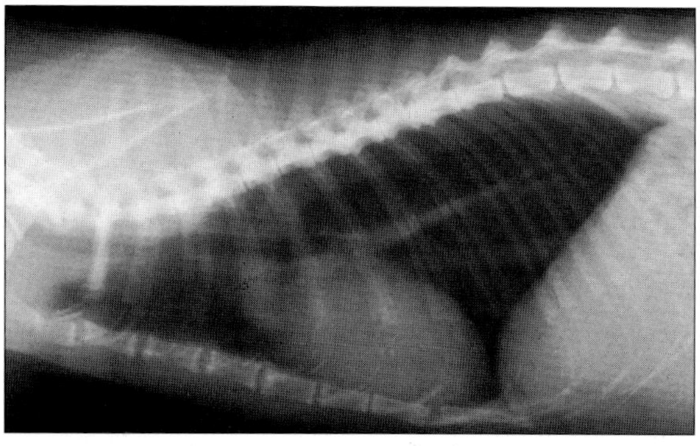

4.5 Radiograph from an aged cat showing the horizontal axis of the heart and tortuous aorta seen in many ageing animals.

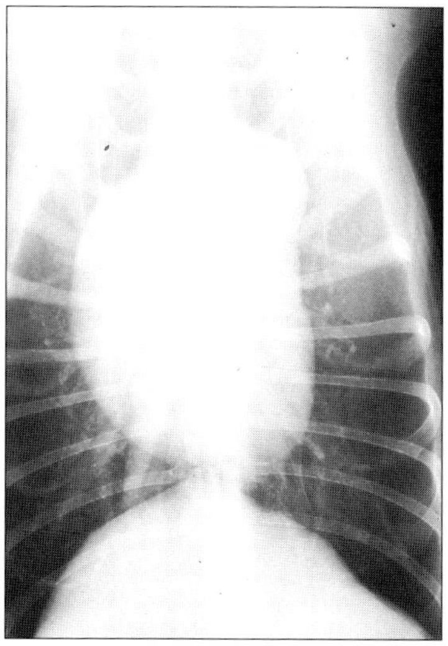

4.6 Ventrodorsal radiograph from a young dog with congenital pulmonic stenosis. The right ventricular hypertrophy is evident as rounding of the right cardiac border. A prominent post stenotic dilatation of the main pulmonary artery is observed along the left cranial border of the heart. Pulmonary vascularity is normal-to-reduced.

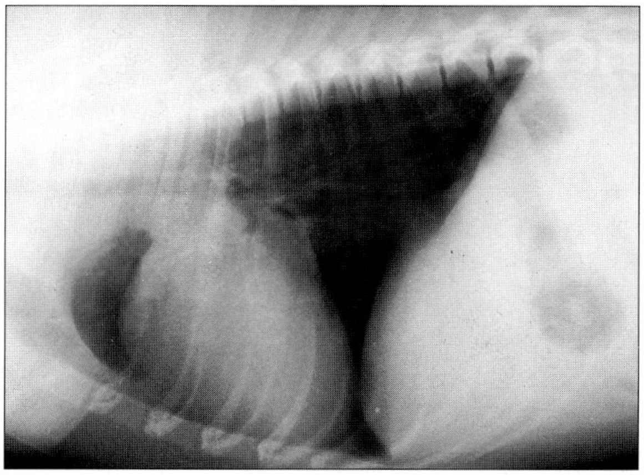

4.7 Lateral radiograph from an 8-month-old boxer dog with pulmonic stenosis, showing marked right atrial enlargement that can be associated with tricuspid regurgitation in pulmonic stenosis. The caudal vena cava is also enlarged.

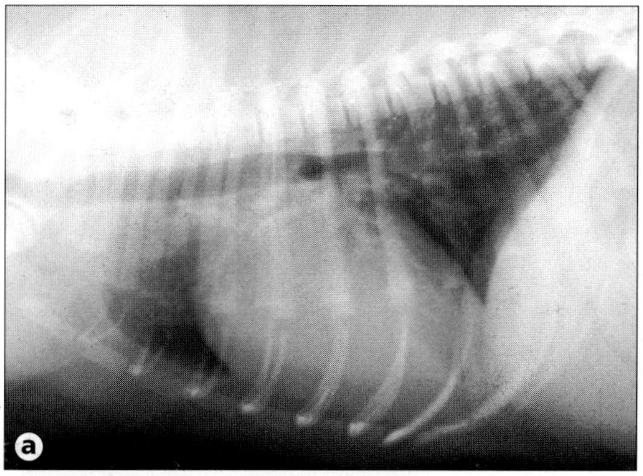

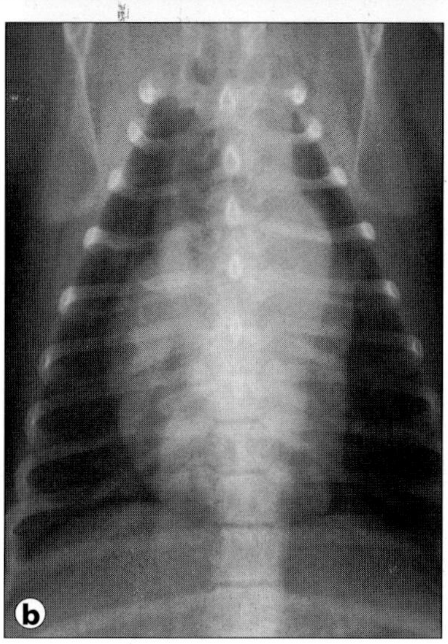

4.8 Radiographs from a West Highland white terrier with patent ductus arteriosus. Note the elongation of the cardiac shadow on the lateral film (**a**) and bulges in the region of the aorta and left atrium on the ventrodorsal film (**b**). Pulmonary vessels also appear rather overperfused. These are all features commonly seen in this disorder.

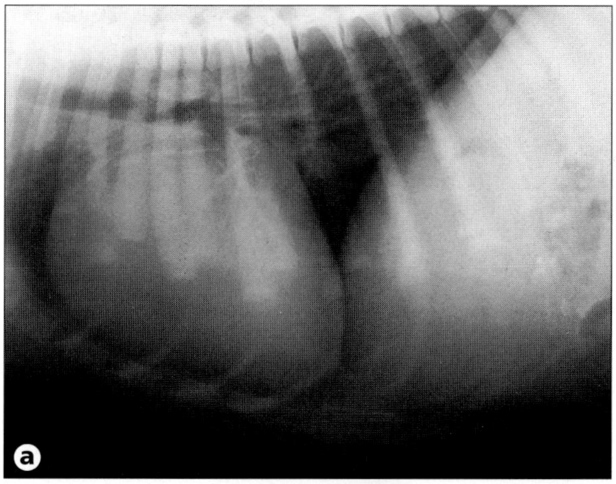

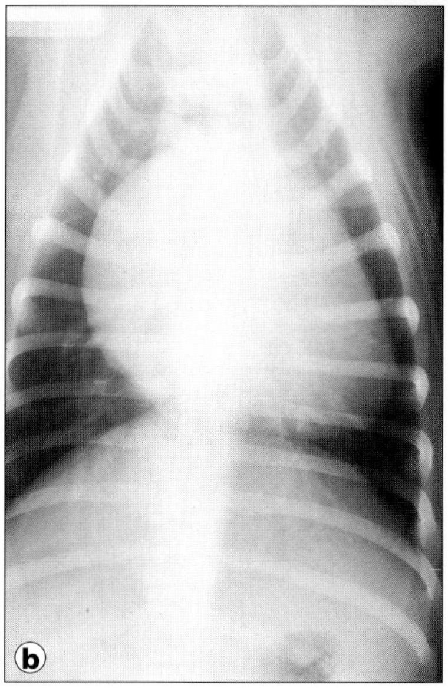

4.9 Radiographs from a 5-month-old golden retriever with severe tricuspid regurgitation due to Ebstein's anomaly. There is widening and increased sternal contact on the lateral view (**a**), and displacement of the cardiac apex to the left with gross rounding of the right side of the heart on the dorsoventral view (**b**).

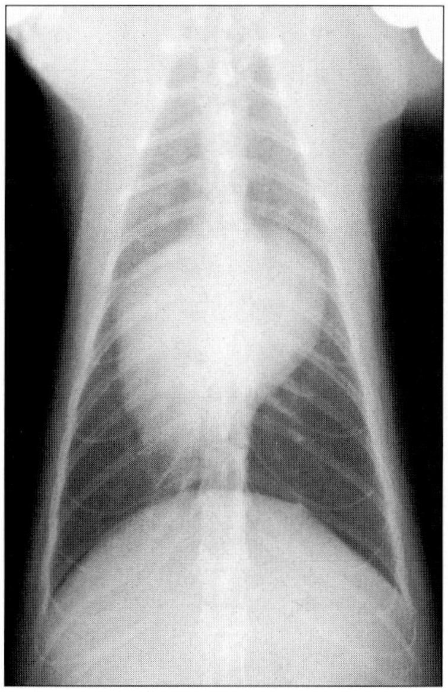

4.10 Ventrodorsal view of a cat with hypertrophic cardiomyopathy, showing left atrial enlargement, a pointed cardiac apex, and the displacement of the apex to the right.

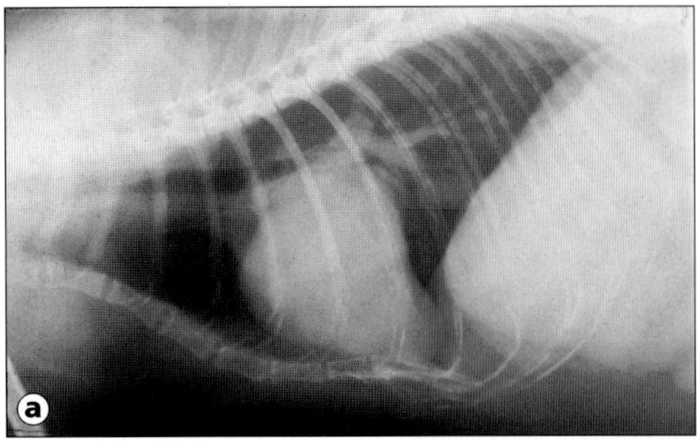

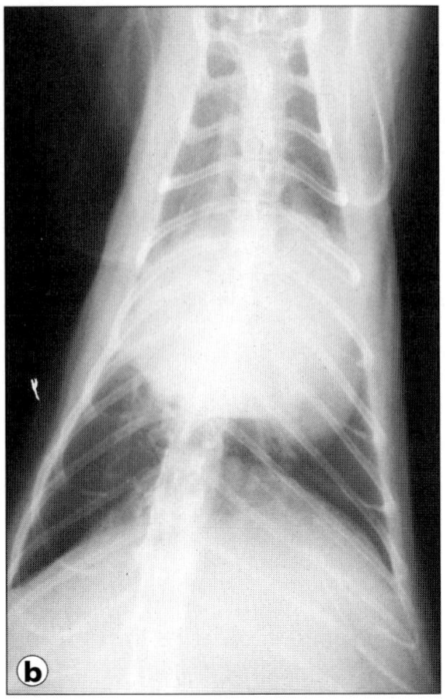

4.11 a, b Radiographs from a Siamese cat with hypertrophic cardiomyopathy and iliac thrombosis. There is massive left atrial enlargement, and probably some enlargement of the right atrium as well. There is also enlargement of the caudal vena cava.

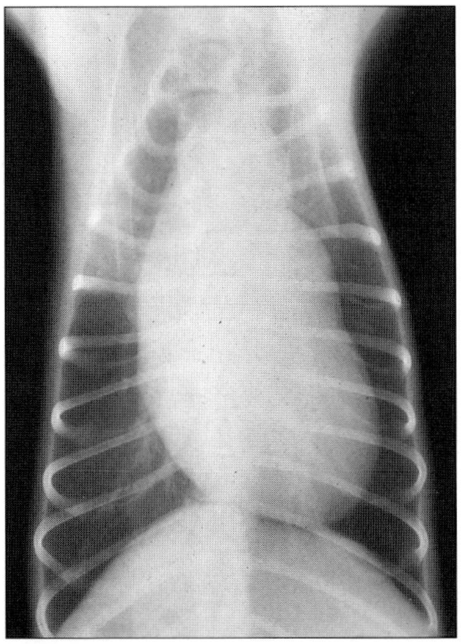

4.12 Ventrodorsal radiograph from a young poodle with aortic stenosis and aortic insufficiency. The left ventricle is enlarged leading to cardiac elongation and to some rounding of the apical border. The ascending aorta and aortic arch are widened owing to post stenotic dilatation. This causes the bulge in the cranial aspect of the mediastinum.

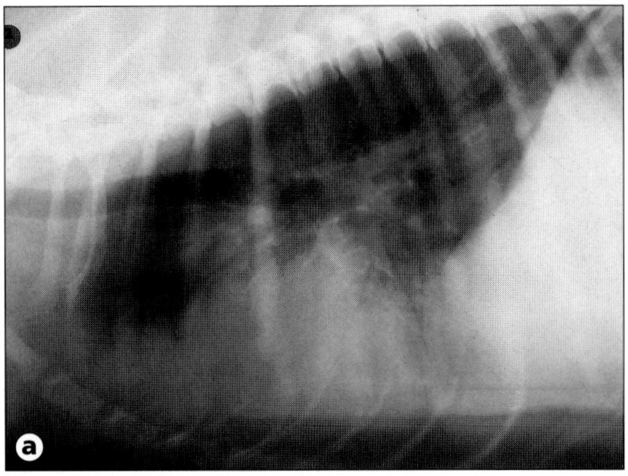

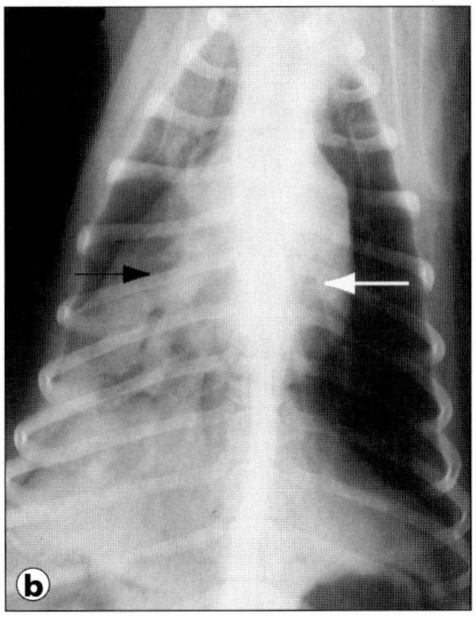

4.13 a, b Radiographs from a golden retriever with acute pulmonary thromboembolism following surgery for a splenic tumour. Note the alveolar pattern of oedema throughout the ventral left lung lobes, and the enlarged and radiodense pulmonary arteries (arrows).

5. Electrocardiography

Electrocardiography is an essential part of thorough case evaluation, yet the clinical information to be gained from the electrocardiogram (ECG) is inevitably limited by the fact that this study records only the electrical activity of the heart. This often has little relation to the mechanical function of the cardiac pump or valves, and the ECG usually provides limited information about severity or aetiology of disease.

Information to be gained from the ECG includes a permanent record of the heart rate and rhythm, a specific diagnosis of most cardiac dysrhythmias and conduction disturbances and, frequently, useful evidence of cardiac chamber enlargement. Furthermore, there may be subtle evidence of the effect of metabolic or electrolyte disturbances on the myocardium.

It is essential that the quality of the ECG be as good as can be obtained with the cooperation of the animal. Electrodes should be placed carefully (using alcohol or other surgical spirit or an ECG conducting gel as necessary) to be in positive close contact with the skin. No person or conducting material should be in contact with the electrodes, nor should electrodes be in electrical contact with one another. The animal should be as still as possible with manual restraint, and it should have a dry coat and be placed on an insulated dry surface. In using Einthoven's triangle, standard recording positions include right lateral recumbency for small animals (with legs extended perpendicularly to the body axis) or, in large animals, standing with the legs square to the body. Standard calibration is 10 mm/mV, with paper speeds of 25 and 50 mm/sec. Further details of ECG recording are beyond the scope of this book, but are richly detailed in the references provided.

The ECG is subject to artifacts if care is not taken over the recording. Movement of the animal is likely to cause displacement of the baseline; muscle potentials of 50 or 60 Hz AC interference (which is most frequently associated with poor electrode contact with the skin), grounding of the animal through wet feet or a damp coat, electrical contact of electrodes one with another, or external contact with the electrodes will all cause baseline noise.

The ECG should be examined systematically. Artifacts should be evaluated, the paper speed and calibration markings noted, and the heart rate should be calculated. The ECG is then assessed for cardiac rhythm before evaluating the waveform for signs of cardiac enlargement or metabolic disturbance. To determine the cardiac rhythm, the entire trace should be examined carefully for P waves, QRS-T complexes, and their coordination. A simple starting point is to assess the tops of the R waves (as in lead II) for regularity. The morphology of these complexes should not vary significantly through the trace. The time intervals of the ECG should be measured and checked against normals to identify conduction delays.

The morphology of waveforms and complexes should be examined in detail for deviations from normal. In small animals, prolongation of the P wave suggests atrial enlargement (usually left), while prolongation of the QRS complex is consistent with left ventricular enlargement or some intraventricular conduction disturbance. Increased amplitude of P waves also suggests atrial enlargement (usually right), while increased amplitude of R waves (with normal frontal axis) is typical of left ventricular enlargement. Low voltage QRS complexes are compatible with a diagnosis of obesity, pericardial effusion, pleural effusions, hypothyroidism, or subcutaneous oedema. Alterations in the frontal axis to the right, combined with terminal negativity of the QRS complex in leads I, II and aVF, suggest right ventricular hypertrophy or, if prolonged, right bundle branch block (see Chapter 23). Left axis deviation, with prominent QR complexes in leads aVL and I and RS complexes in leads II, aVF, and III, suggests left ventricular concentric hypertrophy or left anterior fascicular block.

T-wave abnormalities can be primary or secondary. Primary disturbances include ST segment elevation and depression and enlargement of the T waves; these are usually signs of epicardial or subendocardial injury (ischaemia, pericarditis, hypoxia or electrolyte disturbance – usually potassium or calcium). Secondary ST–T changes are consequences of abnormal depolarization, and therefore any abnormal QRS complex should be followed by an abnormal ST–T wave. The most common example is the ventricular ectopic beat, but secondary changes are also observed in cases of ventricular enlargement and in conduction disturbances.

The clinician must recognize that the lead orientation, the species differences in the atrial and ventricular size, and the various types of cardiac activation processes result in ECG complexes that vary within and between species.

Maximum Normal ECG Intervals					
Animal	**P** (s)	**PQ(R)** (s)	**QRS** (s)	**QT[1]** (s)	**Heart rate** (beats/minute)
Dog	0.040[2]	0.130[2]	0.050–0.060[3]	0.250	60–180
Cat	0.035	0.080	0.040	0.220	140–220[4]
Horse	0.160	0.380[4]	0.140	0.575	28–40[5]
Cow	0.134	0.190	0.124	0.390	40–80

[1] QT is inversely related to heart rate
[2] May be longer in giant breeds (0.055 = P; 0.140 = PR)
[3] 0.05 = small breeds, 0.06 = larger breeds
[4] Varies with different studies, longer when there is high vagal tone
[5] Higher in colts, to 80/min

5.1 Maximum normal ECG intervals (in seconds) in various domestic animals.

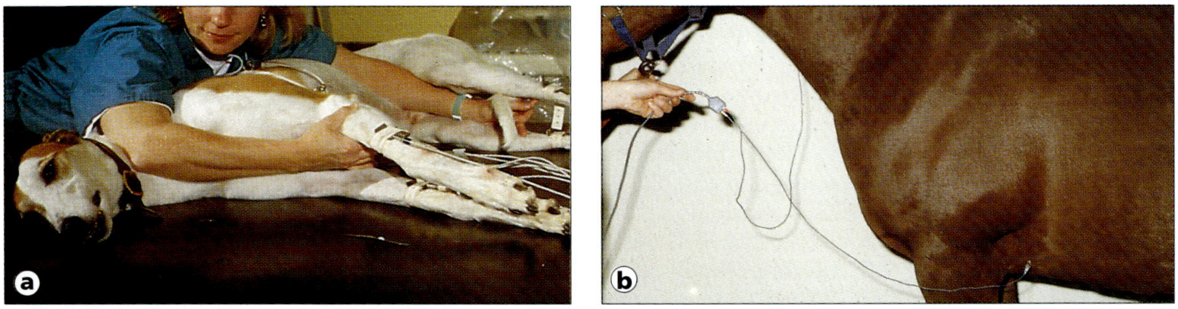

5.2 (**a**) Recording the electrocardiogram in a dog. Electrodes are attached to the four limbs, and additional electrodes may be attached to the precordium (chest or V-leads). Individual leads are recorded by adjusting the lead selector switch. (**b**) A modified lead is often used to record the rhythm in horses or cattle. This involves moving the left forelimb (left 'arm') electrode to the left apex and the right forelimb (right 'arm') electrode to the mid-cervical jugular furrow. Selecting lead I on the recorder will generate a so-called base–apex lead.

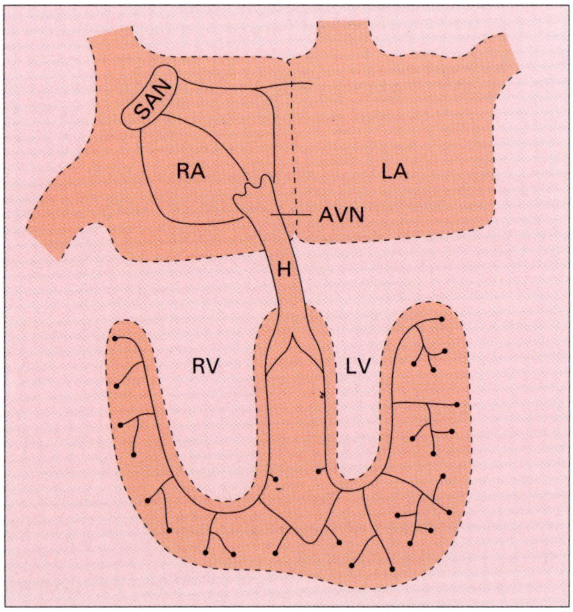

5.3 Schematic of the cardiac-impulse forming and conduction systems; SAN – sinoatrial node (pacemaker), AVN – atrioventricular node, H – bundle of His. (Drawing courtesy of Dr. Robert L. Hamlin).

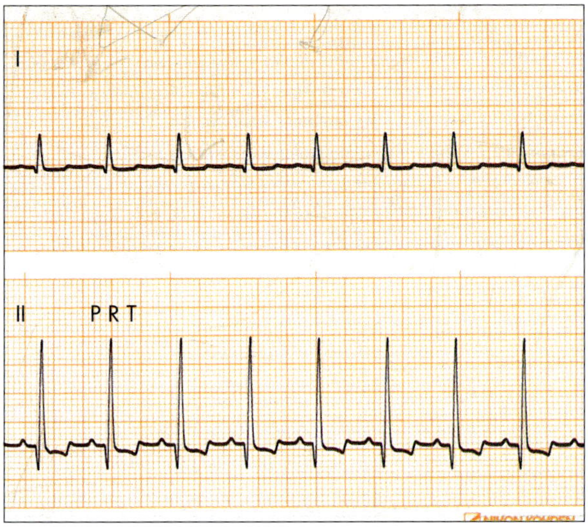

5.4 Normal sinus rhythm, recorded in an anaesthetized cross-bred dog in leads I and II at 25mm/sec. Normal sinus rhythm is not often seen in dogs in daily practice: sinus arrhythmia is more common.

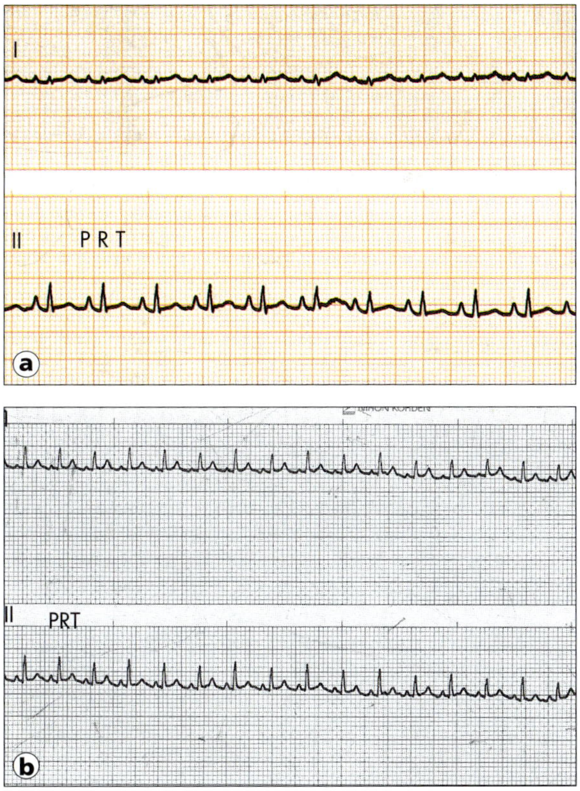

5.5 a, b ECGs from two cats in normal sinus rhythm recorded in leads I and II at 25 mm/sec. Note the low voltages seen in many normal cats. There is slight variation in QRS waveform in **b**, probably associated with the effects of respiration.

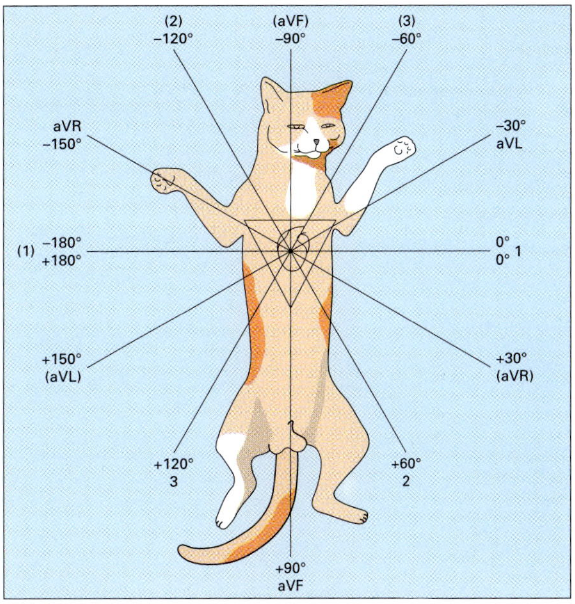

5.6 The frontal plane axis which demonstrates the orientation of leads I, II, III, aVR, aVL and aVF to the dorsoventral (frontal) plane. The animal's left is to the viewer's right. The frontal axis can be quickly estimated by finding the lead with the greatest net positive area under the QRS complex waveforms. Typically, this will be evident in leads II and aVF. Left-axis deviations in small animals are characterized by dominant positive depolarization forces in leads aVL and I. Right-axis deviations in small animals are characterized by dominant positive depolarization forces in leads III and aVR. Axis deviations are difficult to assess in large animals owing to the different methods of ventricular activation among the species.

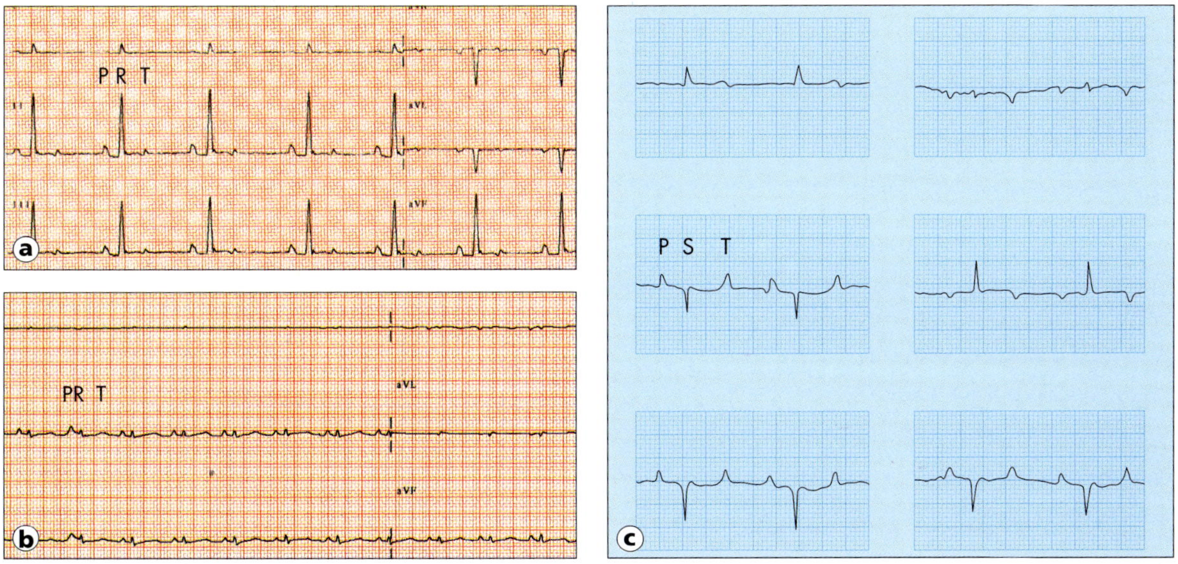

5.7 Normal electrocardiograms. Multiple frontal plane leads recorded from a large breed of dog (**a**), cat (**b**), and a horse (**c**). (50 mm/sec; 10 mm/mV.)

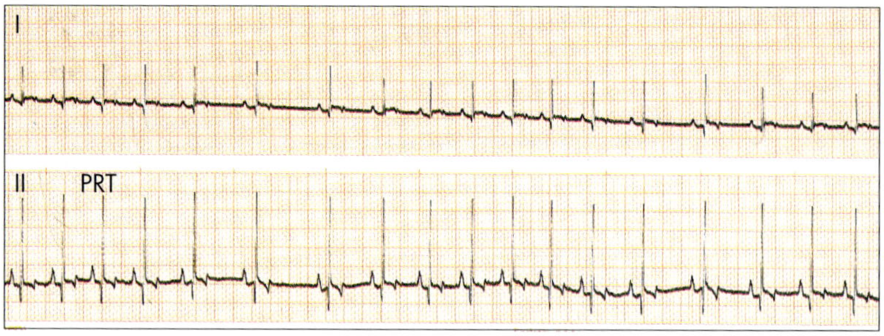

5.8 Sinus arrhythmia in a clinically normal beagle at a heart rate of about 110 beats/min. (Recorded at 25 mm/sec in leads I and II.)

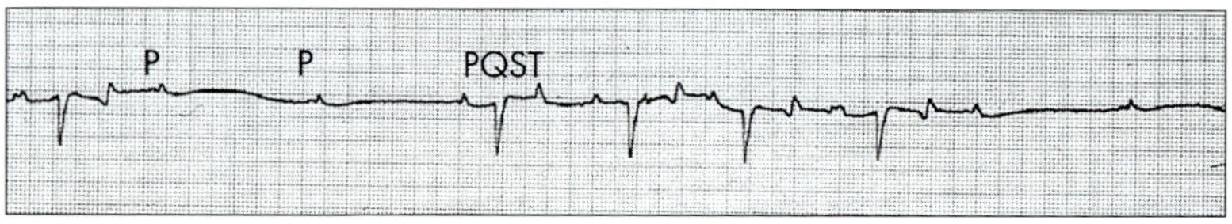

5.9 Base–apex lead recording from a standing normal horse. The trace is characterized by non-conducted P waves which are typical of physiologic second degree AV block.

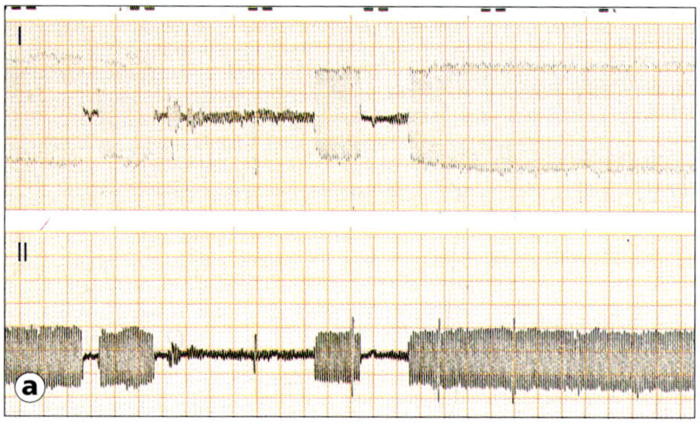

5.10 ECG artifacts. (**a**) Intermittent 50 Hz AC in a boxer dog, due to varying contact with ECG electrodes by the handler. (**b**) The effects of tremor on the trace in the same dog as in **a** (lead II at 25 mm/sec). Although there is a hint of atrial fibrillation, the dog has sinus rhythm with atrial premature beats. (**c**) The effects of purring in a 12-year-old Siamese cat with aortic thrombosis and hypertrophic cardiomyopathy. The cat has atrial fibrillation, but this is not easily diagnosed from this trace; the tall R wave also suggests left ventricular hypertrophy. (Leads I and II at 25 mm/sec.)

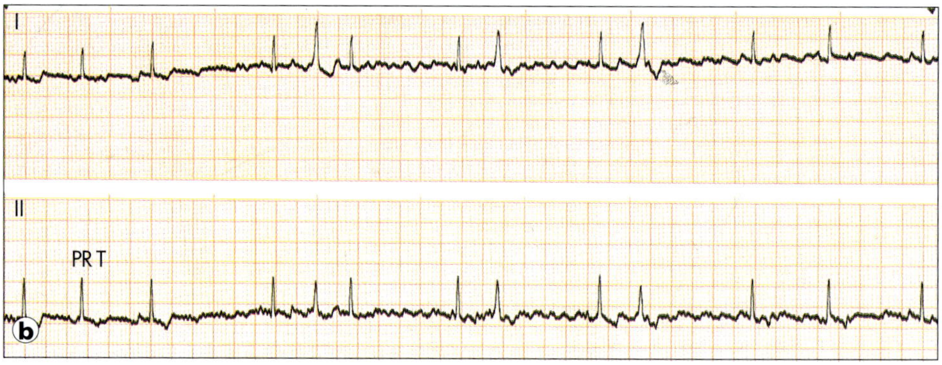

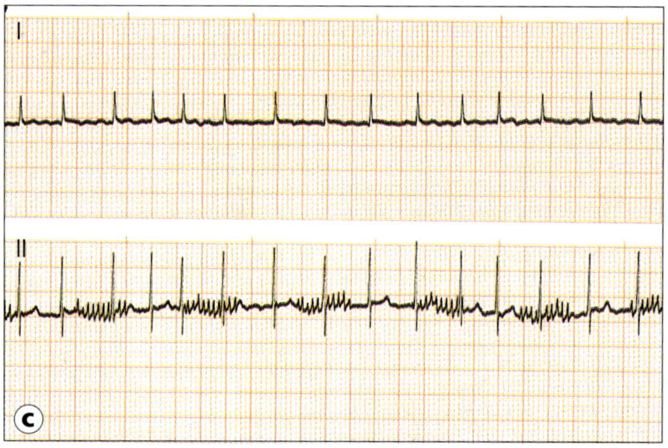

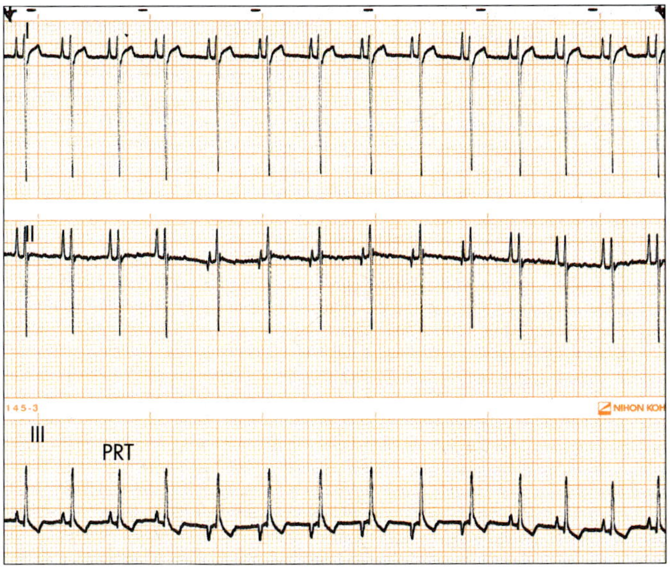

5.11 Right ventricular hypertrophy in a 3-month-old Bichon frise with pulmonic stenosis. There is right-axis deviation, with a deep S wave in leads I and II, and P pulmonale (0.6 mV), indicating right atrial enlargement, as well as marked wandering pacemaker. (Recorded in leads I, II and III at 5 mm/mV; 25 mm/sec.)

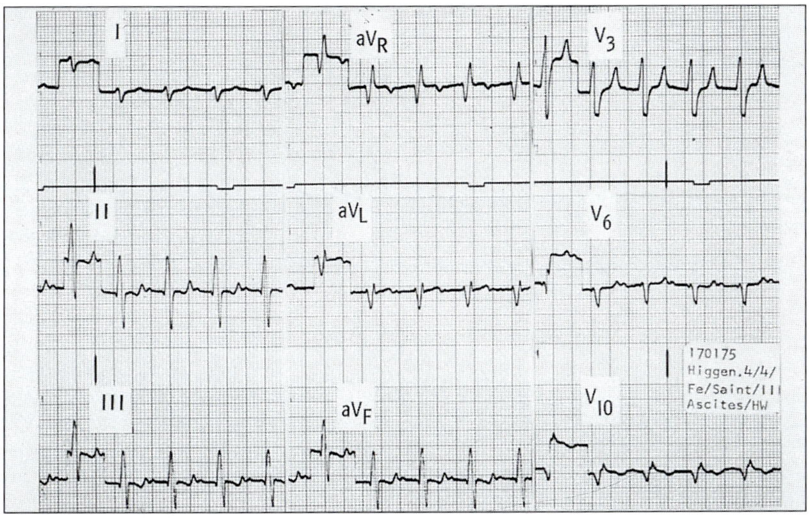

5.12 Right ventricular hypertrophy in a Saint Bernard with severe heartworm disease. Prominent S waves in leads I, II, III, aVF, and V_3 (left lower precordium) are indicative of abnormal, rightward depolarization forces. In this case, the frontal axis is indeterminate.

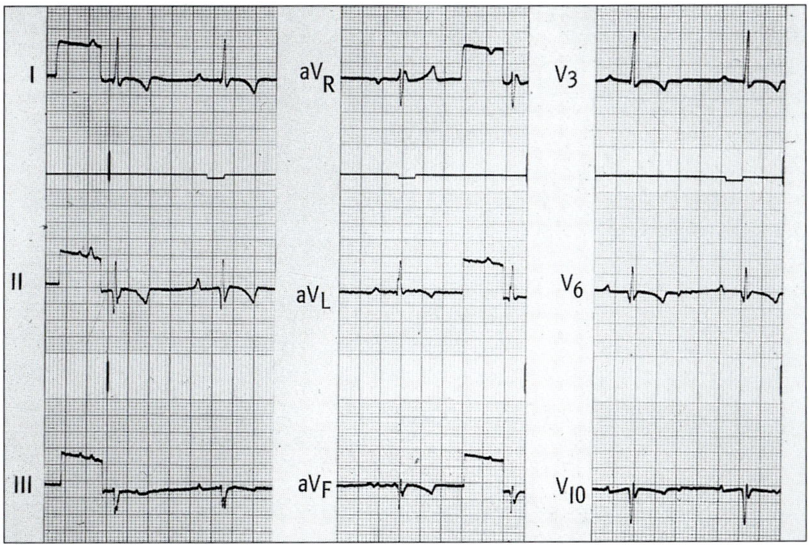

5.13 Left-axis deviation in an old miniature schnauzer. While this finding can be a normal variant, it is also compatible with either left ventricular hypertrophy or left anterior fascicular block. The frontal axis is deviated to the left cranial quadrant (see **5.6**) with prominent R waves in leads aVL and I. The small terminal S waves in leads I and aVF may indicate a minor, intercurrent, right ventricular conduction delay.

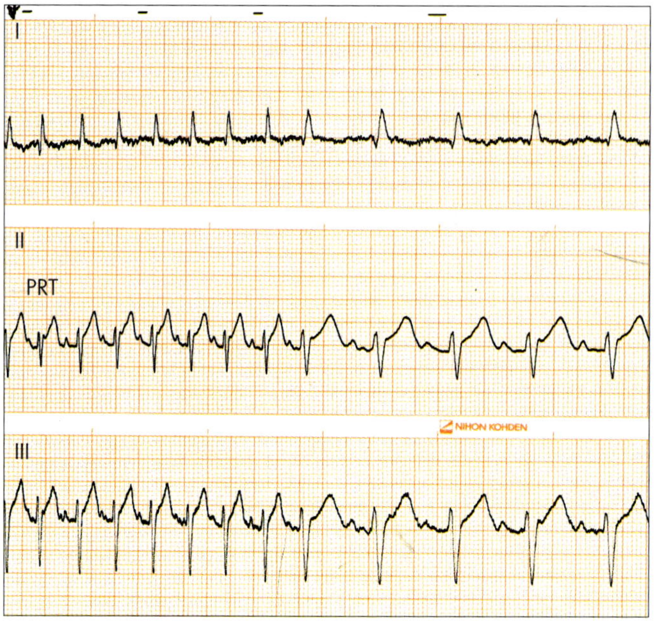

5.14 Marked left-axis deviation and prolongation of the QRS complex, representing left ventricular hypertrophy and probable left anterior fascicular block in a young cat with hypertrophic cardiomyopathy. (Leads I, II and III at 25 and 50 mm/sec.)

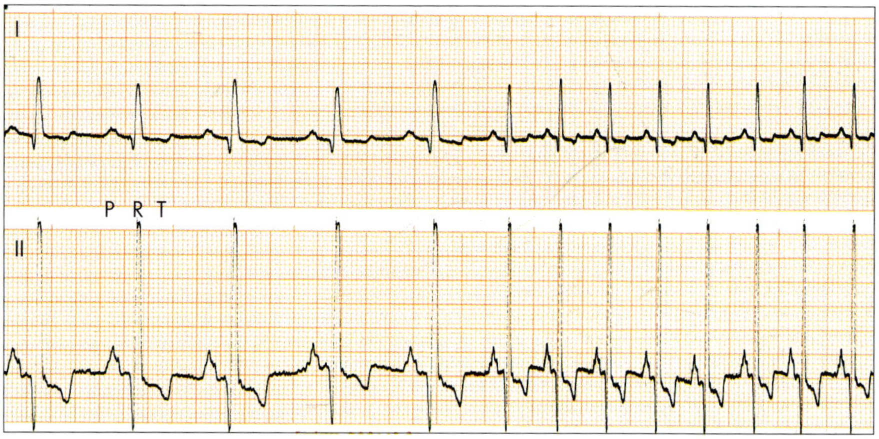

5.15 Evidence of left atrial and left ventricular enlargement in a German shepherd dog with subaortic stenosis, mitral regurgitation and congestive heart failure. There is marked enlargement and widening of the P wave (nearly 0.06 sec), consistent with atrial dilatation, together with a tall R wave (> 3.0 mV), probably indicating left ventricular hypertrophy. (Leads I and II at 50 and 25 mm/sec.)

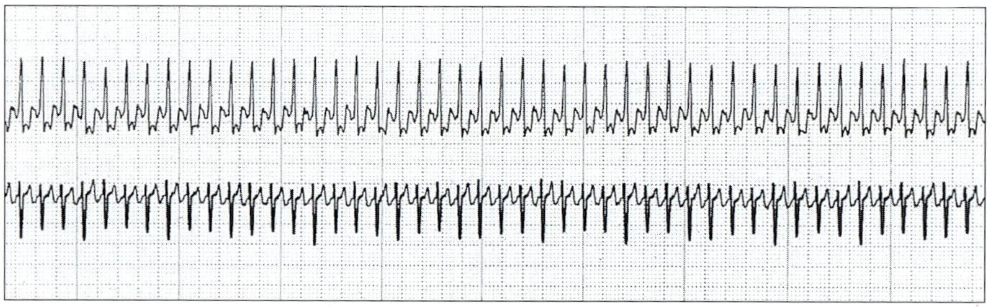

5.16 Printed sample from a 24-hour tape-recorded (Holter) ECG from a dog with subaortic stenosis. Two simultaneous precordial leads are recorded. Severe ST segment depression is observed during the period of exercise-induced sinus tachycardia recorded here. (Paper speed is 25 mm/sec.)

6.

Echocardiography

Conduction of ultrasound is favoured by fluids and inhibited by bone and gas (e.g. air in the lungs). For successful echocardiography therefore, the investigator must find 'windows' between the ribs and ventral to the lungs so that no air lies between the patient's heart and the ultrasound equipment. The examination is operator-dependent as both the sensitivity and specificity of diagnosis are related in part to experience and technical expertise. The full echocardiographic study provides information about the structure, size and function of the heart. When combined with Doppler studies, the direction and velocity of blood flow in the heart and circulation can also be evaluated. Echocardiography complements radiography as it differentiates soft tissues from fluids (which conventional radiography does not), and therefore provides images from within the heart.

The anatomic detail provided by echocardiography is exceptional. The heart valves, the heart chambers and the great vessels can all be examined in detail. Measurements of the size of cardiac chambers and of the thickness of ventricular walls can be achieved accurately, enabling an objective diagnosis of hypertrophy or dilatation. The motion of the ventricular myocardium, which represents the force of myocardial contraction, can also be studied in detail. Valvular lesions such as malformations, bacterial endocarditis, nodular endocardiosis and rupture of chordae tendineae can all be demonstrated by echocardiography. Endocardial thrombi and cardiac tumours can be identified. Pericardial effusions are very readily detected. Congenital lesions such as subaortic stenosis, ventricular and atrial septal defects and, in some cases, patent ductus arteriosus, can also be demonstrated. Valvular dysplasia can present more of a diagnostic challenge, but moderate-to-severe lesions are usually evident with careful imaging.

Even without Doppler studies, the combination of findings from the clinical examination with enlargement of cardiac chambers – whether dilatation or hypertrophy – or of major vessels, lesions, and functional disturbances, can guide an alert clinician to most cardiac diagnoses. However, some minor lesions, including mild subaortic stenosis, are not diagnosed reliably by imaging. Furthermore, the clinician must be careful not to misdiagnose areas of normal echo drop-out as a septal defect.

An echocardiographic study is best carried out with the animal prepared well and gently restrained. The hair should be clipped over the transducer site, and ultrasound coupling gel is used to provide good acoustic contact with the thorax. Sedation, as described for radiography, is useful when performing examinations in very young or fractious animals. In small animals, the transducer should be applied to the chest from below, with the animal in lateral recumbency on a table with precut imaging ports. This method helps to collapse the lungs adjacent to the transducer, thus enhancing the echocardiographic image of the heart. In large animals, echocardiography is readily carried out with the animal standing, often with the forelimb drawn forwards on the side under study.

Echocardiography can include two-dimensional, M-mode and contrast studies, as well as colour-flow, pulsed-wave and continuous-wave Doppler examinations (see Chapter 7). Most echocardiographic studies begin with routine two-dimensional echocardiography and a guided M-mode study of the ventricles, mitral valve, aortic root and left atrium (**6.13**). These studies permit most structural diagnoses and also allow the operator to estimate cardiac dimensions and ventricular systolic function. The image planes used for two-dimensional echocardiography are defined as long-axis (viewing structures in sagittal planes), short-axis (using coronal sections of the heart), apical (orientated from the left ventricular apex) or angled (some characteristics of multiple views). Views are usually named by the positioning of the transducer and the structures that are optimally examined. The M-mode study is very valuable for quantitation. Mensuration should be related not only to body size, but also to breed and age (see references). The left ventricular fractional shortening provides a general estimate of left ventricular systolic function, although it is affected by numerous factors (including sedatives) and is not a particularly accurate method for studying the effects of therapy.

Routine echocardiographic studies should always be interpreted in the light of the physical examination, especially that information derived by auscultation, and should be accompanied by routine radiographic and ECG examinations.

Legends for figures used throughout this chapter: RA – right atrium; RV – right ventricle; LA – left atrium; LV – left ventricle; LVOT– left ventricular outflow tract; Aur – auricle; Ao or AO – aorta; PA – pulmonary artery; IAS – interatrial septum; IVS or VS – ventricular septum; PW – posterior wall of the left ventricle; TV – tricuspid valve; MV – mitral valve; PM – papillary muscle.

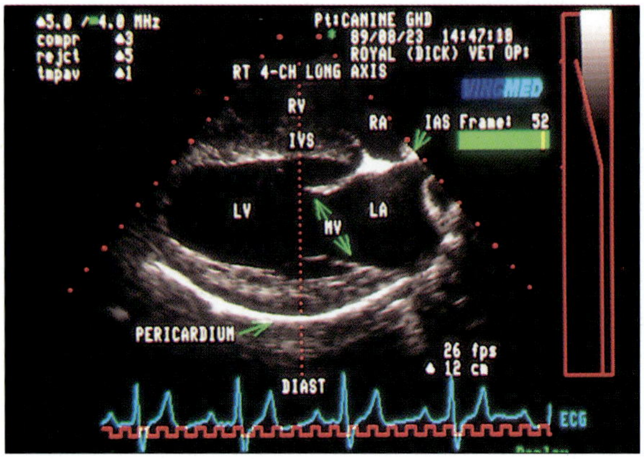

6.1 Long-axis, 4-chambered image of the heart, recorded from the right hemithorax, in a clinically-normal greyhound. The plane is optimized for the left ventricular inlet.

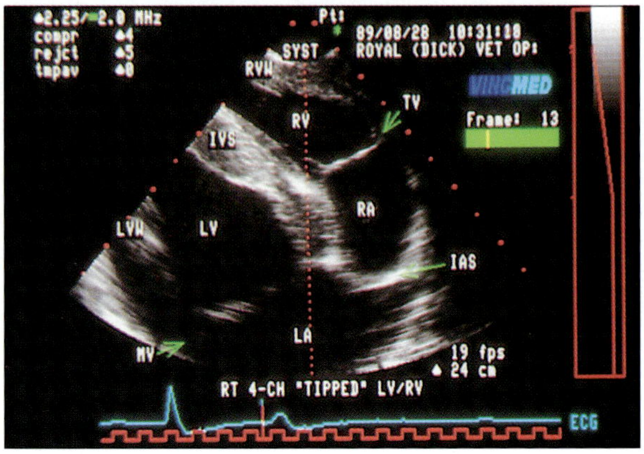

6.2 Long-axis, 4-chambered image from the right, recorded from a horse. The image plane is optimized for the right ventricular inlet. The transducer was placed more ventrally and angled more dorsally than for the usual 4-chambered image.

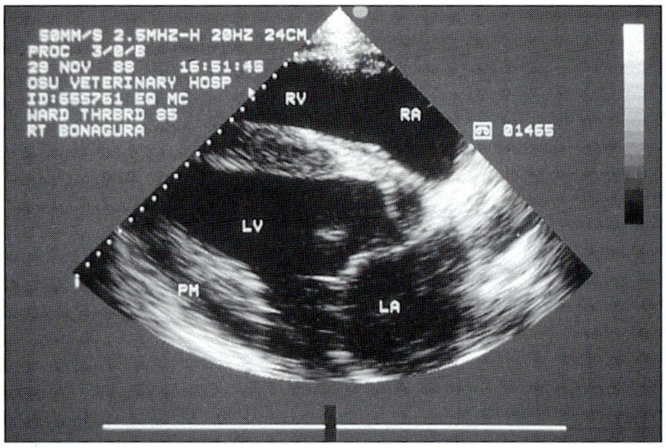

6.3 Long-axis, 4-chambered image from the right, obtained from a thoroughbred gelding. The ventricular septum is evident between the right and left ventricles. A prominent mural (posterior) papillary muscle (PM) also is evident.

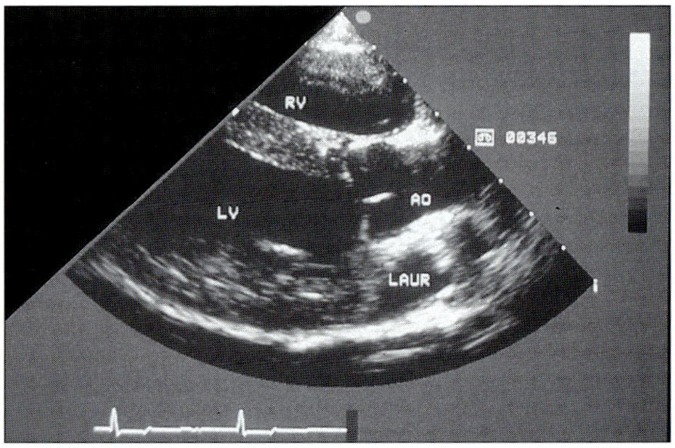

6.4 Long-axis image from the right, optimized for the left ventricular outlet and ascending aorta, recorded from a dog. The closed aortic valve is evident.

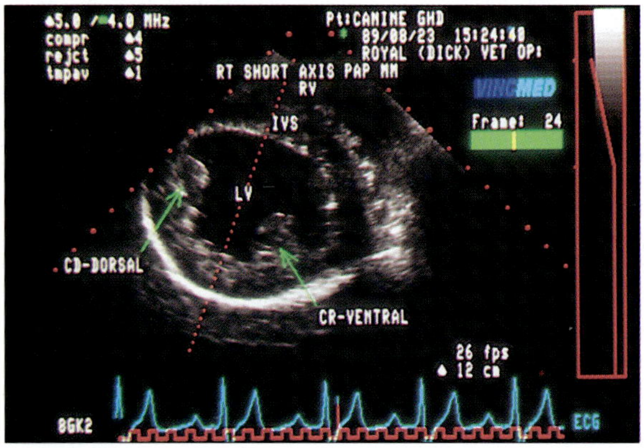

6.5 Short-axis image of the ventricles from the right, at the level of the papillary muscles, recorded from a dog. (CD – caudal; CR – cranial)

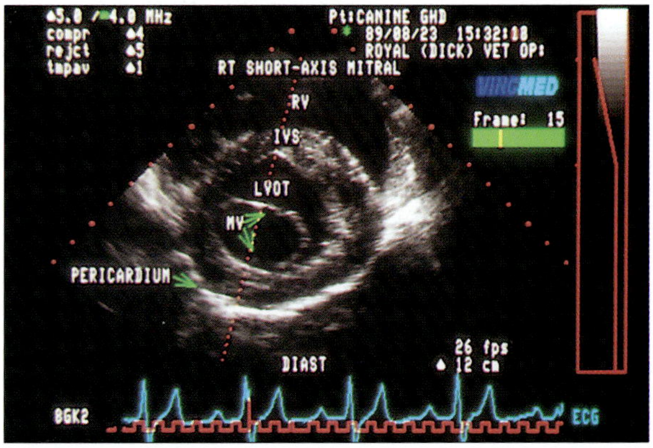

6.6 Short-axis image of the ventricles recorded at a level just dorsal to that of **6.5**. The mitral valve orifice (MV) is open, as recorded during diastole.

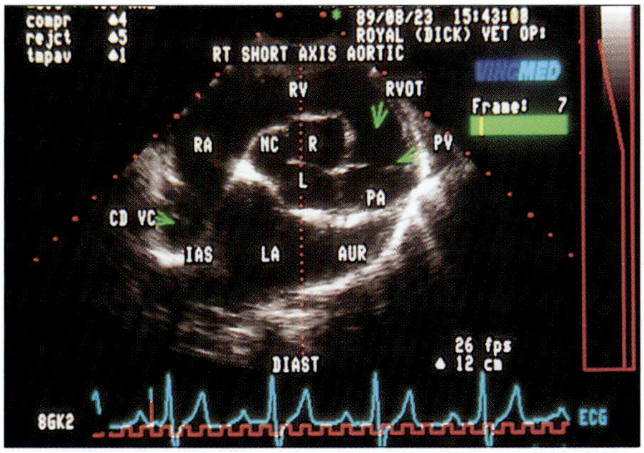

6.7 Short-axis image recorded dorsal and slightly cranial to that of (**6.6**). Structures at the base of the heart (at the level of the aortic valve) are evident. (CD VC – caudal vena cava; NC, R, L – non-coronary, right and left aortic valve cusps).

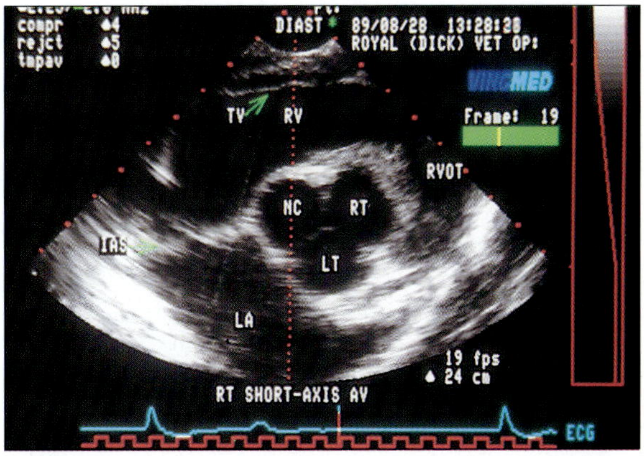

6.8 Short-axis image of the base of the heart recorded from a horse. The right ventricular outflow tract (RVOT), and left atrium and auricular appendage are readily seen in this view. The right (RT), left (LT), and non-coronary (NC) aortic valve sinuses can be appreciated as well.

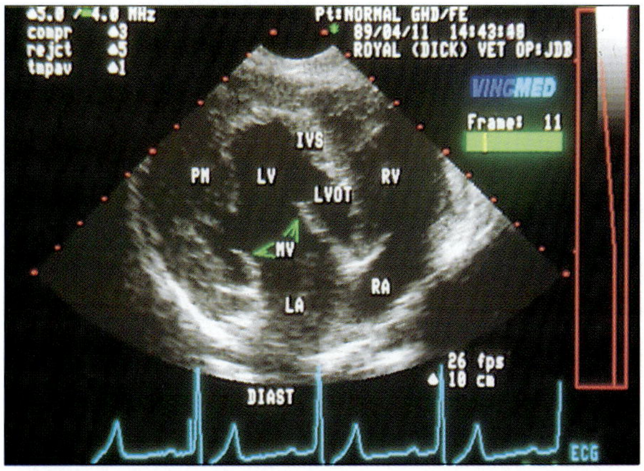

6.9 Apical, 4-chambered image of the heart recorded from the left apex of a dog. The format of this figure is a mirror-image of the convention now used to demonstrate apical 4-chamber images of the heart.

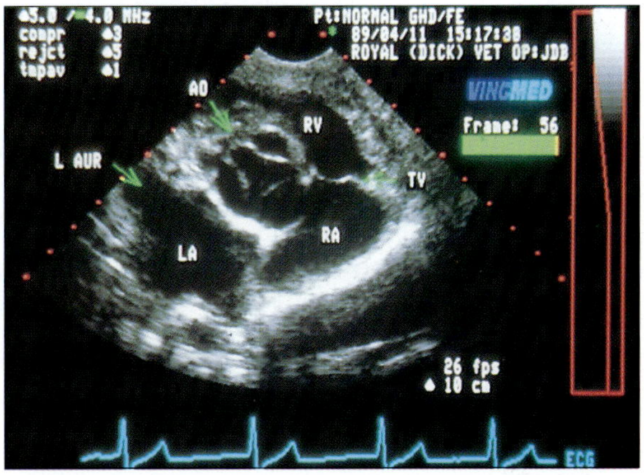

6.10 Short-axis image of the base of the heart recorded from the left cranial hemithorax of a dog. The heart is recorded during systole, as evidenced by the open aortic valve leaflets (arrow).

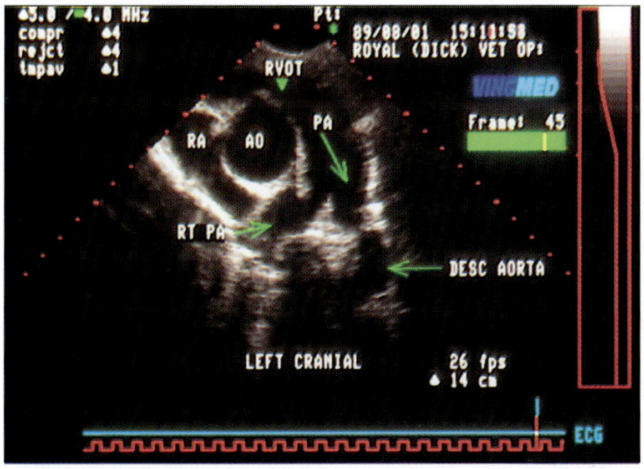

6.11 View from the left cranial position of the pulmonary artery (PA) and descending aorta (DESC AO) of a dog.

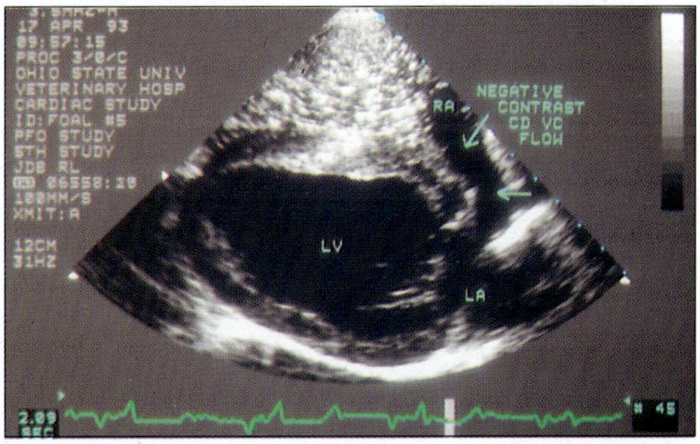

6.12 Example of a contrast echocardiogram recorded from a full-term foal. Saline was injected into the jugular vein and resulted in a clouding of the right atrium and right ventricle with echodense targets. The saline contrast was diluted (negative contrast – arrow) by blood returning from the caudal vena cava along the atrial septum.

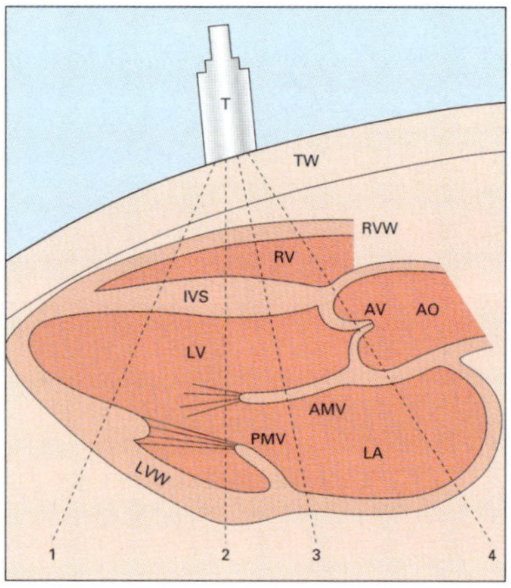

6.13 Standard cursor positions used to derive the M-mode echocardiogram. The cursor positions are indicative of papillary (1), chordal/ventricular (2) mitral valve (3), and aortic–left atrial (4) positions. Either long-axis (shown) or short-axis image planes can be used. (AMV – anterior mitral leaflet; PMV – posterior mitral leaflet; TW – thoracic wall)

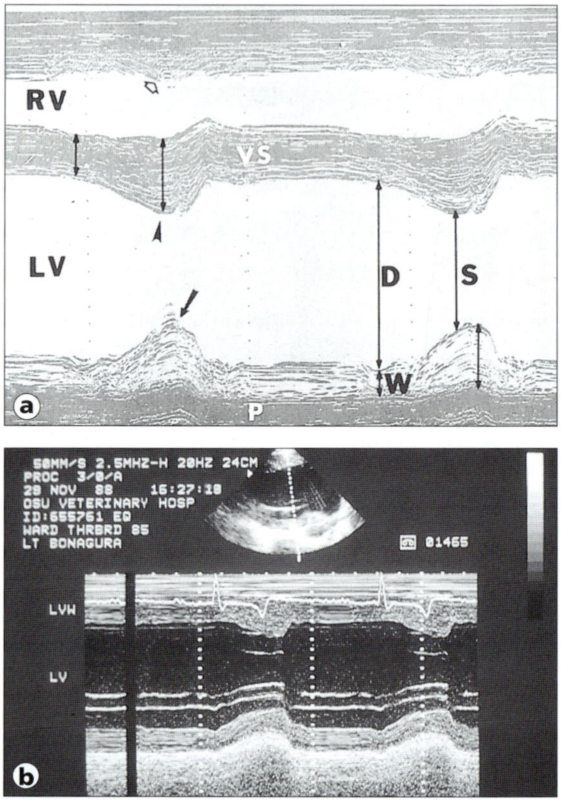

6.14 M-mode echocardiograms of the left ventricle in two horses. (**a**) The ventricles are imaged from the right hemithorax. Diastolic (D) and systolic (S) dimensions are indicated (W – posterior left ventricular wall). (**b**) Often the left ventricle must be imaged from the left hemithorax in order to include the entire chamber. In such cases, the left ventricular wall is now closest to the transducer and the ventricular septum is in the far field. Echoes of chordae tendineae are evident in the lower portion of the recording. The brightest echo is from the interface of the pericardium.

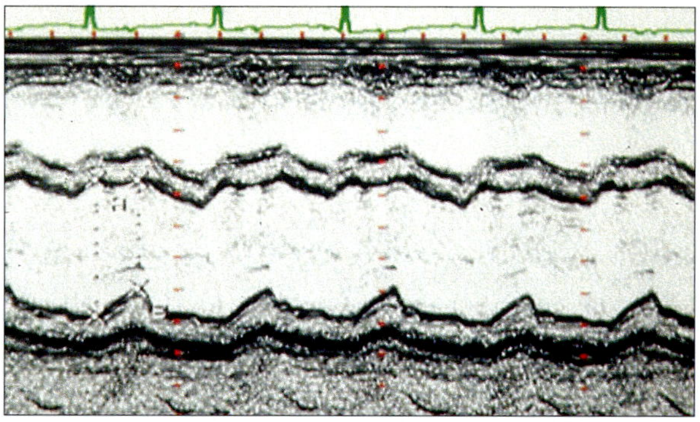

6.15 M-mode echocardiogram of the right and left ventricles recorded from a dog with dilated cardiomyopathy. The method for measuring the internal left ventricular dimensions is shown. Shortening fraction is calculated as: (ventricular diastolic dimension – ventricular systolic dimension)/ ventricular diastolic dimension ×100.

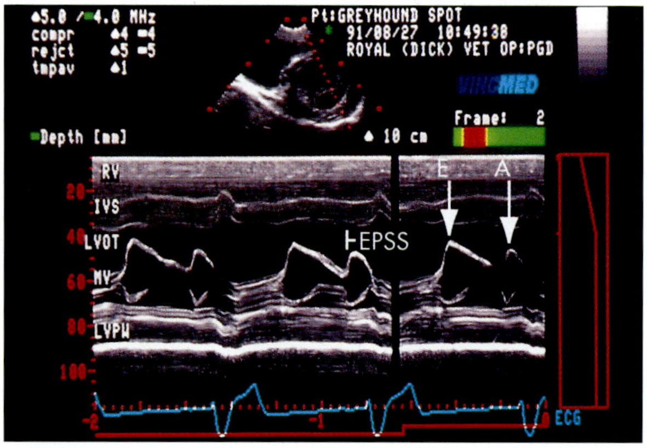

6.16 M-mode echocardiogram at the level of the mitral valve recorded from a greyhound (E – E point; A – A point; EPSS – E point to septal separation).

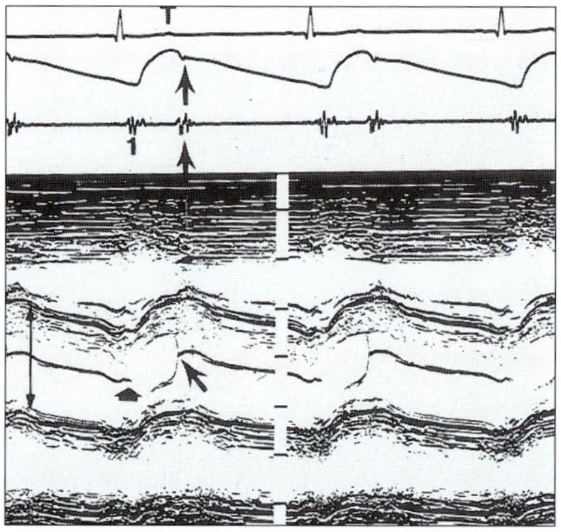

6.17 M-mode at the level of the aortic root and left atrium recorded from a dog. The opening of the aortic valve can be observed (broad arrow) and the closure of the valve coincides with the second heart sound and incisura of the aortic pressure curve (arrows). Traces at the top are ECG, arterial pressure and phonocardiogram.

7. Doppler Echocardiography

Doppler ultrasound has added a new aspect to cardiac diagnosis. Applying the Doppler principle to ultrasound imaging, the frequency of a reflected signal will differ from that of the signal emitted by the transducer whenever reflected by a moving object. This Doppler frequency shift can be analyzed by modern echocardiographic equipment to reveal the velocity and direction of blood movement at almost any site within the heart and great vessels. This provides the clinician with a noninvasive and very powerful means of assessing the circulation. Doppler information is displayed in two basic formats: colour-flow imaging and spectral traces.

The two-dimensional colour-flow image ('colour-flow mapping') can be likened to a colour angiogram, although the information obtained is not always quantitatively equivalent. Essentially, flow rate and direction are displayed by a colour coding that is overlaid onto the two-dimensional echocardiogram. Flow towards the transducer is coded in red, while flow away from the transducer is coded in blue. Colour-flow information can also be combined with an M-mode study to produce a colour M-mode echocardiogram; the principal benefit of this mode is the high temporal resolution of flow across a single line of ultrasound.

Spectral Doppler recordings display flow rate and direction versus time as a graph. Flow towards the transducer is coded positive (above the baseline) while flow away from the transducer is coded negative (below the baseline). The ECG permits accurate timing within the cardiac cycle along the x-axis, while a velocity scale on the y-axis permits accurate measurement of flow velocity. Flow velocities are obtained from within a specific sample range cell or 'sample volume' (with pulsed-waved Doppler) or at any depth along a line of ultrasound through the heart (with continuous-wave Doppler). Typical normal patterns of flow involve a single-peaked, triangular, negative trace from the aorta and pulmonary artery in systole (**7.8** and **7.14**), and a double-peaked, 'M-shaped', positive trace from the mitral and tricuspid valves in diastole (**7.3** and **7.12**).

Colour-coded Doppler studies display high-velocity or turbulent flow as a mosaic of colours, often with hues of yellow or green added. Pulsed-wave Doppler displays turbulence as a widening or dispersion of the spectral tracing; however, this mode cannot display high-velocity flow accurately, and an ambiguous signal direction (signal *aliasing*) results (**7.16**). Signal aliasing is also common in colour-coded Doppler because this is derived from multiple pulsed-wave sample volumes (**7.6** and **7.7**). Continuous-wave studies provide accurate measurements of high-velocity flow which are not encumbered by aliasing. High-pulsed-repetition frequency Doppler is an intermediate form available in some instruments. The various modes each have strengths and limitations and the interested reader is directed to the references for details about the technology, study methods and interpretation of these studies.

The presence of abnormal flow patterns such as valvular regurgitation, shunting across septal defects or a patent ductus arteriosus can be detected readily by Doppler techniques. The increased velocity and turbulence of flow through a stenotic lesion, regurgitant valve or restrictive left-to-right shunt can be easily demonstrated with either spectral or colour techniques.

In addition to such *qualitative* information, there are important quantitative clinical uses for Doppler-derived measurements. Foremost is the estimation of pressure gradients. In the normal heart, the peak systolic and diastolic pressures measured at either side of a cardiac valve are equal, though they do not occur at precisely the same time. Thus, while the normal *peak-to-peak* pressure gradient is zero, an *instantaneous* pressure gradient can be detected. Such gradients drive blood through the circulation, but they are typically small, usually between 2 and 8 mmHg. These normal gradients can be estimated by using Doppler-derived velocity data and generally correspond to red blood cell velocities of between 0.5 and approximately 1.8 m/sec. Abnormal pressure gradients and high-velocity flow develop in many cardiac conditions, including valve stenoses or outflow tract obstruction. A large pressure gradient also drives blood across a restrictive ventricular septal defect or an incompetent cardiac valve; these are simply reflections of differences in normal pressures developed in the heart during the cardiac cycle (see Chapter 8). A pressure gradient and high-velocity flow pattern can be readily identified and measured by Doppler techniques. This information is useful for both diagnosis and management.

Gradients can be estimated using Doppler by employing the modified Bernoulli equation:

$$\text{gradient (mmHg)} = (\text{maximal velocity})^2 \times 4$$

where the maximal velocity is in m/sec.

The Bernoulli relationship works very well for clinical evaluation of subaortic stenosis, pulmonary stenosis, ventricular septal defect, hypertrophic cardiomyopathy, pulmonary hypertension and valvular insufficiency. Accurate assessment of the pressure drop across a stenosis, shunt or incompetent valve enhances clinical decision-making, and minimizes the need for cardiac catheterization.

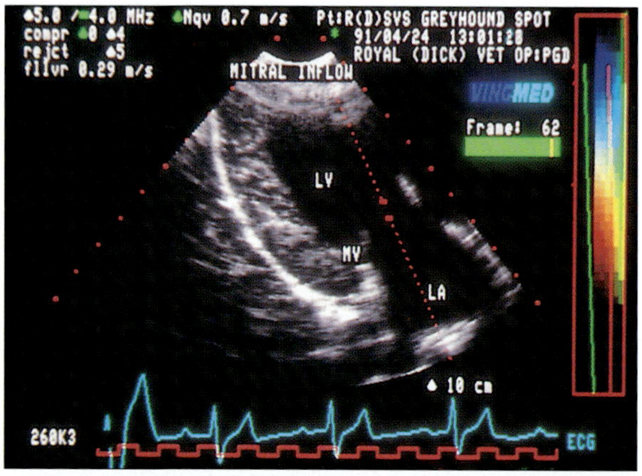

7.1 Long-axis, 2-chambered view of the heart from the left apex, showing ideal alignment with left ventricular inflow through the mitral valve for Doppler studies.

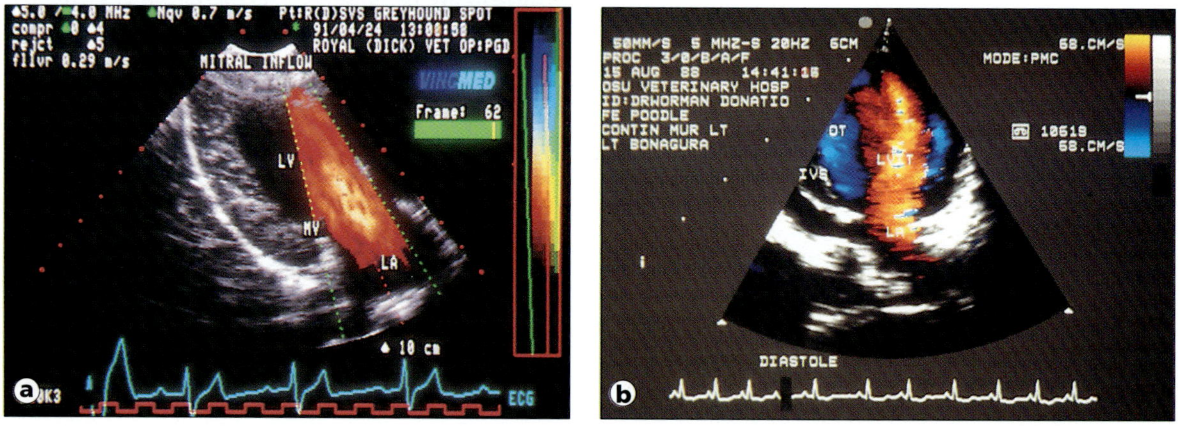

7.2 (**a**) The same view as in **7.1**, with colour-flow Doppler, showing normal left ventricular inflow (coded red – towards the transducer). The highest velocity in the central core of flow is demonstrated by the brightest colour. (**b**) Mitral valve inflow demonstrated by different equipment. The red/orange pattern of flow indicates blood moving from the left atrium into the left ventricle; the blue pattern of flow is blood curling up from the left apex towards the basilar portion of the ventricle and the left ventricular outflow tract (OT). The fastest moving red cells are coded in the brightest colours in this map.

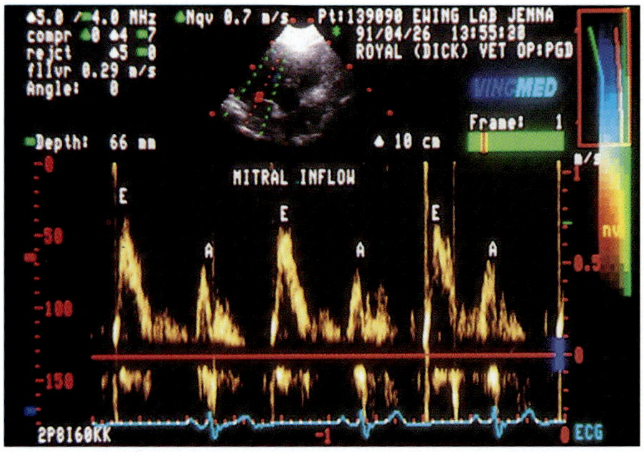

7.3 Pulsed-wave spectral Doppler recording of mitral valve inflow from a normal Labrador retriever. Note the greater velocity of flow in early diastole (E wave), and the lesser velocity (A wave) following atrial contraction.

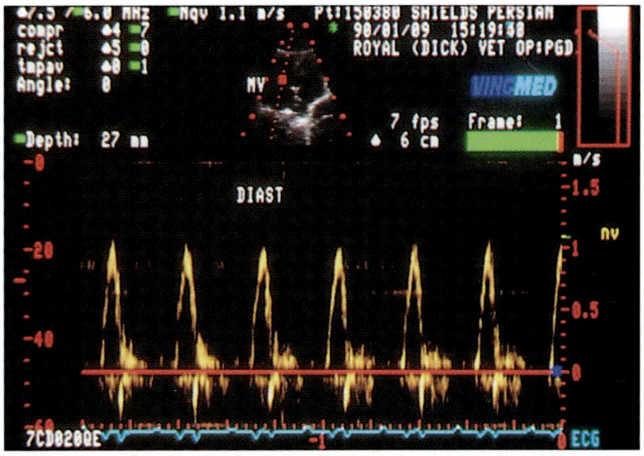

7.4 Pulsed-wave spectral Doppler recording of mitral valve inflow in a Persian cat. At the normal fast heart rate in this species, the E wave and A wave coincide, with summation of the waves.

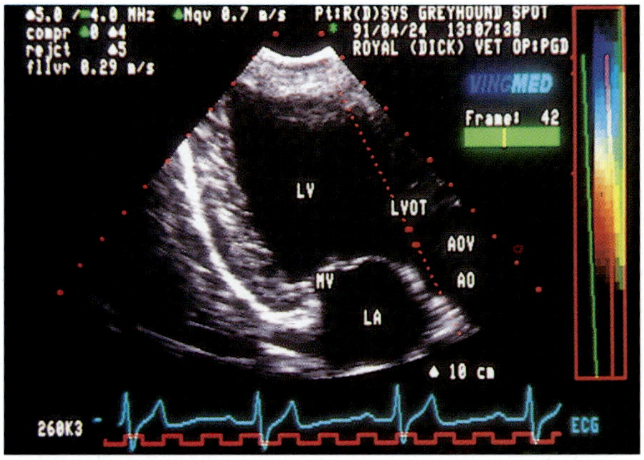

7.5 Long-axis, 2-chambered view of the heart from the left apex in a normal dog , optimized for alignment with left ventricular outflow.

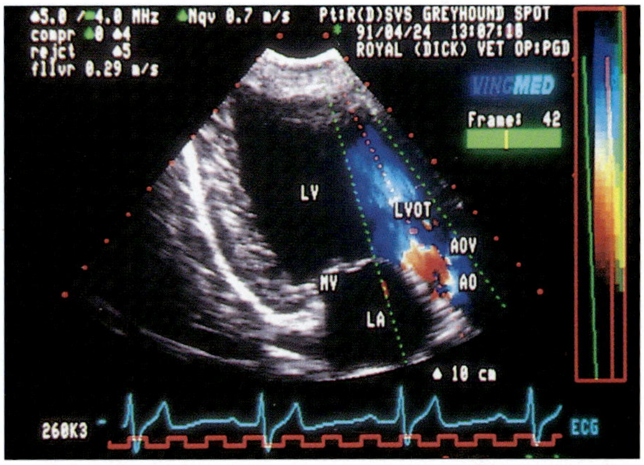

7.6 Colour-flow recording from the same dog and view as in **7.5**. Note the laminar flow (coded blue – away from the transducer) and the aliasing of the signal to red when blood velocities exceed the brightest central core velocity that can be demonstrated by pulsed-wave Doppler.

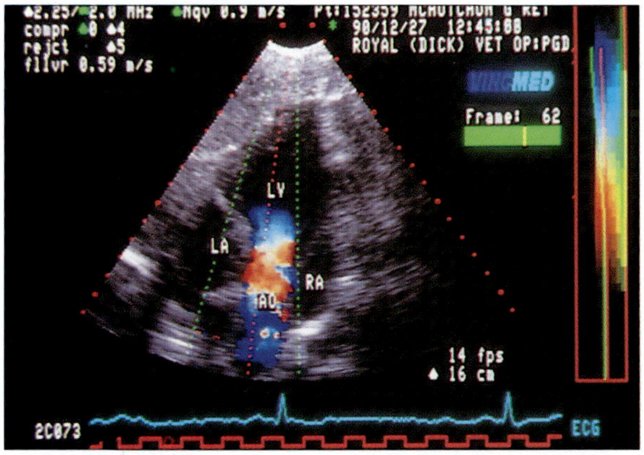

7.7 Subcostal view of the heart with normal left ventricular outflow in a golden retriever, as demonstrated by colour-flow Doppler. There is aliasing of the signal from blue to red. The best alignment with aortic flow in dogs is usually obtained from this site.

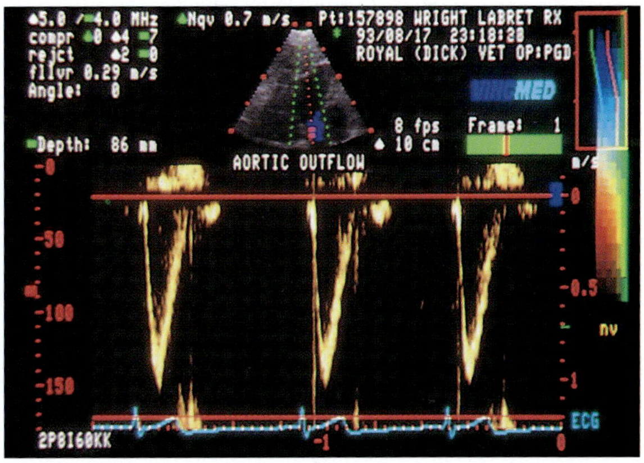

7.8 Pulsed-wave spectral Doppler recording of normal aortic outflow in a Labrador retriever. Note the normal maximal velocity (1.1 m/sec), and laminar flow indicated by a clear and triangular 'envelope'; there is little 'spectral dispersion'.

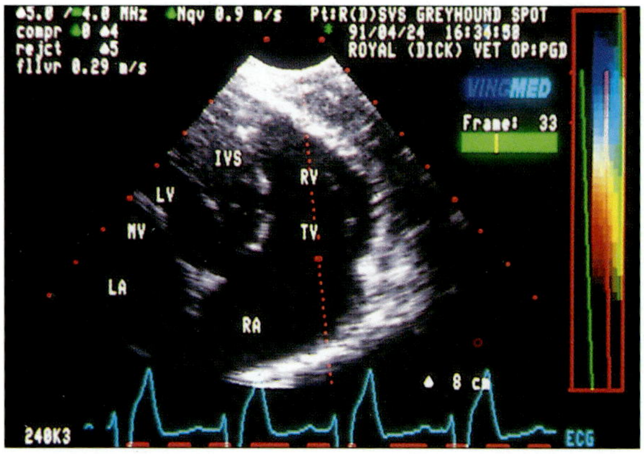

7.9 Four-chambered view of the heart of a dog from a site cranial to the left apex, optimized for alignment with tricuspid inflow.

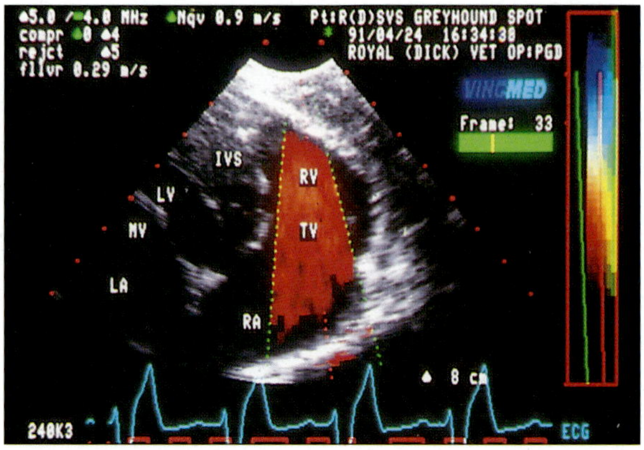

7.10 Colour-flow Doppler recording from the dog in **7.9**, showing normal laminar right ventricular inflow (coded red – towards the transducer).

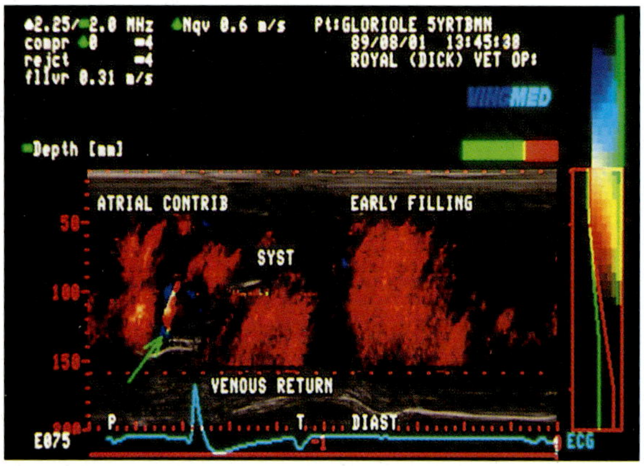

7.11 Colour M-mode view of flow on the atrial side of the mitral valve in a thoroughbred horse, showing the duration of flow during various components of the cardiac cycle.

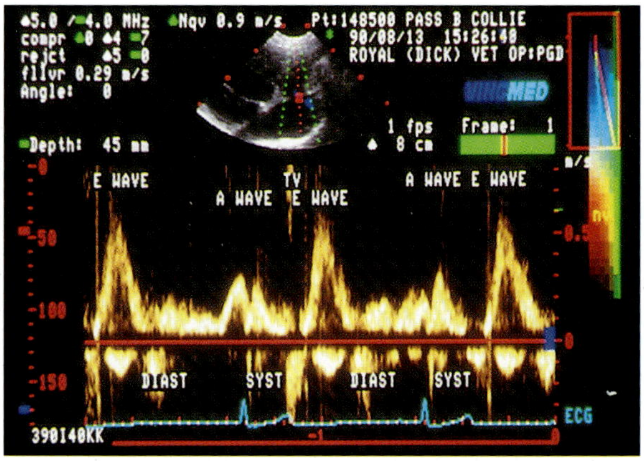

7.12 Pulsed-wave spectral Doppler recording of normal tricuspid inflow in a border collie. Note that the early filling (E wave) is greater than the atrial contraction (A wave).

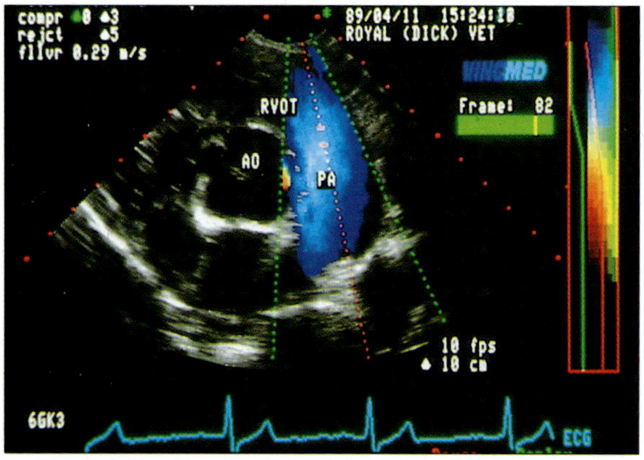

7.13 Normal flow in the pulmonary artery of a greyhound demonstrated by colour-flow Doppler, recorded from the cranial site on the left side of the thorax. The flow is away from the transducer (coded blue) and laminar.

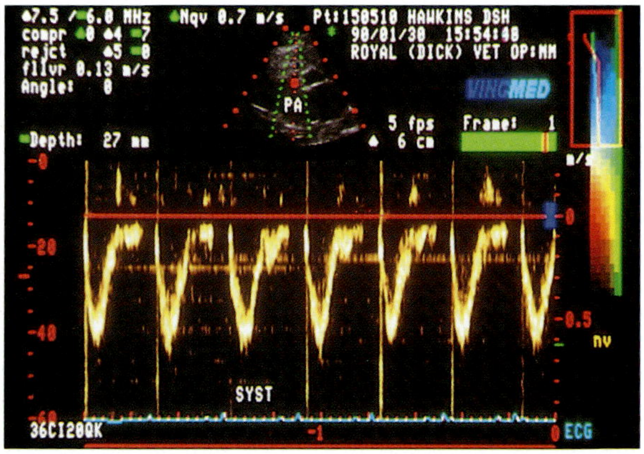

7.14 Pulsed-wave spectral Doppler recording from the pulmonary artery of a cat. Note the normal laminar flow indicated by the clear 'envelope', with a maximal velocity of flow of about 0.6 m/sec.

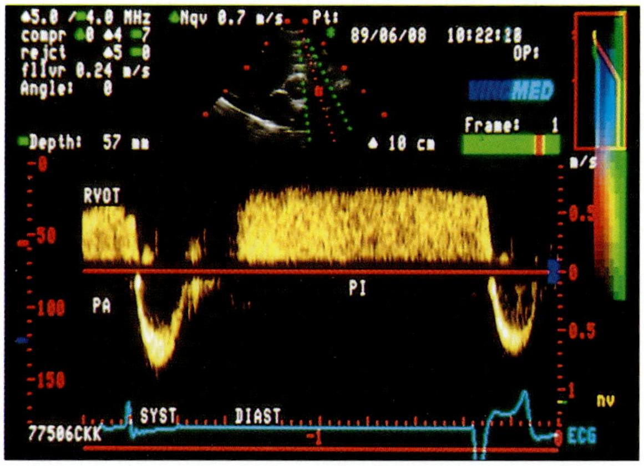

7.15 Pulmonary insufficiency recorded from a normal dog. The systolic flow signal is triangular and below the baseline. The disturbed flow of regurgitation across the pulmonic valve is evident. Pulmonary regurgitation is found in many normal dogs. In cases where the regurgitant velocity is higher than normal, pulmonary hypertension can be diagnosed.

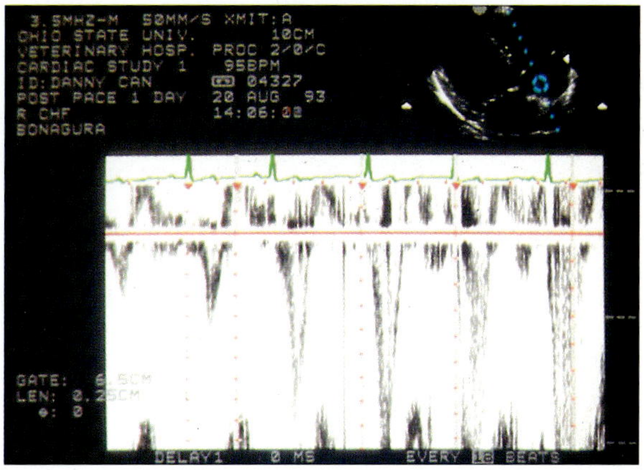

7.16 Pulsed-wave Doppler mapping of a tricuspid regurgitant jet in a dog. The sample volume was moved progressively towards the tricuspid orifice. At the level of proximal flow convergence into the orifice (left), a negative triangular flow pattern is observed. As the regurgitant jet gains velocity nearer to the orifice (centre), the signal becomes higher in velocity, and disturbed. A signal alias is evident at the far right.

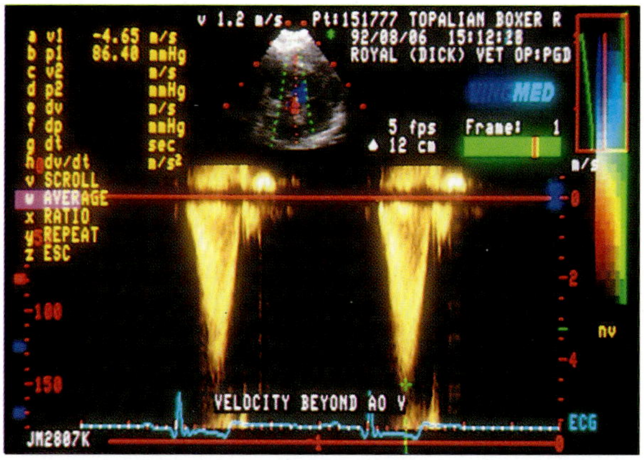

7.17 Pulsed-wave HPRF spectral Doppler recording from the ascending aorta of a boxer dog with severe supravalvular aortic stenosis. There is high-velocity flow (4.65 m/sec), and flow is turbulent, as indicated by the loss of the clear 'envelope' of the flow. Compare this with the laminar aortic flow in **7.8**.

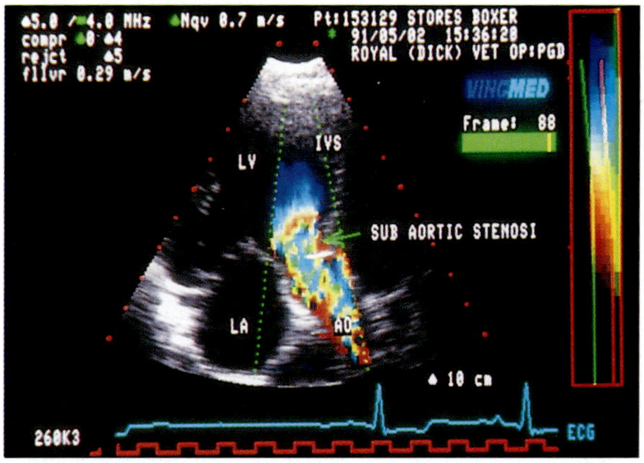

7.18 High-velocity disturbed aortic flow recorded as colour variance (yellow/green) by colour-flow Doppler in a boxer with subaortic stenosis. Compare this with the laminar flow in **7.6**.

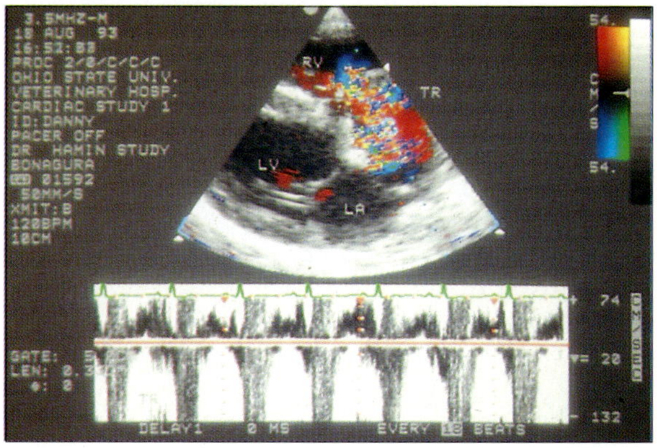

7.19 Tricuspid regurgitation recorded in the same dog as in **7.16**. The upper panel demonstrates the turbulent mosaic of the regurgitant jet colliding with normal (i.e. red and homogeneous) venous return. The derived pulsed-Doppler recording is shown below with a high-velocity, disturbed, aliased signal of tricuspid regurgitation evident during systole.

8. Cardiac Catheterization and Angiocardiography

Cardiac catheterization can be used to study congenital and acquired diseases of the heart and circulation, to assess the haemodynamic significance of cardiovascular (CV) lesions, to biopsy the myocardium, to pace the heart, and to perform and monitor therapy. Procedures are commonly carried out in conjunction with angiocardiography which requires the exposure of closely-timed, sequential, radiographic films or video-tape recordings following the injection of water-soluble radiopaque media into the heart or blood vessels. Optimal results with cardiac catheterization require familiarity and expertise, the availability of fluoroscopy to guide the catheter to the chosen site, a good image recording system, and the monitoring of blood pressure and oxygen saturation. It is therefore demanding in time, expertise and equipment.

Catheters are typically introduced into the circulation through either the jugular vein or carotid artery, or the femoral vein or artery. Various guide wires, introduction sheaths, and specialized catheters are available. With experience, an operator can navigate the heart and vascular system using fluoroscopic guidance (in small animals) or by using intravascular pressure waveforms as a guide. In addition to pressure wave forms, haemoglobin oxygen saturation (oximetry) can assist in calculation of cardiac output and shunting fractions. Increasingly, diagnostic cardiac catheterization has been replaced by Doppler echocardiography; however, new indications for catheterization (cardiac pacing and therapeutic balloon dilatation of stenotic lesions and coil/device occlusion of cardiac shunts) have been developed in recent years.

Intracardiac and intravascular pressures and haemoglobin oxygen saturation vary with location, body position, physiologic state, and species. Since the systemic vascular resistance is approximately 5–6 times greater than the pulmonary vascular resistance, peak systolic pressures recorded in the aorta and left ventricle are generally about 120 mmHg in the resting animal. Diastolic aortic pressure is usually about 80 mmHg. Diastolic left ventricular pressures usually range from subatmospheric in early diastole (due to active ventricular relaxation) to a maximum of 10–12 mmHg at end diastole (after the atrial contraction). Left atrial and pulmonary venous pressures are quite low in normal animals, usually between 0–12 mmHg throughout the entire cardiac cycle. Corresponding pressures on the right side of the circulation are as follows: pulmonary artery (systolic/diastolic) = 22–30 / 8–12 mmHg; right ventricle = 22–35 / 0–8 mmHg; right atrium = 0–8 mmHg. Right-sided pressures in large animals tend to be at the higher end of this range. Intracardiac pressures can change significantly with physiologic state.

Congestive heart failure is characterized by inadequate cardiac output with exercise or at rest, and by elevated venous, atrial and ventricular end-diastolic pressures. Stenotic cardiac lesions cause a pressure gradient to develop across the narrowed zone. This gradient is proportional both to the severity of obstruction and to the flow volume traversing the lesion. An incompetent atrioventricular valve increases the atrial pressure in systole. An incompetent semilunar valve elevates the ventricular diastolic pressure on the affected side. Shunting lesions alter the normal oximetry findings; a left-to-right shunt, for example, increases the haemoglobin oxygen saturation at the level of the shunt and beyond.

The angiographic series of recordings is used to evaluate cardiac anatomy, blood flow patterns, and to estimate cardiac function. Injections are usually made in the left and right ventricles and the ascending aorta. A left ventricular injection can be used to diagnose mitral regurgitation, various forms of aortic stenosis or left-to-right shunting through a ventricular septal defect. An aortic injection may demonstrate aortic regurgitation, patent ductus arteriosus, malformations of the aortic arch, or anomalous coronary arterial anatomy. A right ventricular injection can identify tricuspid regurgitation, forms of pulmonic stenosis, or right-to-left shunting through a ventricular septal defect as observed with the tetralogy of Fallot.

Ventricular size, geometry and systolic function may be estimated by observing the ventricular dimensions and wall movements throughout the cardiac cycle. Examples of angiography can be found throughout this Atlas.

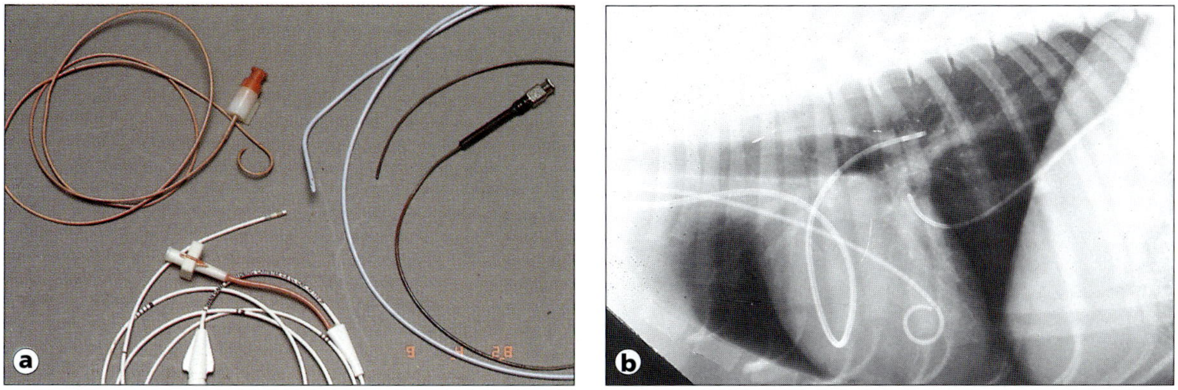

8.1 (**a**) Examples of various catheters used for cardiac catheterization and angiocardiography. The different shapes permit the operator to navigate the vascular system effectively. (**b**) Radiograph of a dog demonstrating various cardiac catheters. A 'pigtail' catheter has been advanced from the carotid artery into the left ventricle. A flow-directed pulmonary artery catheter was introduced into the jugular vein and traverses the cranial vena cava, right atrium, right ventricle and pulmonary artery, producing the characteristic 'loop' on the lateral film. A multipurpose curved catheter has been advanced from the femoral vein into the caudal right atrium.

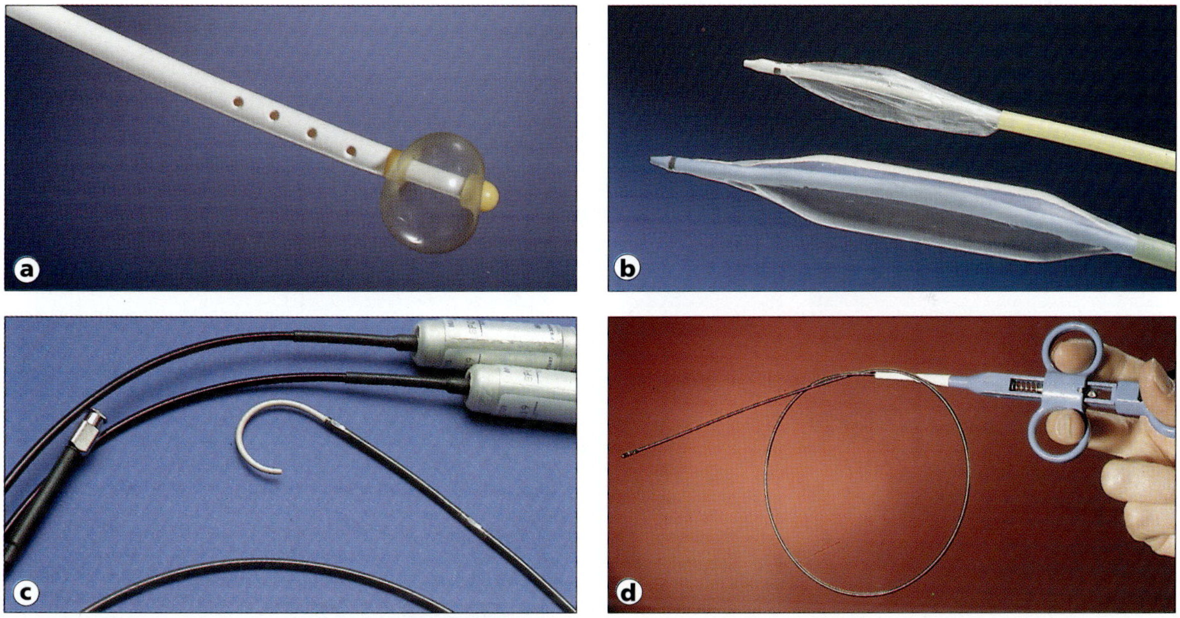

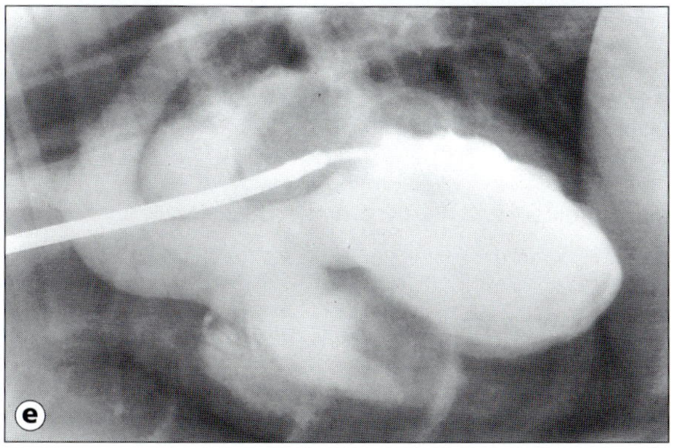

8.2 Special-purpose catheters. (**a**) A balloon-tipped angiographic (Berman) catheter. The balloon protects the myocardium and helps to keep the catheter in the ventricle. (**b**) Catheters used for balloon valvuloplasty and dilation of stenotic regions. (**c**) A micromanometer-tipped catheter used for high fidelity pressure recordings. (**d**) An endomyocardial biotome used for percutaneous biopsy of the right ventricle muscle via the jugular vein. The catheter is looped for photography. (**e**) Lateral radiography of a transeptal catheterization. A special rigid catheter was advanced from the jugular vein, through the atrial septum, and is now used to permit an angiographic catheter to be passed into the left atrium and left ventricle. An injection of contrast medium demonstrates a left-to-right shunt across a ventricular septal defect.

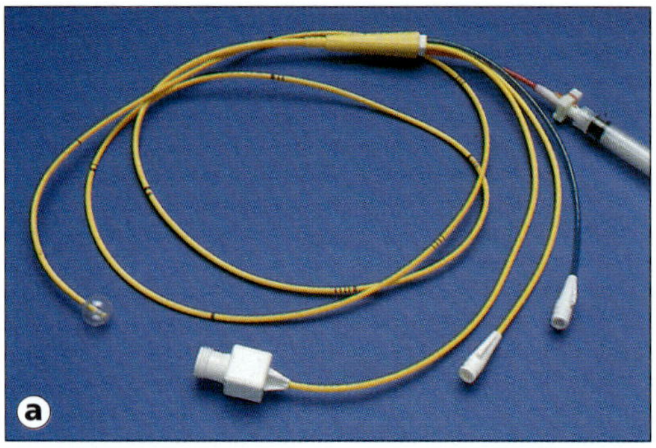

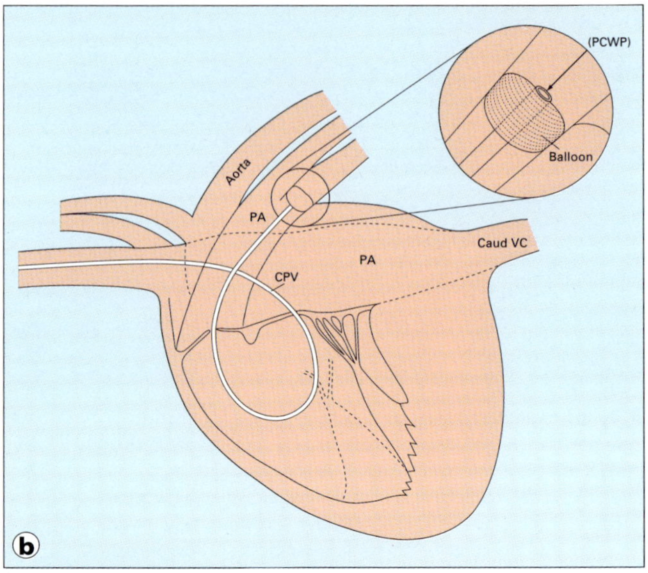

8.3 Swan–Ganz catheters. (**a**) Inflated balloon-tipped (Swan–Ganz) catheter used for monitoring pulmonary artery and pulmonary artery capillary wedge pressures (PCWP). (**b**) Diagram of the method for recording capillary wedge pressure. Once inflated, the balloon samples pressure in the distal pulmonary capillary bed, while preventing transmission of pressures from the proximal pulmonary artery.

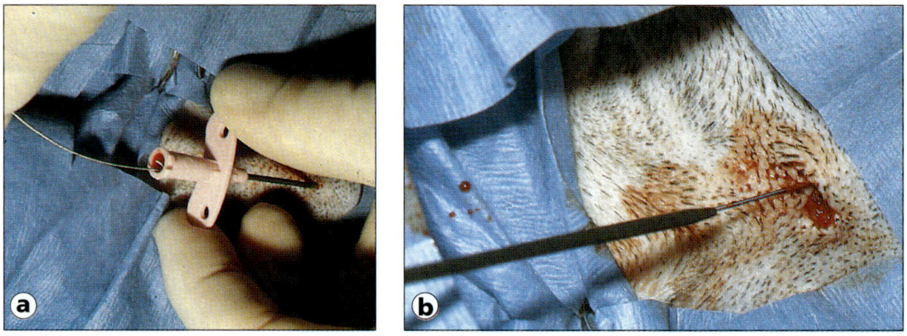

8.4 Percutaneous cardiac catheterization. (**a**) A flexible guide wire is advanced into the vessel. (**b**) After removing the cannula, a vessel dilator is placed over the wire which has previously been advanced into the vein.

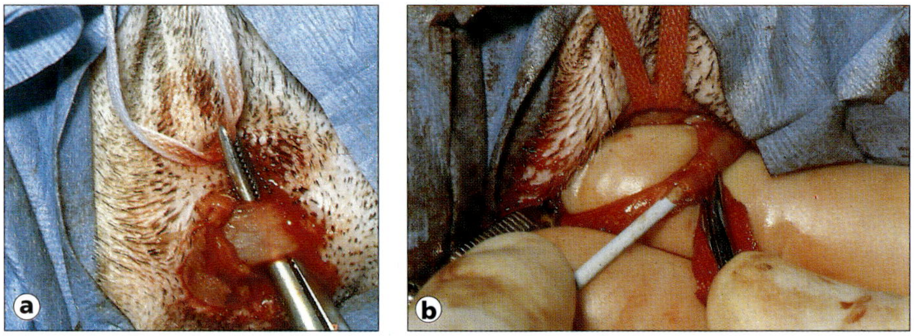

8.5 Surgical cut to exposure the jugular vein. (**a**) Blunt dissection and elevation of the vein. (**b**) Placement of a catheter into the jugular venous lumen.

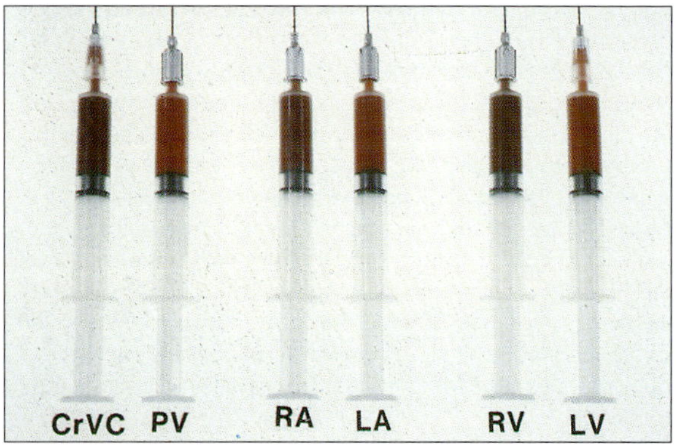

8.6 Oximetry. Samples of blood are obtained from various locations, from left to right, cranial vena cava, pulmonary vein, right atrium, left atrium, right ventricle, left ventricle. Note the difference in colour. Precise measurement of haemoglobin oxygen saturation is useful for estimation of cardiac output and detection and quantitation of cardiac shunts.

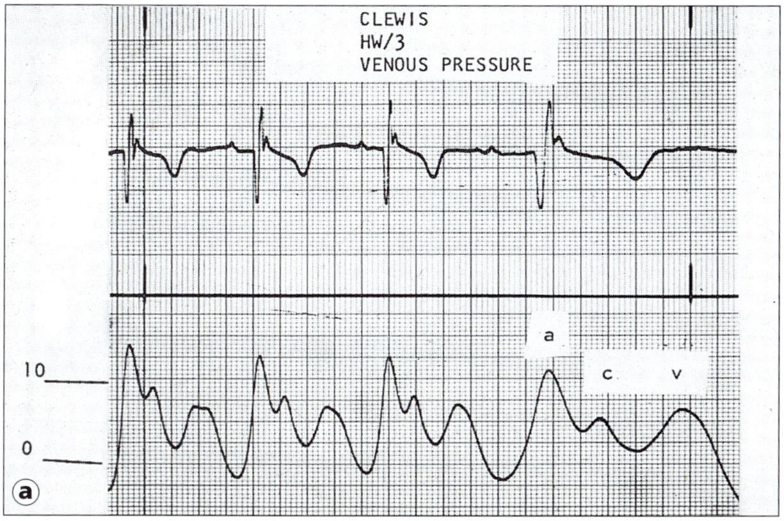

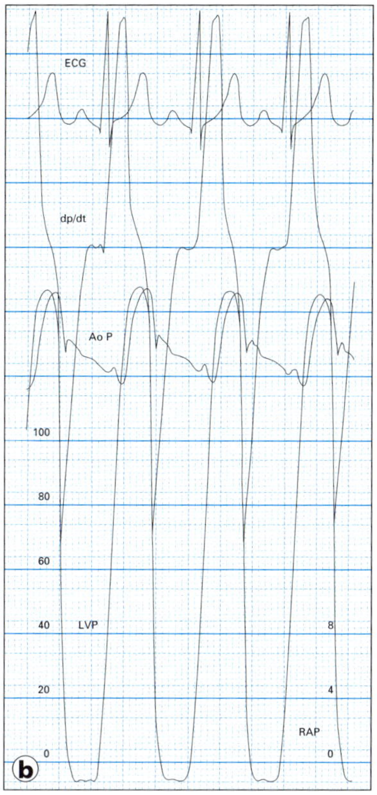

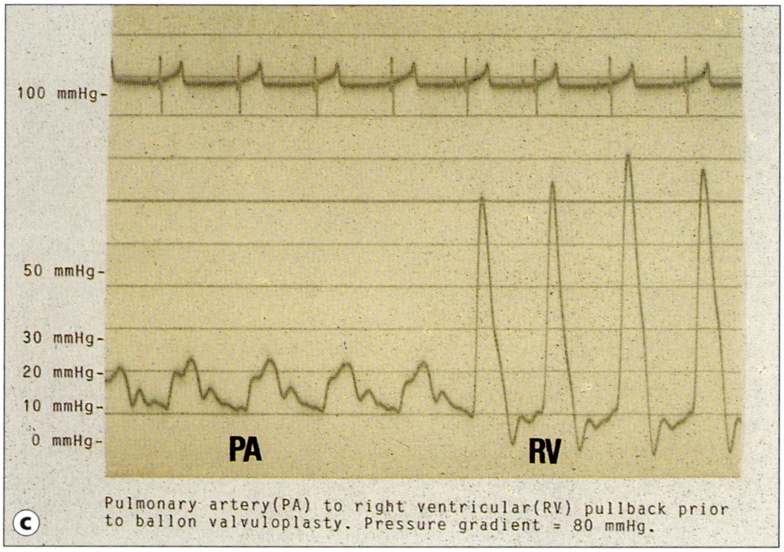

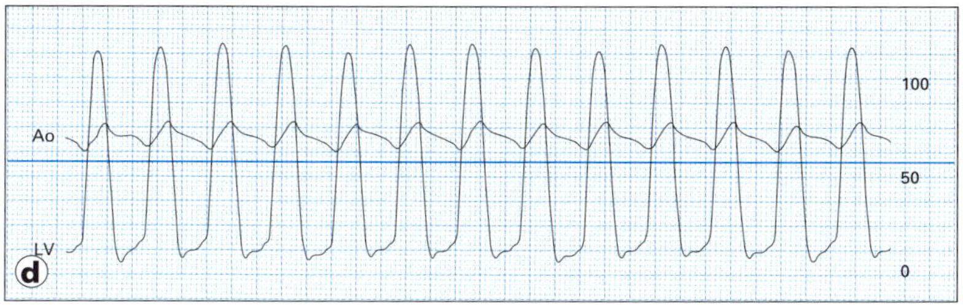

8.7 Measurement of intracardiac and intravascular pressures. (**a**) ECG (top) and right atrial pressure curves from a dog with heartworm disease and first degree AV block. (Paper speed is 50 mm/sec.) The A, C and V waves are noted (the last cycle is recorded at a paper speed of 100 mm/sec). The overall venous pressure is increased (the scale on the left is in mmHg). The prominent A-wave indicates right ventricular stiffness and vigorous atrial contraction. (**b**) Aortic and left ventricular pressures and left ventricular dp/dt recorded with a high-fidelity manometer catheter. Note the near superimposition of the normal systolic aortic and left ventricular pressures. (RAP – right atrial pressure) (**c**) Typical 'pull-back' pressure recording from a dog with pulmonic stenosis. The recording is from the pulmonary artery (PA) and then the right ventricle (RV). Note the systolic pressure gradient between the two areas, which is indicative of a stenotic pulmonary valve. (**d**) Simultaneous aortic (Ao) and left ventricular (LV) pressures recorded from a dog with congenital subaortic stenosis. The pressure gradient is the area between the two traces during systole.

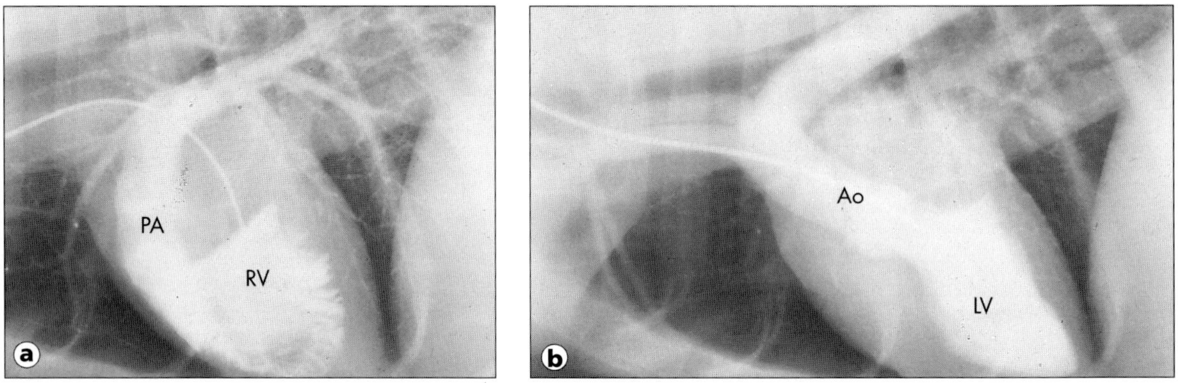

8.8 Angiocardiograms. (**a**) Normal right ventricular injection. (**b**) Normal left ventricular injection.

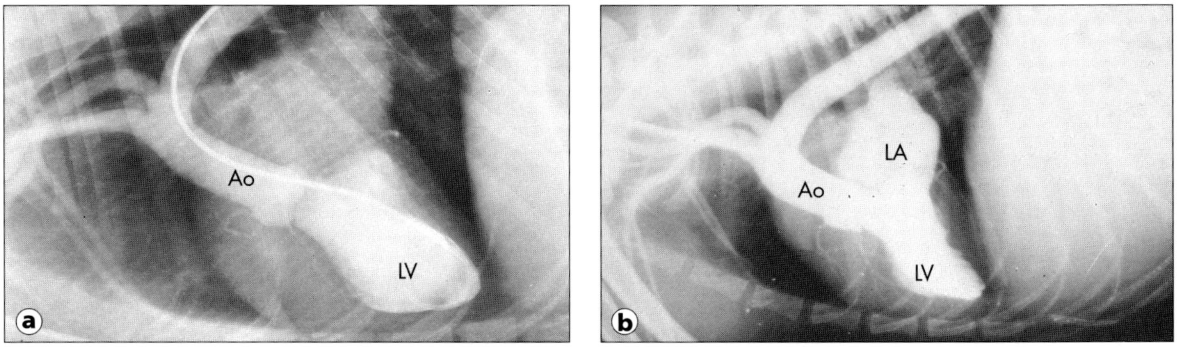

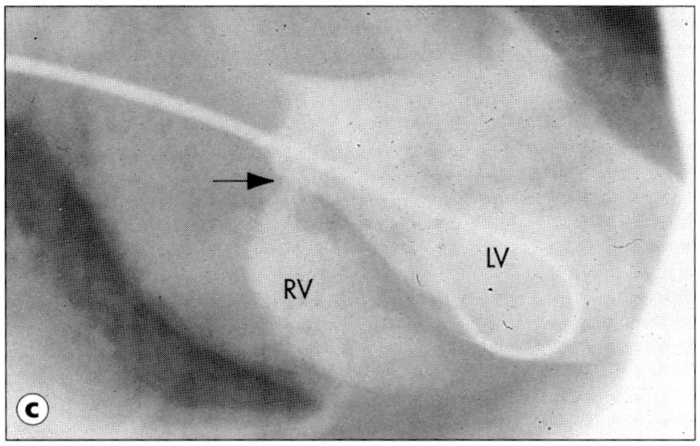

8.9 Direct angiograms in disease. (**a**) Injection into the left ventricle from a catheter introduced from the femoral artery. This dog had mitral stenosis and a dilated left atrium is evident; however, there was minimal if any mitral regurgitation. (**b**) Example of mitral regurgitation which is evident following injection of contrast medium into the left ventricle. (**c**) Example of a left-to-right shunt across a ventricular septal defect. Contrast medium was injected into the left ventricle and opacifies the right ventricle via a 'high' ventricular septal defect (arrow).

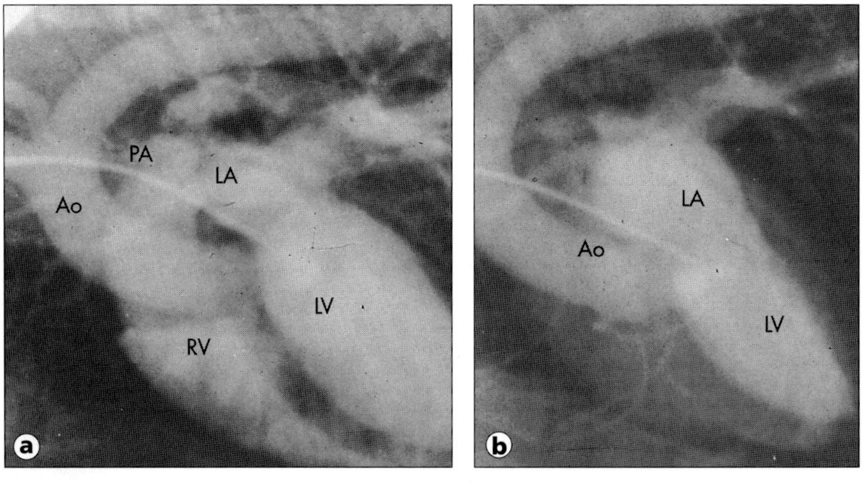

8.10 Nonselective angiocardiography. (**a**) Normal, nonselective angiocardiogram from a cat. Contrast medium was injected in the right atrium and subsequently opacifies the atrium, right ventricle, pulmonary arteries and veins, left atrium, left ventricle, and aorta. (**b**) Later in the study, contrast media has been cleared from the right side of the heart, but still opacifies the left side. This is a systolic frame and the left atrium is larger (venous return) while the left ventricle is smaller (ejection).

9. Mitral Valve Disease

The mitral valve is best considered as part of a valve apparatus which includes the leaflets and slightly thicker cusps (free edges), atrial wall, valve annulus, and the supporting chordae tendineae and papillary muscles. The mitral valve comprises two major leaflets which are designated anterior (septal) and posterior (mural). Incomplete commissures are contained witin the posterior mitral leaflet in horses, and these 'accessory leaflets' are often the site of ruptured chordae tendineae. Mitral regurgitation (MR) is the most commonly encountered valvular disorder in general veterinary practice. Mitral valve regurgitation can be considered the functional consequence of valve dysfunction. There are numerous potential causes of mitral (and tricuspid) valve regurgitation (**9.1**), but most cases stem from valve degeneration, cardiomyopathy, chordal rupture, endocarditis (see Chapter 13), or congenital malformation. Frequently, MR is a sequel to dilatation of the valve annulus with a volume-overloaded left ventricle.

Congenital malformations are usually termed *mitral valve dysplasia*. The disease is commonly encountered in dogs, especially in the Great Dane, English bull terrier, German shepherd, mastiffs, and in various retrievers; it is also seen in cats. There may be malformed valve leaflets or cusps, abnormal chordae tendineae (e.g. short, absent or elongated), or abnormal papillary muscles (e.g. fused or malpositioned). Valvular lesions or foreshortened chordae may lead to concurrent mitral stenosis.

Mitral valve degeneration (endocardiosis) is most common in dogs. It involves nodular (myxomatous) thickening and shortening of the valve leaflets characterized histologically by deposition of acid-staining glycosaminoglycans and fibrous tissue. Chordae tendineae are often involved; these may become thickened, stretched or ruptured. The effects of mitral valve degeneration are not generally observed until the animal ages and the murmur of MR becomes evident. However, degenerative changes may begin shortly after maturity in some dogs and, in cavalier King Charles spaniels, there is premature valve degeneration. Intramural coronary arteriosclerosis is observed commonly in older dogs with endocardiosis, and may cause myocardial ischaemia or microscopic infarction.

Mitral valve disease is less well-defined in other species. Congenital malformations are common in cats but, although degeneration may occur in aged cats, are not often recognized. By far the most important cause of MR in cats is myocardial disease (**9.1**). Horses can develop peracute MR due to ruptured chordae tendineae or endocarditis. Fibrous thickening of the valve is not uncommon in middle aged to older horses. Idiopathic, noninfective valvulitis has been recognized in some horses with relatively severe MR, including young animals. Mitral disease in ruminants is not clinically important.

The pathophysiology of MR and the resultant clinical signs depend on the cause and severity of the mitral dysfunction. Rate of onset, cause, regurgitant volume and left atrial distensibility are the key factors influencing clinical signs and prognosis. In rapidly progressive MR, as with ruptured chordae tendineae or acute bacterial endocarditis, there is little time for left atrial dilatation. Accordingly, peracute MR causes a sudden increase in left atrial pressure and may precipitate left-sided congestive heart failure with alveolar oedema. More slowly developing MR, or a case caused by congenital malformation, permits progressive left atrial dilatation and tolerance of a large regurgitant volume. Coughing or dyspnoea may occur intermittently in such cases from left-mainstem bronchial compression or exercise-related increases in left atrial pressure; however, pulmonary oedema may not be evident at rest. Chronic cases of MR can predispose to pulmonary hypertension and right-sided heart failure; this situation occurs in dogs with intercurrent lung disease and tricuspid endocardiosis. Cats and horses also develop substantial elevations in pulmonary arterial pressure from chronic MR. With progressive left atrial dilatation, regardless of cause, the heart is predisposed to atrial arrhythmias. Dogs with severe left atrial dilatation may experience endocardial tears and even rupture of the atrium with resultant cardiac tamponade.

Significant MR causes volume overload of the left side of the heart, together with an eccentric form of left ventricular hypertrophy. Myocardial systolic function is relatively well preserved in most dogs with MR, although numerous experimental studies have demonstrated an inherent reduction in myocardial contractility related to the chronic volume overload. The dilated left ventricle also becomes less compliant. Cardiac output may be limited as well, especially during sudden exertion or with excitement, predisposing to exercise intolerance and episodes of collapse or syncope.

The hallmark of MR is a systolic murmur that is best heard over the left apex and radiates dorsally and to the right. The direction of the regurgitant jet may result in a cranially directed murmur that may be confused with aortic murmurs in dogs and horses. In cases of chronic mitral valve disease, the flow disturbance is first detected as a brief, localized, protosystolic murmur, which gradually becomes more prolonged and eventually holo- or pansystolic. The typical murmur of severe MR is louder and radiates more widely than that of mild MR. The first sound may become very loud and the third sound prominent or even confused with the second, which is often obscured by the murmur. Musical murmurs or systolic whoops are occasionally heard; they often indicate a ruptured chorda tendinea. A unique variant of the MR murmur, detected almost exclusively in horses (and human beings), is the mid-to-late systolic crescendo murmur of mitral valve prolapse. This murmur is caused by stretched or ruptured chordae tendineae. The murmur of MR in cats with hypertrophic cardiomyopathy may not be holosystolic (see Chapter 17) and it may be very soft in animals with underlying dilated cardiomyopathy.

Definitive diagnosis of MR is readily made by Doppler echocardiography in all species, or by angiography in dogs and cats. The aetiology is usually suggested by the species, breed, age and clinical circumstances. Two-dimensional echocardiography assists in differentiating anatomic lesions. In cases of moderate-to-severe MR, the two-dimensional or M-mode echocardiogram demonstrates a dilated, hyperdynamic left ventricle as ejection of the regurgitant volume into the low-pressure left atrium assists rapid emptying. Myocardial failure can be recognized echocardiographically as an increased end-systolic volume, indicating incomplete emptying of the chamber. Heart failure often precedes overt myocardial failure. Left atrial size correlates relatively well with the regurgitant volume in pure mitral valve disease. Radiographic signs of both left atrial and ventricular enlargement and of pulmonary congestion and oedema are easily recognized in dogs and cats, and thus form a practical basis for evaluating these conditions. The ECG may demonstrate left-sided cardiac enlargement and repolarization changes, as well as cardiac dysrhythmias (typically atrial premature beats or atrial fibrillation).

The initial therapy for severe mitral regurgitation should involve diuresis (e.g. using furosemide), with venodilatation (using nitroglycerine ointment) if pulmonary oedema is present, and reduction of mitral regurgitant fraction with arterial vasodilators such as hydralazine. Chronic treatment of MR in small animals typically involves use of maintenance diuretics, angiotensin-converting enzyme inhibitors (e.g. enalapril), digoxin and a sodium-restricted diet. Antiarrhythmic therapy may be required (see Chapter 23). Cough suppressants may be needed to control the cough caused by left bronchial compression. Treatment of heart failure is discussed in Chapter 3 and in the Appendix.

Common Causes of Atrioventricular Valvular Regurgitation	
• Mitral valve dysplasia (MR) • Tricuspid valve dysplasia (TR) • Myxomatous valvular disease (endocardiosis causing MR, TR) • Bacterial endocarditis (MR) • Ruptured chorda tendinea (MR) • Avulsion of the papillary muscle (MR, TR) • Transmural myocardial infarction (MR)	• Ventricular or atrial dilatation (MR/TR) e.g.: • Patent ductus arteriosus (MR) • Myocardial diseases (MR/TR) • Pulmonary hypertension (TR) • Causes of left ventricular hypertrophy (MR) • Causes of right ventricular hypertrophy (TR) • Cardiac arrhythmias
MR – mitral regurgitation	TR – tricuspid regurgitation

9.1 Common causes of atrioventricular valvular regurgitation.

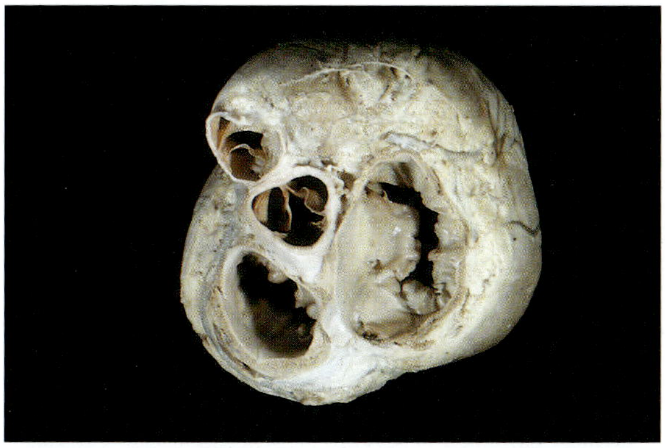

9.2 Heart valves of a normal dog viewed from the dorsal and a slightly caudal perspective. The aortic valve is in the centre; the tricuspid is the largest valve on the right; the pulmonic is left and cranial; the mitral valve is the most caudal. The tricuspid valve in the dog and cat is characterized by only two leaflets, while three are present in the horse and cow.

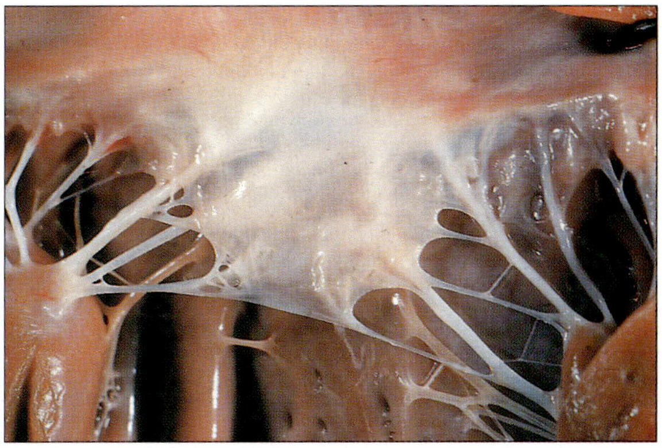

9.3 Normal canine mitral valve cusp, showing the relatively uniform, thin and transparent connective tissue.

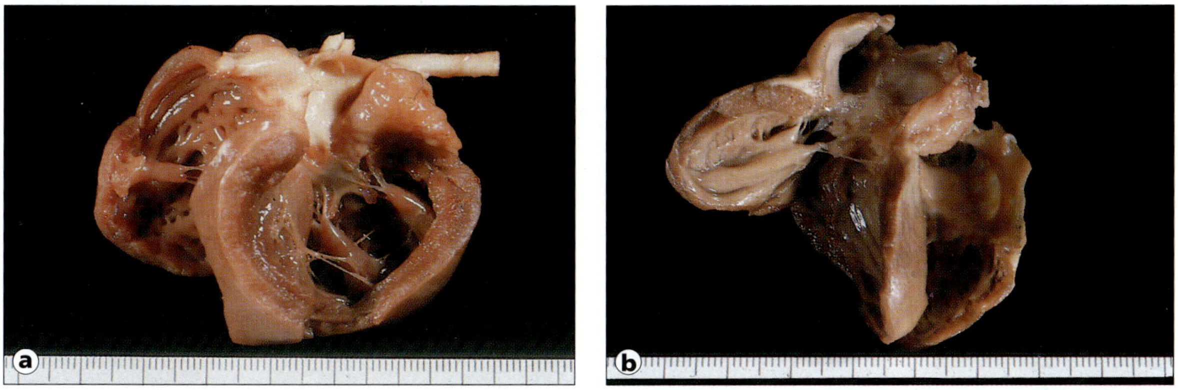

9.4 Mitral dysplasia in two cats. (**a**) Both mitral leaflets in this specimen were characterized by opposing 'C-shaped' notches in the cusp leading to an oval-shaped defect when the valve leaflets were apposed in systole. (**b**) Caudoventral view of the heart demonstrating a single, multiheaded, papillary muscle.

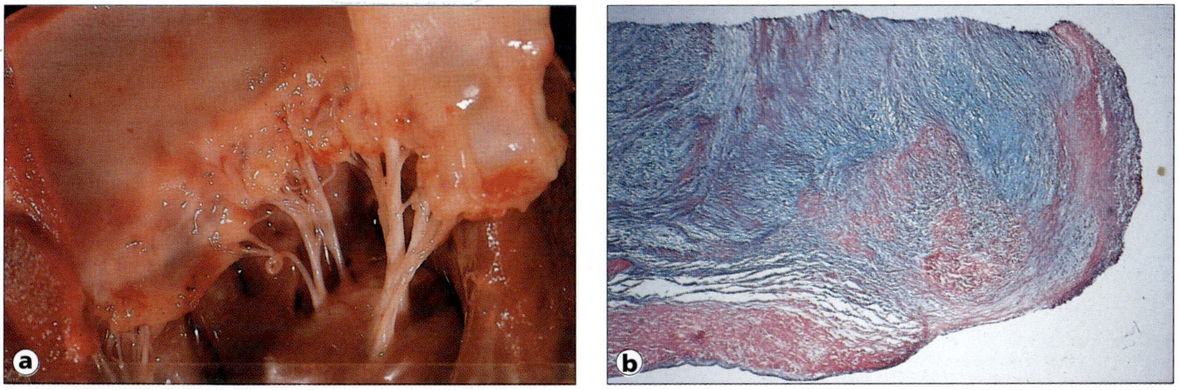

9.5 (**a**) Mitral nodular endocardiosis in a 10-year-old German shepherd dog. The mitral valve cusp is irregularly thickened and nodular, contributing to valvular incompetence. (**b**) A section of canine mitral valve, showing the accumulation of intracellular glycosaminoglycans that thickens and distorts the cusp, contributing to incompetence.

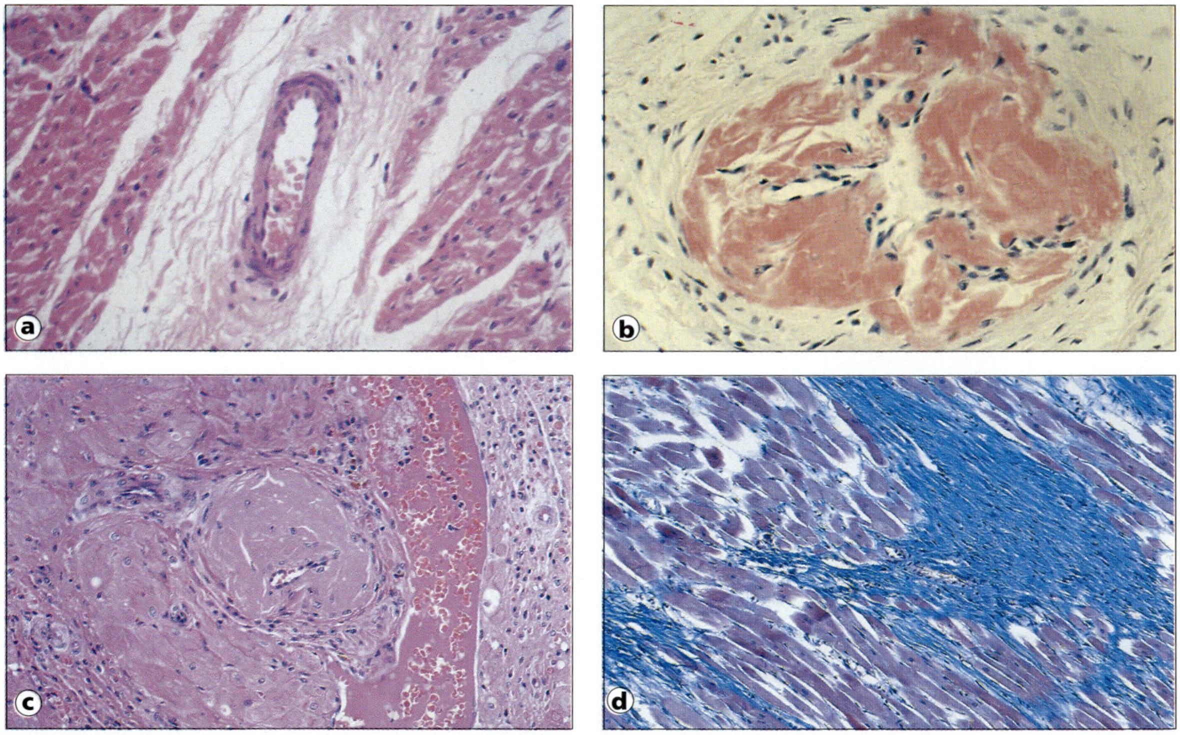

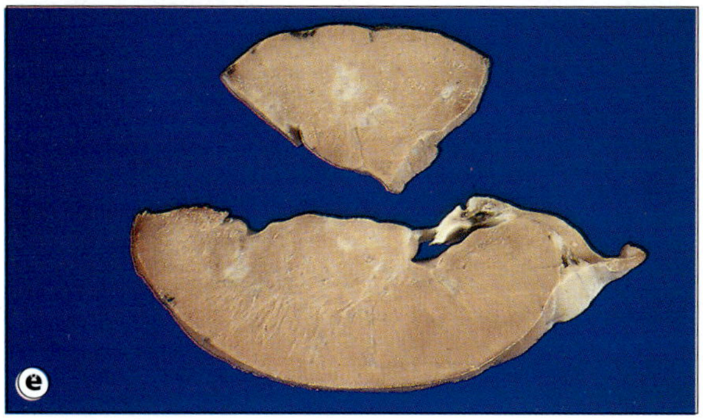

9.6 (**a**) Photomicrograph of a normal, intramural coronary artery in a dog. (**b**) Photomicrograph showing intramural coronary arteriosclerosis in a 15-year-old cross-bred dog. The lumen of this artery is narrowed by accumulation of amorphous hyaline material in the tunica intima. There is also partial atrophy of the tunica media. (**c**) Photomicrograph showing that the material accumulating in the arterial wall (same dog as in **b**) is amyloid (sirius red stain).
(**d**) Photomicrograph showing myocardial scarring in the papillary muscle of a 12-year-old cross-bred dog. Such lesions result from ischaemic atrophy of the myocardium because of progressive stenosis of intramural coronary arteries (MSB stain). (**e**) Occasionally, such ischaemic atrophy and scarring can be recognized macroscopically, as in the papillary muscle of the same dog as in **d**.

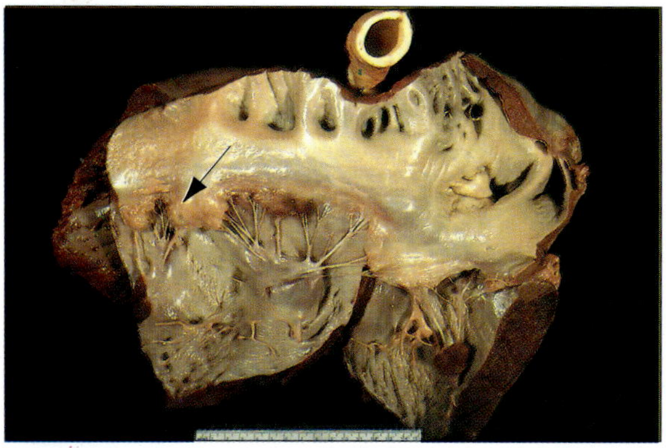

9.7 (**a**) Degenerative mitral valve in a horse viewed from the caudal aspect. The left atrium and ventricle are dilated. Jet lesions are evident above the valve, particularly above the accessory cusp (arrow). The mitral valve is mildly thickened.

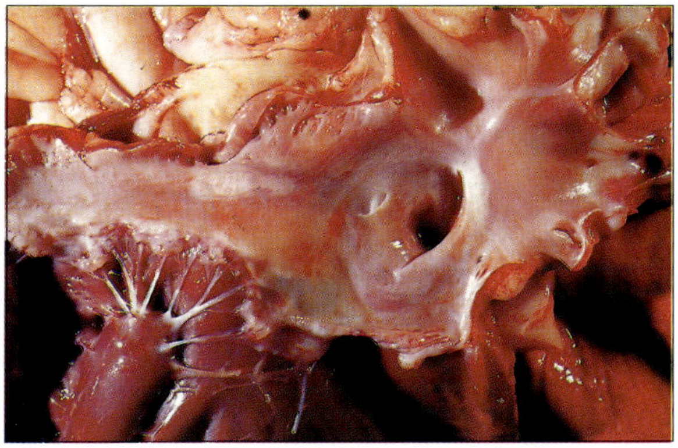

(**b**) Chronic mitral regurgitation in a 3-year-old Samoyed dog which has caused the formation of plaques of atrial endocardial thickening known as *jet lesions*.

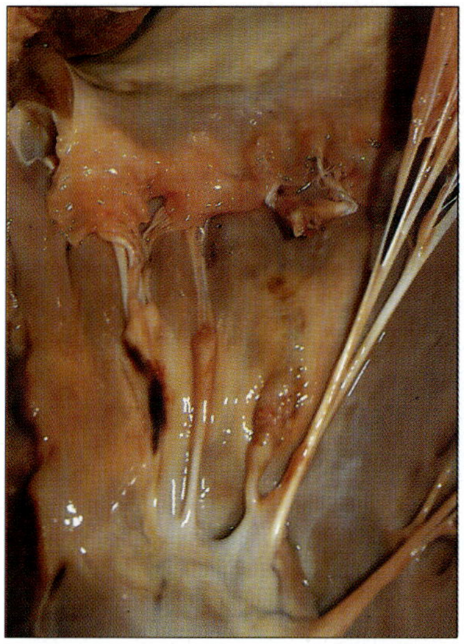

9.8 Ruptured chorda tendinea with contraction of the ruptured segments is evident in this equine specimen. The chords on the left are abnormally thickened but have not ruptured. The chords to the right of the rupture appear normal.

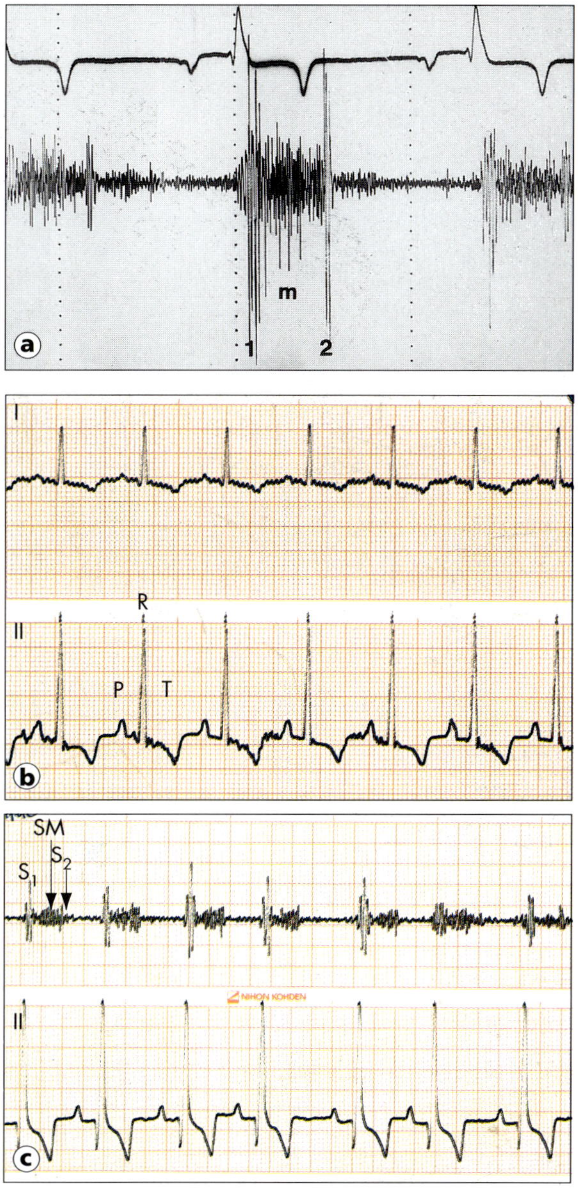

9.9 (**a**) Phonocardiogram of a horse with mitral regurgitation (m); first and second heart sounds are indicated. (**b**) ECG (50mm/sec) from a short-haired domestic cat with mitral regurgitation due to valve dysplasia. Although the cat had left atrial enlargement, the P wave is slightly tall (0.3 mV); the R wave is also tall (2.7 mV) in lead II, indicating left ventricular enlargement. (**c**) Phonocardiogram (medium frequency) and ECG lead II from an 8-year-old cavalier King Charles spaniel with mitral regurgitation. A pansystolic murmur is seen in the medium frequency waveband. (S_1 – first heart sound; S_2 – second heart sound; SM – systolic murmur).

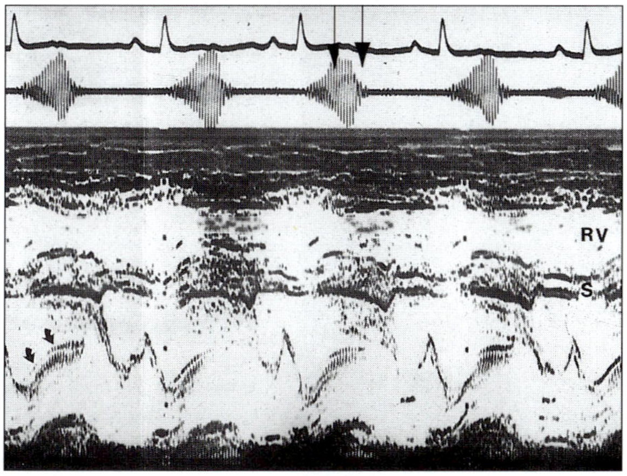

9.10 Recording of a musical systolic murmur in a dog with a minor rupture of a chorda tendinea. The phonocardiogram recording represents high frequency systolic vibrations of the anterior mitral valve leaflet (arrows).

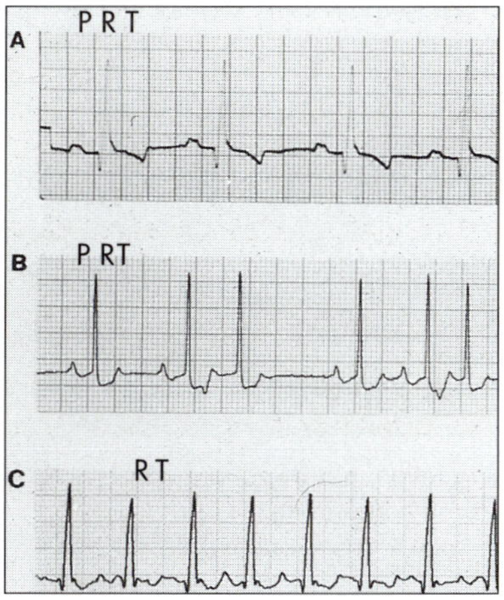

9.11 ECGs demonstrating abnormalities observed with mitral valve disease.
(**a**) Widened P and R waves with increased amplitude suggestive of left atrial and left ventricular enlargement.
(**b**) Atrial premature complexes.
(**c**) Atrial fibrillation.

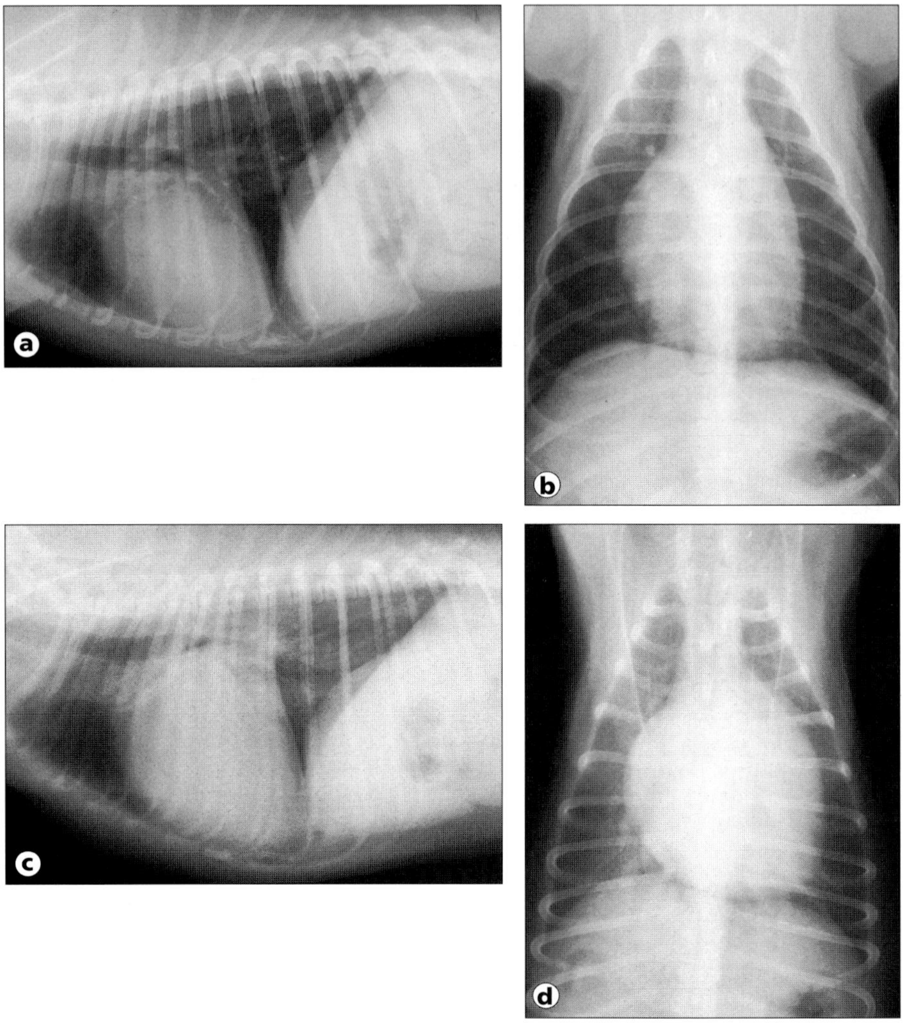

9.12 (**a** and **b**) Radiographs of a cross-bred, 8-year-old dog with mitral regurgitation; at this time the dog was asymptomatic, and these radiographs show a cardiac outline and vascular perfusion that are essentially within normal limits. (**c** and **d**) Radiographs of the same dog two years later. The dog had developed exercise intolerance and a persistent cough. These radiographs show many of the classic changes associated with mitral regurgitation, which should be compared with the films in **a** and **b**. Visible, are marked left atrial enlargement, pulmonary congestion, enlargement of the caudal vena cava and hepatic enlargement. There is also partial compression of the mainstem bronchus on the lateral film, which is probably a major factor in the aetiology of coughing. There is also a slight increase in the size of the right side of the heart, with increased sternal contact on the lateral film.

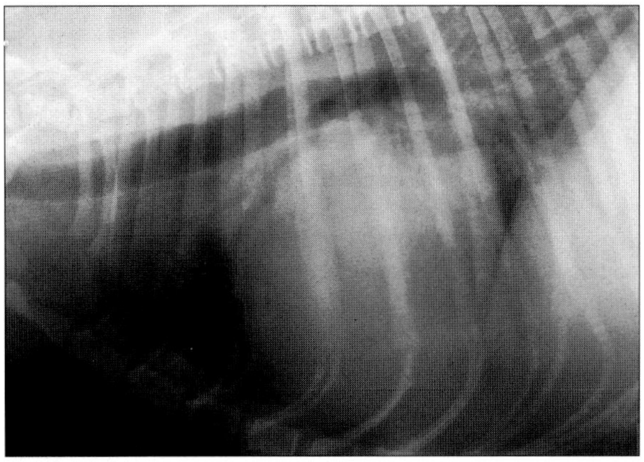

9.13 Lateral radiograph of the thorax of a collie-cross dog with severe mitral regurgitation and congestive heart failure. Note the marked left atrial enlargement, some alveolar oedema, and the enlarged cranial lobe vessels.

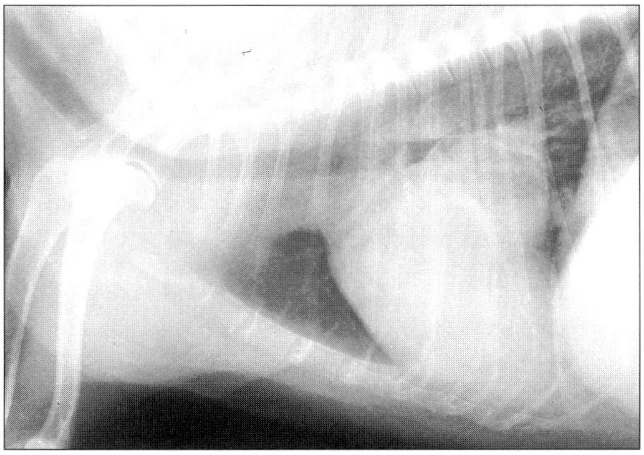

9.14 Radiograph of a dog with chronic and severe mitral regurgitation showing massive left auricular enlargement causing compression of the left mainstem bronchus.

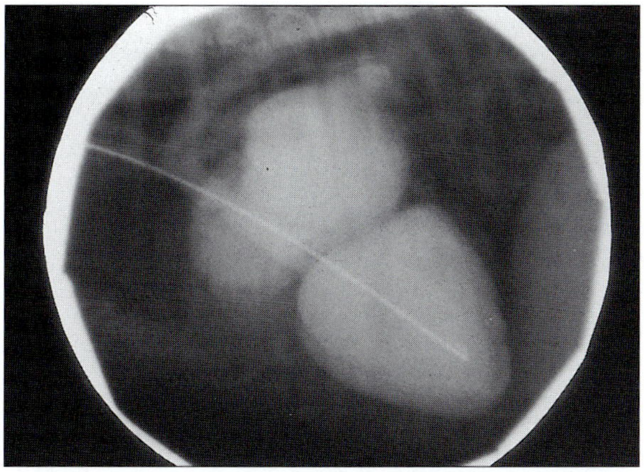

9.15 Left ventricular angiogram from a cat with mitral regurgitation demonstrating regurgitation of contrast medium into a dilated left atrium. The cause in this case was congenital dysplasia.

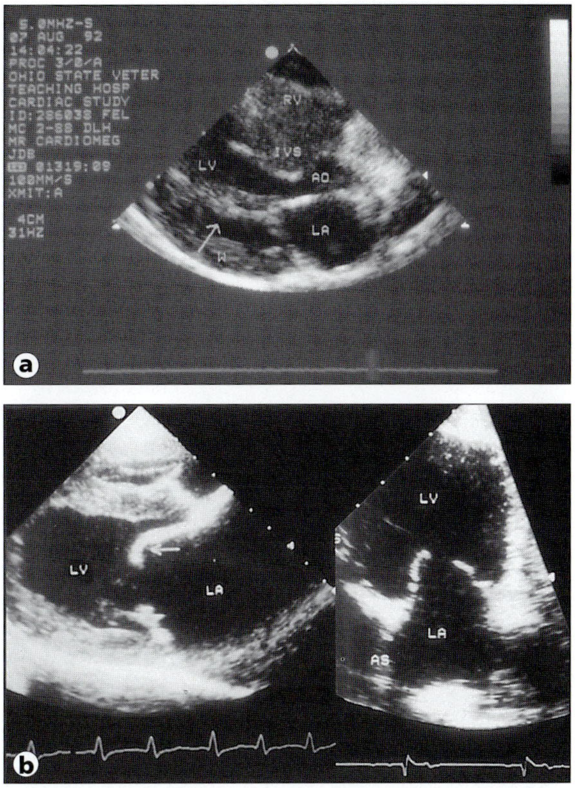

9.16 Echocardiograms in mitral valve dysplasia. (**a**) Single papillary muscle in a cat (arrow). (**b**) Mitral stenosis in a dog observed from the right hemithorax (left) and left apex (right). Note the curving of the anterior leaflet and the limited maximal opening. The curved leaflet is typical of a tethered cusp.

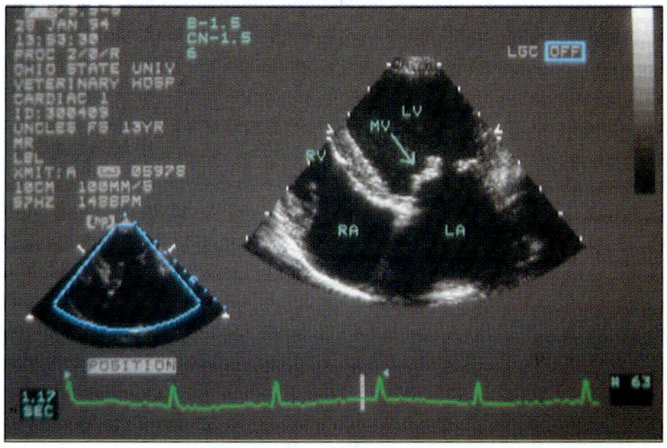

9.17 Echocardiogram from a dog with chronic mitral endocardiosis showing a thickened valve (arrow) and left atrial dilatation.

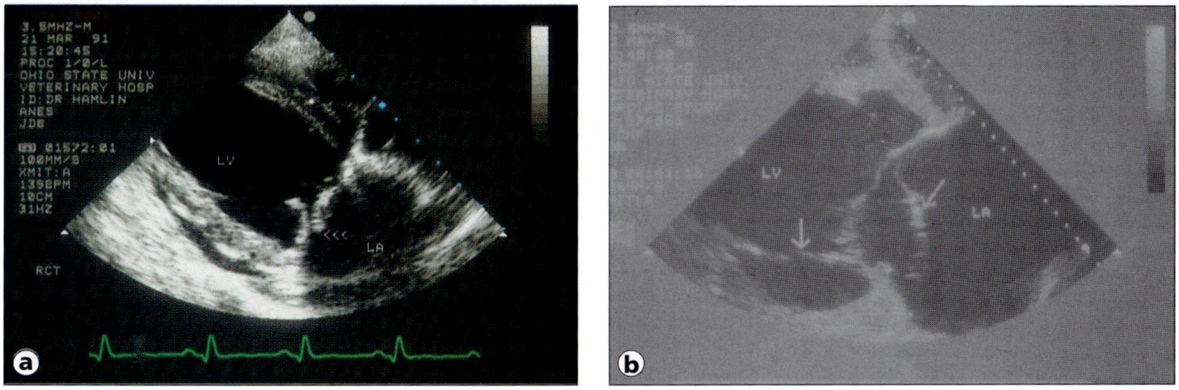

9.18 Prolapsed mitral valve leaflet in a dog (**a**) and a horse (**b**). In **a**, the anterior leaflet prolapsed behind the posterior leaflet. In **b**, a curved echo behind the normal line of closure (right arrow) is typical of a failing leaflet. Both cases were caused by rupture of chordae tendineae. A normal chord is evident as well (left arrow).

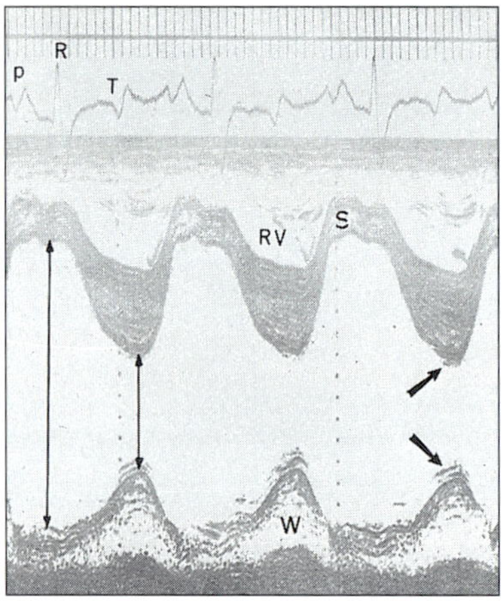

9.19 M-mode echocardiograms from a horse with mitral regurgitation. Note the hyperdynamic contraction of the left ventricle, typical of well-preserved myocardial function and afterload, mismatching to the ventricular systolic pressure. This is a consequence of ejection of blood into the low resistance left atrium.

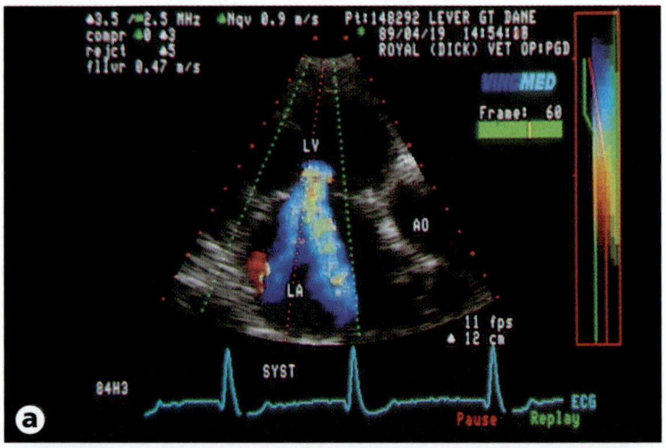

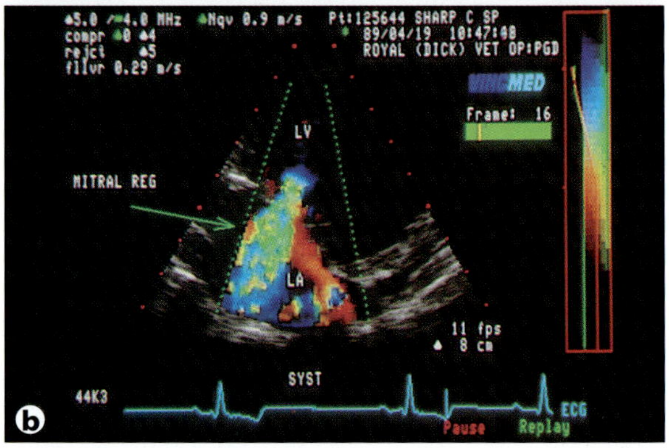

9.20 (**a**) Colour-flow Doppler recording from the mitral valve of a Great Dane with dilated cardiomyopathy, showing two jets of mitral regurgitation (coded blue – away from the transducer), one with a high-velocity core. The large cross-sectional area at the origin of the jet (at the valve) suggests moderate-to-severe regurgitation. (**b**) Colour-flow Doppler recording from a cocker spaniel with severe mitral regurgitation, showing variance (disturbed flow) indicated by yellow-green colour, and flow towards the mitral valve from the pulmonary veins in systole.

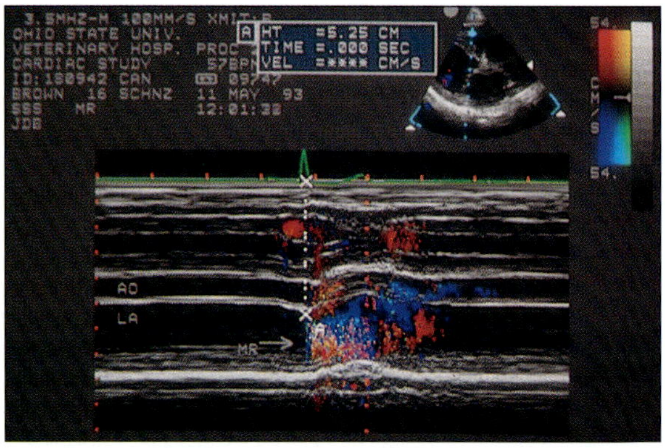

9.21 Colour M-mode of a dog with mitral regurgitation (arrow) demonstrating a prolonged systolic turbulent pattern within the left atrium.

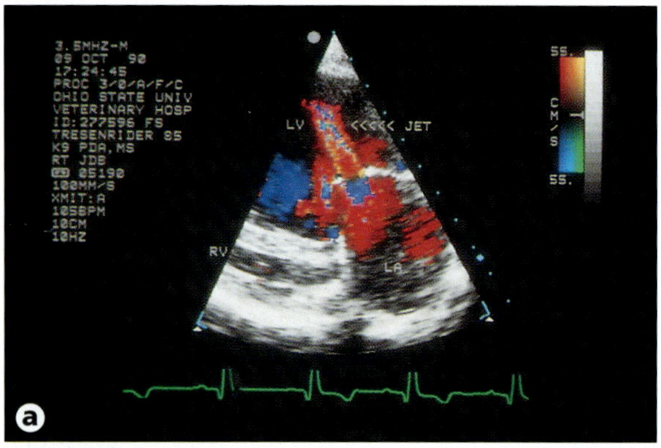

9.22 (**a**) Colour-flow Doppler recording from the mitral valve of a dog with mitral stenosis. The convergence of blood into the narrowed orifice results in an alias from red to blue at the region of proximal flow convergence. A 'candle flame' jet of diastolic turbulence is observed in the left ventricular inlet as blood enters the ventricle at high velocity.

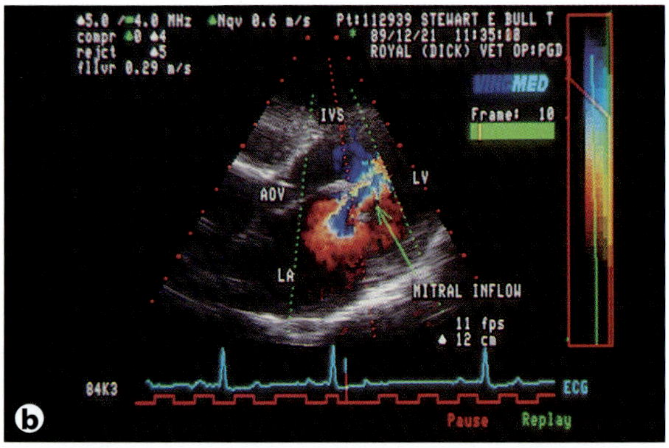

(**b**) Colour-flow Doppler recording from an English bull terrier with congenital mitral valve stenosis. The inflow is coded red (towards the transducer) with a central core of aliased flow (coded blue) representing higher-than-normal flow velocity. (Courtesy of Mrs J. Dukes McEwan.)

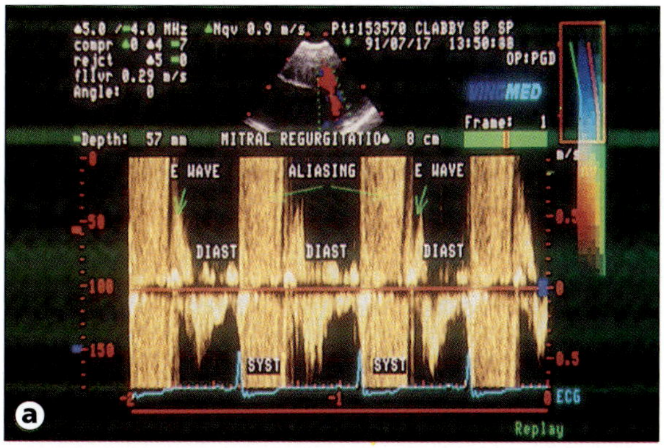

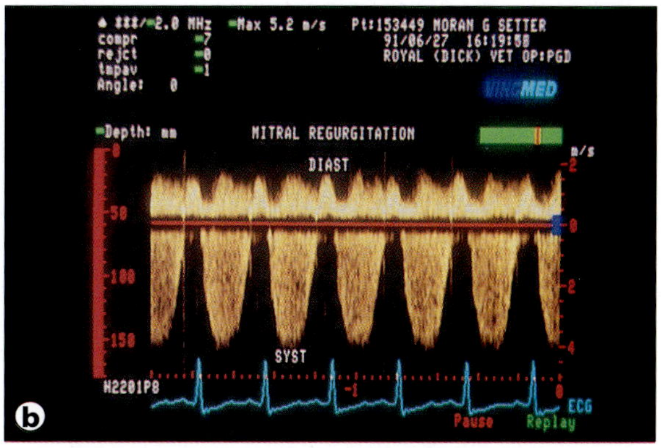

9.23 (**a**) Pulsed-wave spectral Doppler recording from a springer spaniel with dilated cardiomyopathy and secondary mitral regurgitation. The E wave of early inflow can be seen above the baseline, together with an aliased signal, in which the maximal velocity of regurgitant flow (below the baseline) cannot be accommodated by the pulsed-wave recording, and is seen to 'wrap around' the top to occupy all of the trace in systole. (**b**) Continuous-wave spectral Doppler recording from a Gordon setter with dilated cardiomyopathy and secondary mitral regurgitation. The regurgitation (maximum 4 m/sec) extends beyond systole to occupy most of the cardiac cycle. The period of mitral inflow (above the baseline in diastole) is very limited, and the velocity of flow (> 1 m/sec) is increased, partly by the added regurgitant volume.

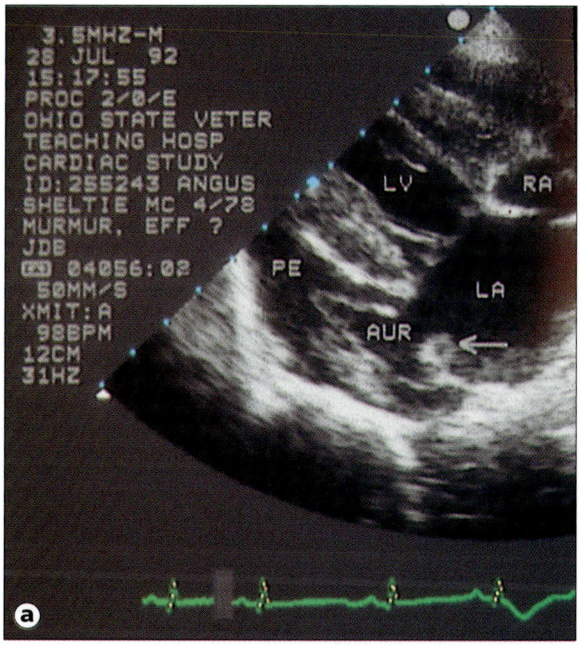

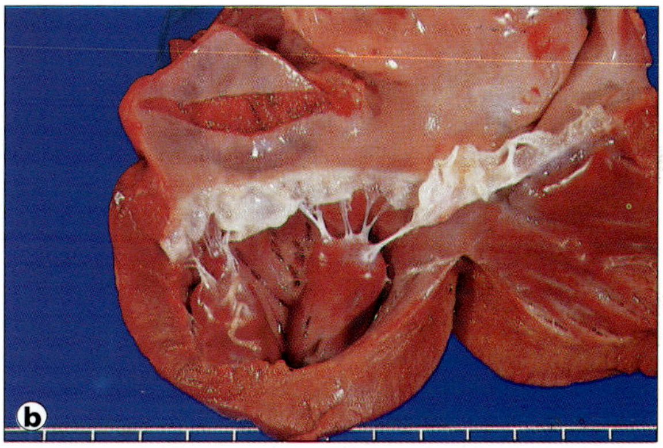

9.24 Ruptured left auricle in two dogs with chronic mitral regurgitation. (**a**) Echocardiogram demonstrating a pericardial effusion (PE) and large thrombus attached to the left auricle. There is also a probable thrombus in the left atrial cavity (arrow). The dog survived for approximately 1 month. (**b**) Large linear endocardial tear and ruptured left atrium in a cross-bred bitch with chronic mitral endocardiosis.

10. Tricuspid Regurgitation

The causes and pathophysiology of tricuspid disease are largely similar to those of mitral regurgitation, except for the pathological and clinical features described below.

Tricuspid regurgitation (TR) can be caused by congenital or acquired disease (see **9.1**). Malformation of the tricuspid valve is most often observed in dogs (and pigs), with larger canine breeds, especially retrievers, being over-represented. Tricuspid anomalies, including severe stenosis of the valve, have been observed in both cats and foals. Acquired tricuspid valve disease caused by valve degeneration is seen mainly in dogs with endocardiosis (usually in association with mitral valve disease), in horses with fibrous thickening, and in cattle and horses with bacterial endocarditis (see Chapter 14). Tricuspid regurgitation may occur secondary to cardiomyopathy. Racing horses often develop TR, though the lesion responsible has not been defined. Dilatation of the poorly defined right atrioventricular ring or hypertrophy of the papillary muscles are often associated with TR. Substantial TR may develop in association with a stenotic pulmonary valve or in pulmonary hypertension caused by left-sided heart failure, pulmonary disease or pulmonary vascular disease (cor pulmonale). Ruminants are particularly susceptible to right-sided heart enlargement induced by pulmonary hypertension, and they can develop TR and congestive heart failure from severe interstitial lung disease, or from the hypoxia of grazing at high altitude (see Chapter 22). Dogs with dirofilariasis, pulmonary embolism or severe, diffuse interstitial lung diseases can also develop TR.

Isolated TR, unless it is severe, does not appear to be as damaging as MR; in severe cases, clinical signs of right-sided cardiac failure (Chapter 3) or atrial fibrillation can ensue. The condition is recognized by a systolic murmur that is best heard over the right side of the thorax. The murmur typically radiates dorsally and less intensely to the left cranial thorax. When related to pulmonary hypertension, a valuable clinical clue is the presence of a loud, tympanic pulmonic component of the second heart sound. Right atrial and ventricular dilatation are responses to haemodynamically significant TR and these findings are useful in assessing the potential significance of TR murmurs. Cardiomegaly can be detected radiographically in small animals, and by echocardiography in all species, though mild enlargement is difficult to discern because of the complex geometry of the right side of the heart. The aetiology of TR can be gauged by considering the species, age, breed and related clinical and laboratory findings. The two-dimensional echocardiogram is very helpful in the differential diagnosis of anatomic lesions (e.g. malformation, thickening and endocarditis). In cases of TR associated with cor pulmonale, an expected finding is dilatation of the main pulmonary artery.

TR can be confirmed by angiography in small animals or by Doppler echocardiography in all species. The TR jet secondary to pulmonic stenosis or pulmonary hypertension will generally be of very high velocity, exceeding 3 m/sec (see Chapter 7).

Therapy for congestive heart failure related to TR involves long-term use of diuretics to prevent excessive sodium and water retention, digitalization and judicious use of angiotensin-converting enzyme inhibitors (usually starting at 10–20% of the daily dosage for left-sided or biventricular heart failure). Combination diuretic therapy may be useful (e.g. furosemide with a thiazide plus spironolactone or triamterene) and malabsorption of cardiac drugs may necessitate parenteral administration of diuretics. Over-diuresis or excessive vasodilator therapy must be avoided to prevent low cardiac output, with syncope, or fatal hypotension. Arrhythmias such as atrial fibrillation should be controlled (Chapter 23). In cases of cor pulmonale, oxygen should be administered and the underlying pulmonary or vascular condition (e.g. heartworm disease) should be treated.

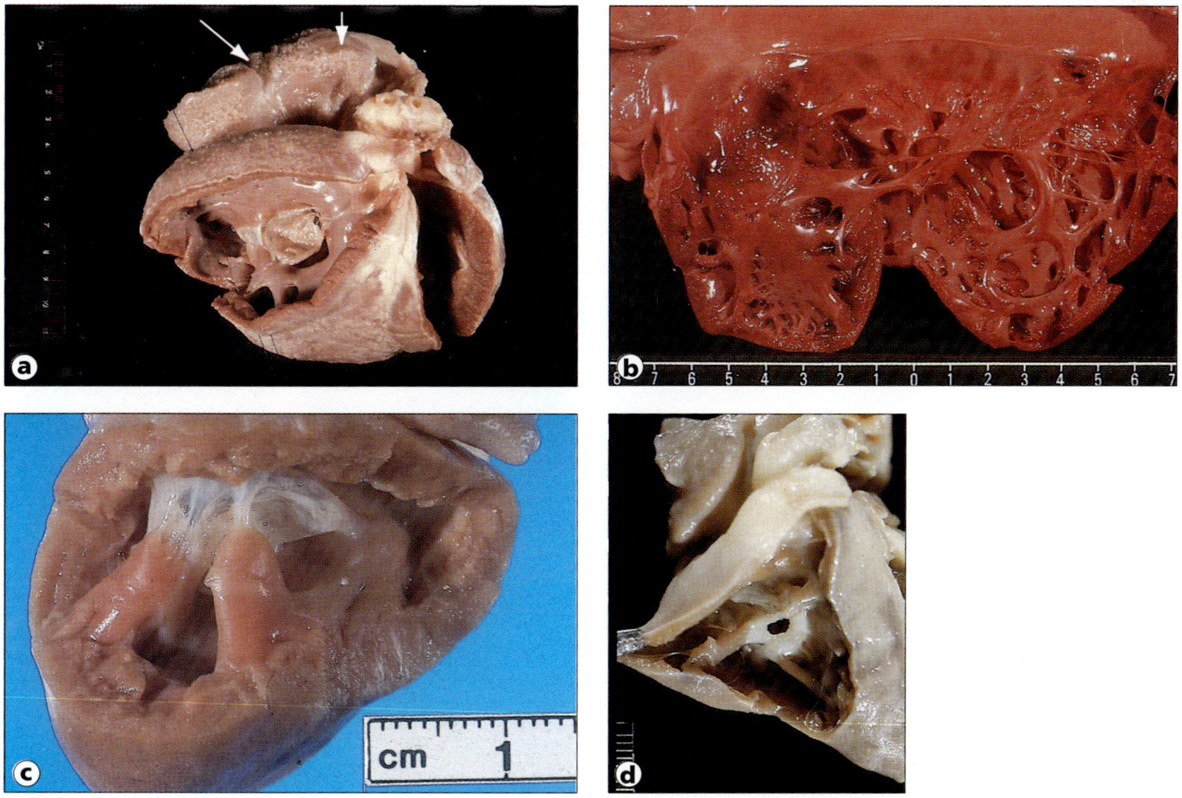

10.1 Tricuspid dysplasia. (**a**) Severe right-sided cardiomegaly in a dog with tricuspid dysplasia. The right auricle (arrows) is severely dilated owing to florid tricuspid regurgitation. The valve is abnormally formed with fused papillary muscles, abnormal leaflets, and some short chordae tendineae. (**b**) Tricuspid valve dysplasia in a 12-month-old German shepherd dog. The right atrium is massively dilated because malformation of the tricuspid valve has caused tricuspid incompetence in early life. (**c**) Tricuspid dysplasia in a Labrador retriever puppy characterized by shortened chordae tendineae and large papillary muscles (courtesy of Dr Matt W. Miller). (**d**) Severe tricuspid valve stenosis and right ventricular hypoplasia in a cat with marked ascites.

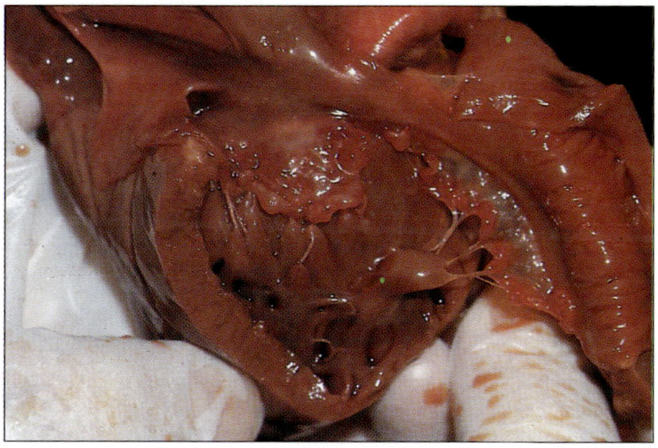

10.2 Endocardiosis of the tricuspid valve in a dog. Both the septal and lateral tricuspid leaflets are characterized by nodular thickening of the valve cusps.

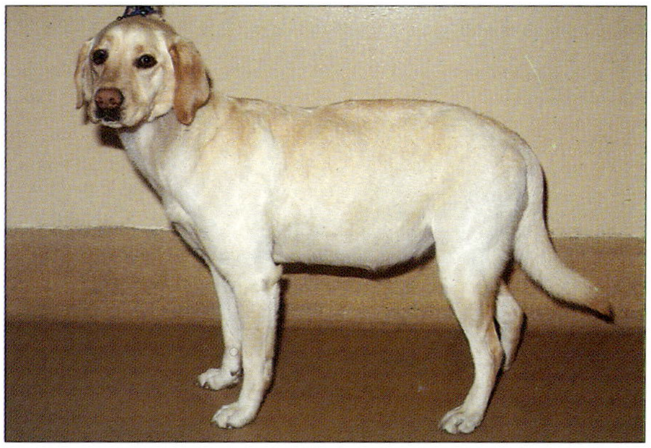

10.3 Ascites in a yellow Labrador retriever dog with tricuspid regurgitation.

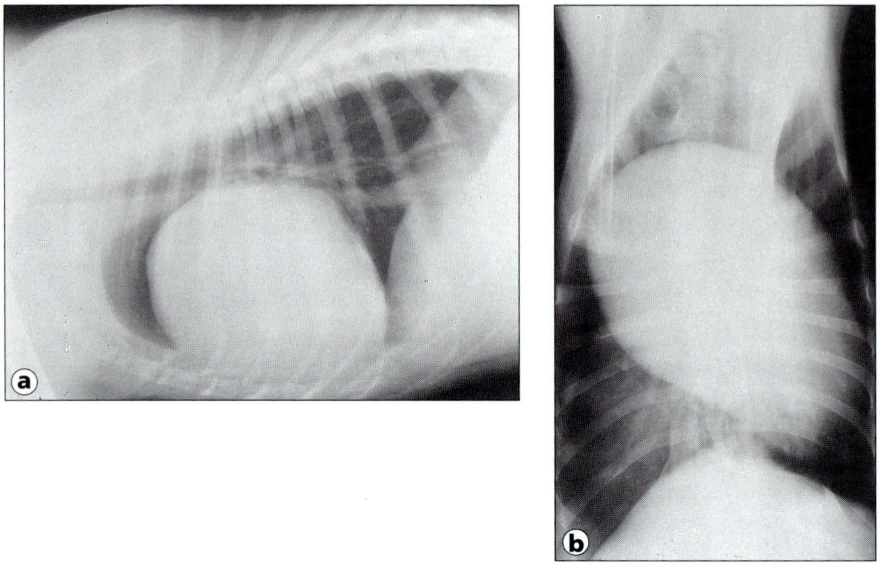

10.4 Radiograph of a dog with tricuspid regurgitation, showing massive right atrial enlargement and right ventricular enlargement. (**a**) The lateral projection demonstrates an absence of any left atrial enlargement, marked elevation of the trachea proximal to the carina, and a cranial bulge attributable to right auricular dilatation. (**b**) The enlarged right side of the heart has caused shifting of the apex to the left on the ventrodorsal view.

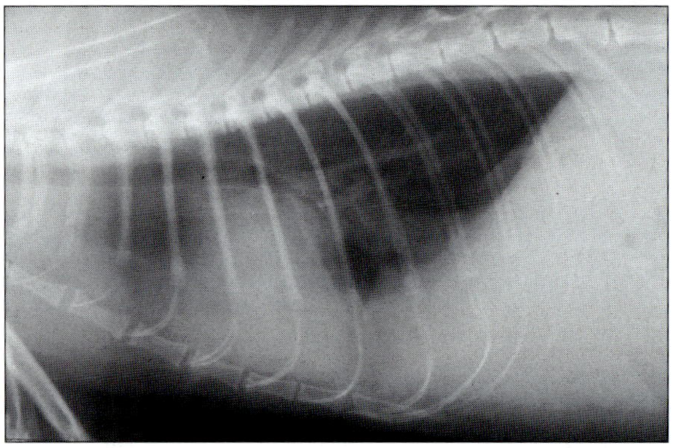

10.5 Thoracic radiograph of a 5-year-old Birman cat with tricuspid dysplasia, showing increased sternal contact, pleural effusion, which partly obliterates the cardiac outline, and a dilated caudal vena cava.

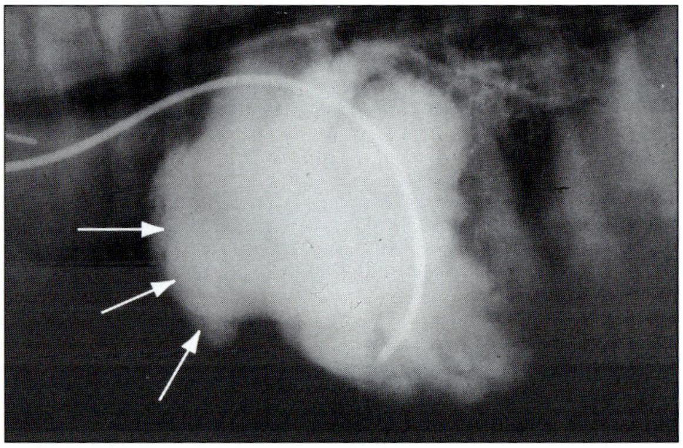

10.6 Angiocardiogram from a dog with tricuspid regurgitation. The contrast medium was injected into the right ventricle and has lead to equal opacification of the right atrium and auricular appendage (arrow).

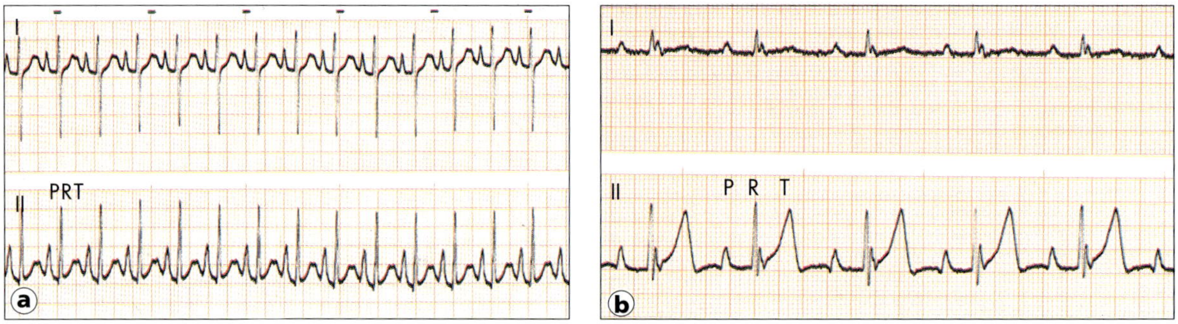

10.7 (**a**) ECG (leads I and II at 25mm/sec) from a 6-month-old boxer with pulmonic stenosis and secondary tricuspid dysplasia, showing a marked S wave in lead I which represents right ventricular hypertrophy, and a very tall and wide P wave, compatible with right atrial enlargement.

(**b**) ECG (leads I and II at 50mm/sec) from a 16-month-old Labrador retriever with tricuspid dysplasia. There is a slightly tall P wave, suggesting right atrial enlargement, but there is also an RSr′ complex intraventricular conduction disturbance that is often seen in this condition.

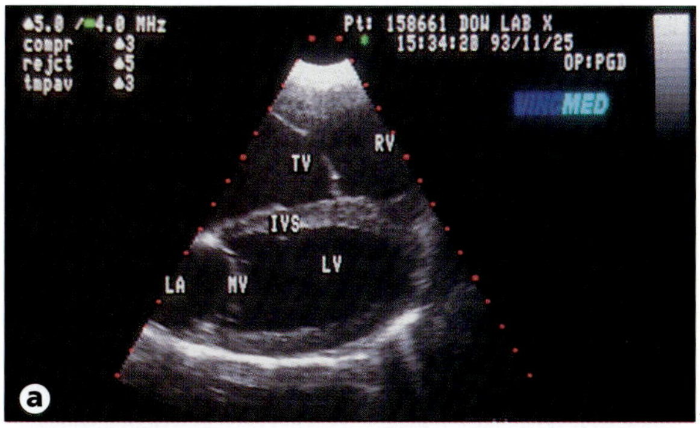

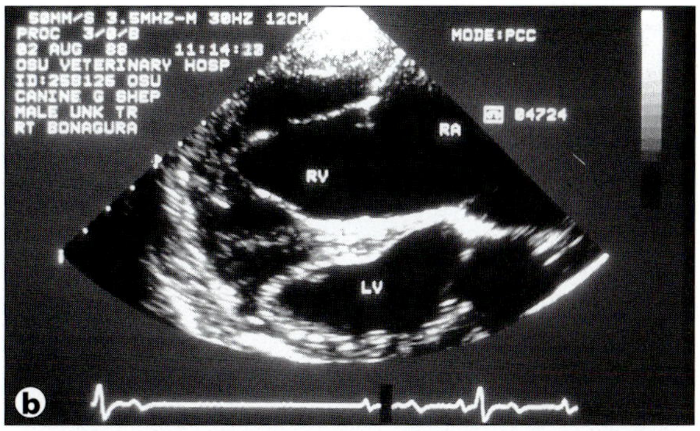

10.8 (**a**) Right paracostal two-dimensional echocardiogram from another Labrador retriever, showing dilatation of the right side of the heart; the position of the tricuspid valve annulus is low in the ventricle (Ebstein's-like anomaly). (**b**) Right paracostal two-dimensional echocardiogram from a German shepherd dog with tricuspid dysplasia. The chordae tendineae are markedly elongated and there is severe right atrial and right ventricular volume overload. The ventricular septum bulges into the left ventricle.

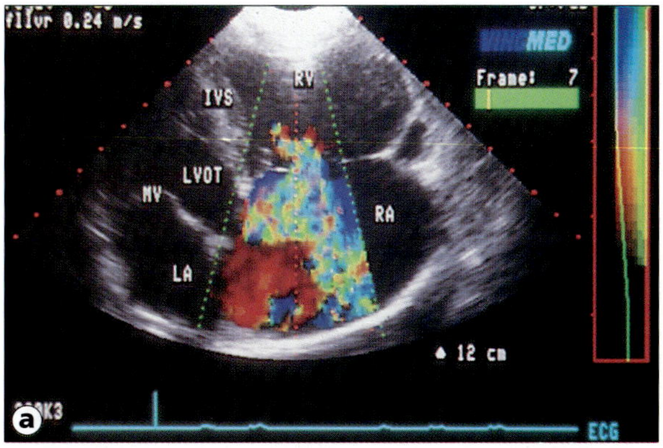

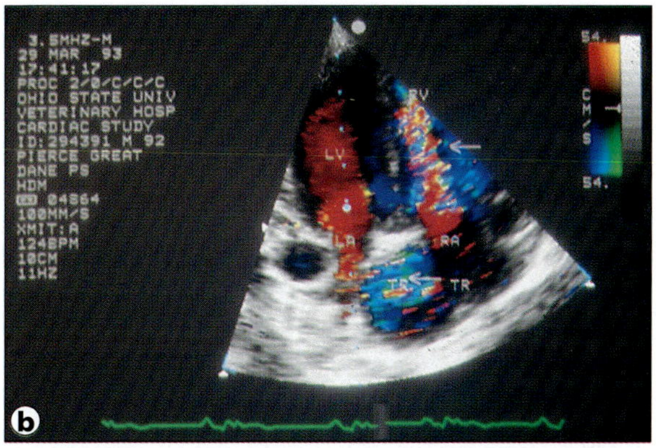

10.9 (**a**) Colour-flow Doppler recording from the dog in **10.8a**, showing massive tricuspid regurgitation with disturbed flow. (**b**) Colour-flow Doppler recording from a dog with tricuspid stenosis due to dysplasia of the valve. The image is a 4-chambered image recorded in early diastole, from the left apex. Normal, non-turbulent inflow is observed in the left ventricular inlet (coded in red), whereas a highly turbulent mosaic of tricuspid stenosis is observed in the right ventricular inlet. The blue flow pattern in the right atrium is a consequence of mapping (and temporal delay in displaying) the tricuspid regurgitant volume at end-systole.

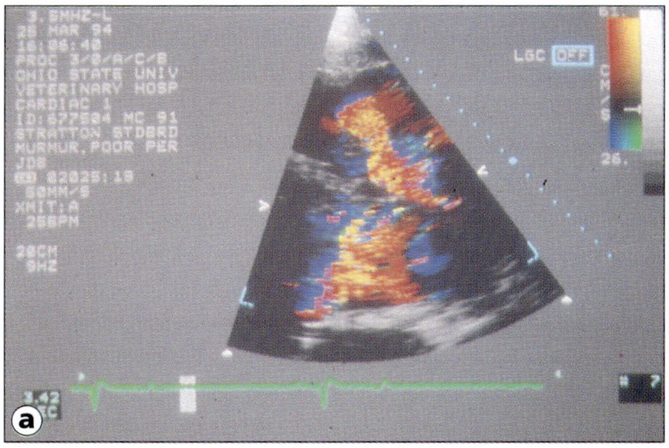

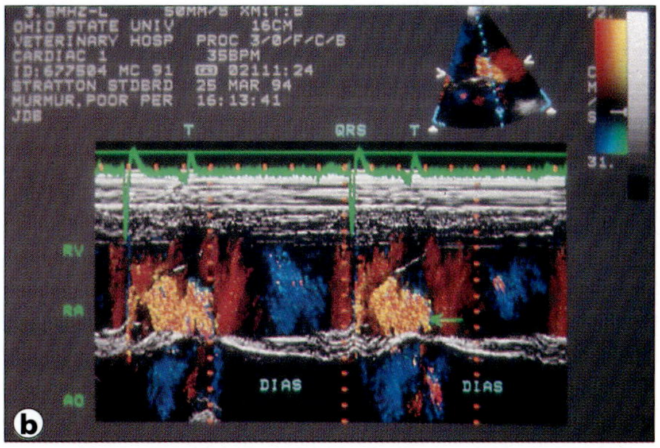

10.10 Colour Doppler studies from a horse with tricuspid regurgitation. (**a**) The tricuspid regurgitant jet is seen in this image taken from the right hemithorax (arrow). The flow at the lower portion of the figure is systolic ejection into the aorta and is normal. (**b**) Colour M-mode demonstrates the method of timing the duration of tricuspid regurgitation. The tricuspid regurgitant jet is the mosaic with yellow added to demonstrate disturbed flow. The blue and red flow patterns are normal. The aortic root is below the right atrium in this image.

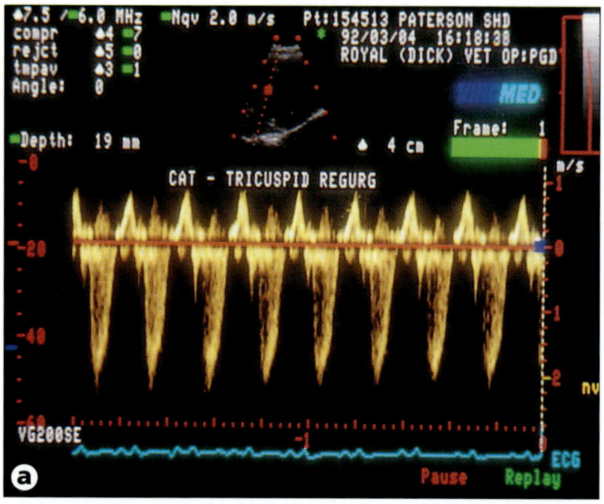

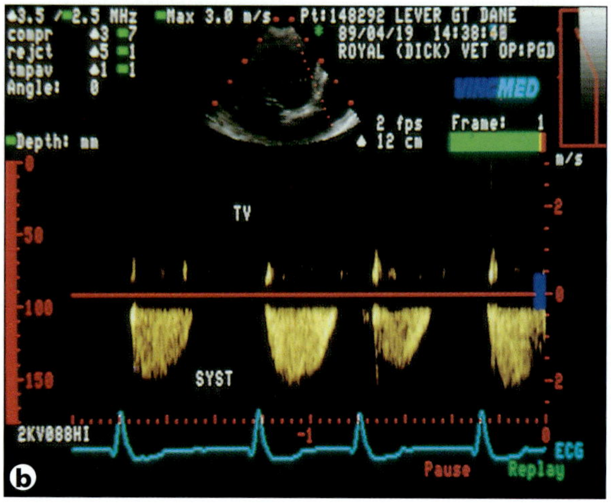

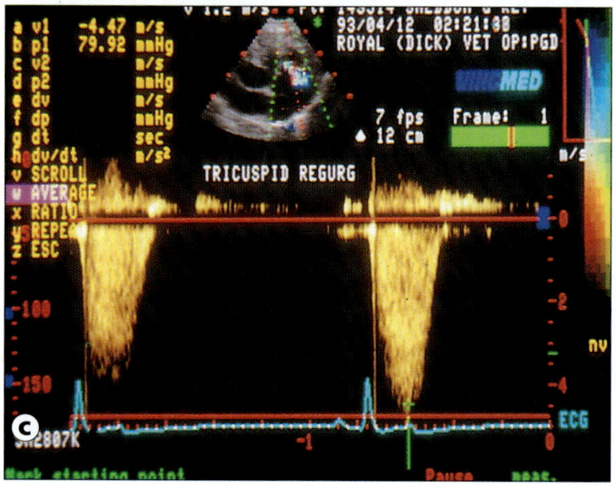

10.11 (**a**) HPRF pulsed-wave spectral Doppler recording from the tricuspid valve of a domestic cat with tricuspid regurgitation associated with ventricular septal defect. The moderate maximum velocity of flow (2.2 m/sec) suggests an absence of elevated right ventricular systolic pressure. (**b**) Continuous-wave spectral Doppler recording from a dog with dilated cardiomyopathy, showing tricuspid regurgitation and atrial fibrillation. The variable flow velocity is related to differences in developed pressure associated with dysrhythmia. (**c**) HPRF pulsed-wave spectral Doppler recording from a golden retriever with tricuspid regurgitation secondary to pulmonic stenosis. The velocity of regurgitant flow (4.47 m/sec) is higher than normal, owing to elevated right ventricular systolic pressure.

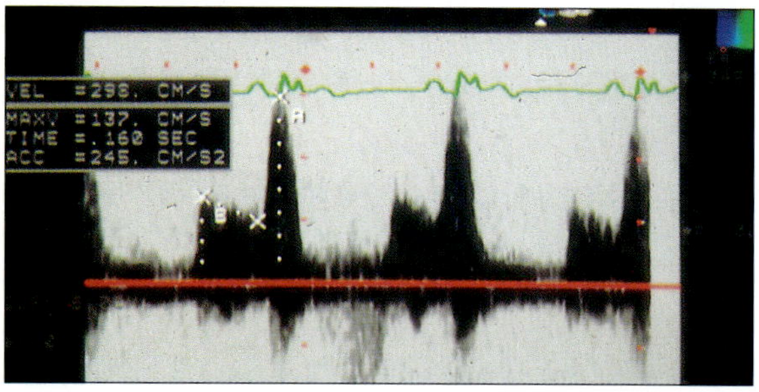

10.12 Continuous-wave spectral Doppler recording from a dog with tricuspid stenosis. Early diastolic filling is prolonged leading to a very flat E–F slope. The atrial contribution to filling (the A wave) has markedly increased velocity, approaching 3 m/sec.

11.

Aortic Stenosis

Aortic stenosis (AS) in animals is almost always related to a congenital malformation. Severe vegetative bacterial endocarditis may cause an acquired stenosis of the aortic valve, though this is uncommon. While malformation of the valve leaflets or supravalvular aorta may be observed, the vast majority of lesions occur in the subvalvular region (subvalvular or subaortic stenosis: SAS). SAS is mainly observed in dogs and pigs; cats are rarely affected, and the condition is insignificance in ruminant or equine practice. Many canine breeds are predisposed to AS, notably the golden retriever, Newfoundland, German shepherd, boxer, Rottweiler and English bull terrier. AS is heritable in most breeds, though the mode of transmission is incompletely understood.

The functional and clinical consequences of SAS vary with the severity of obstruction. Small incomplete subaortic ridges cause minor obstructions, trivial pressure gradients, soft heart murmurs and no overt hypertrophy or clinical signs. However, minor lesions can potentially be propagated in breeding animals. Complete subaortic rings may be discrete, wide or tunnel-like. These cause significant obstructions to flow and induce concentric left ventricular hypertrophy. Subaortic obstructions create a moderate-to-severe systolic pressure gradient between ventricle and aorta (see also Chapter 8). Clinical consequences include a high-velocity flow stream (or jet) in the ventricular outlet and ascending aorta, flow disturbances (turbulence) and post-stenotic dilation of the ascending aorta. The subaortic ridge may envelop the base of the aortic valve, or high-velocity jets may thicken the valve leaflets, a change that predisposes some dogs to mild-to-moderate aortic regurgitation. The hypertrophic left ventricle is poorly perfused through the sclerotic intramyocardial coronary arteries. Abnormal coronary perfusion and myocardial ischaemia have been documented. Ischaemia undoubtedly plays a role in the production of myocardial fibrosis (a change that may be evident at necropsy), and in the generation of ventricular arrhythmias which are often observed clinically.

The clinical features of SAS are summarized in Appendix A3, *Congenital Heart Disease in Animals*. Mildly affected animals are clinically normal, with the exception of a soft, left-sided, localized, systolic murmur. The murmur becomes louder and longer, and it peaks later, with increasing severity of obstruction (and often radiates loudly into the right hemithorax). With severe obstruction, signs of low cardiac output may include exercise intolerance or syncope. Sudden death is common in severe SAS, probably related to ventricular tachycardia or fibrillation. Left-sided cardiac failure can be seen, particularly if there is concurrent MR, myocardial failure, or atrial fibrillation. The ECG is variable but may demonstrate left ventricular hypertrophy, ventricular premature beats, or S–T depression. Thoracic radiographs are often unremarkable in mild cases but, with moderate-to-severe stenosis, elongation of the heart and post-stenotic dilation of the aorta may be seen. Echocardiography can demonstrate most (but not all) obstructions. Left ventricular hypertrophy and hyperechoic subendocardial areas of fibrosis are observed in severe cases.

The diagnosis is confirmed by cardiac catheterization, or preferably by Doppler studies. Either technique can be used to derive the pressure gradient across the stenosis (see Chapters 6 and 8). The gradient is the most useful indicator of the severity of disease, especially when considered with other findings such as clinical signs, concurrent mitral lesions, dysrhythmias and myocardial fibrosis. Though the prognosis is guarded in severe cases (e.g. Doppler gradients > 100–125 mmHg), many mildly affected dogs live normal lives. The authors have documented reduction of ventricular arrhythmias and improvement of exercise-related S–T segment changes with beta blockade (see Appendices), though the effect of beta-adrenergic or calcium-channel blockers on survival has not been critically evaluated. Balloon catheter dilation can be carried out at specialist centres, and this usually reduces the gradient, at least initially. Should congestive heart failure occur, the dosage of any beta blocker should be diminished (to prevent excessive bradycardia) and alternative medical management instituted (Chapter 3). Arteriolar dilators are relatively contraindicated in outlet obstruction, but angiotensin-converting enzyme inhibitors may be used at very low dosages, provided arterial blood pressure is monitored to prevent hypertension. Bacterial endocarditis of the aortic valve is a risk in any dog with SAS, and antibiotic prophylaxis should be undertaken when appropriate.

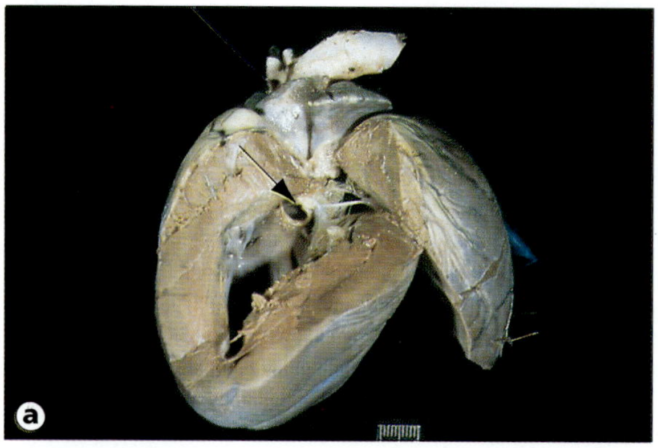

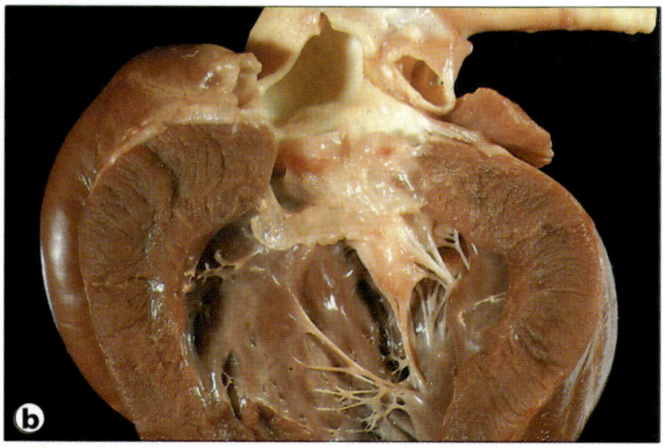

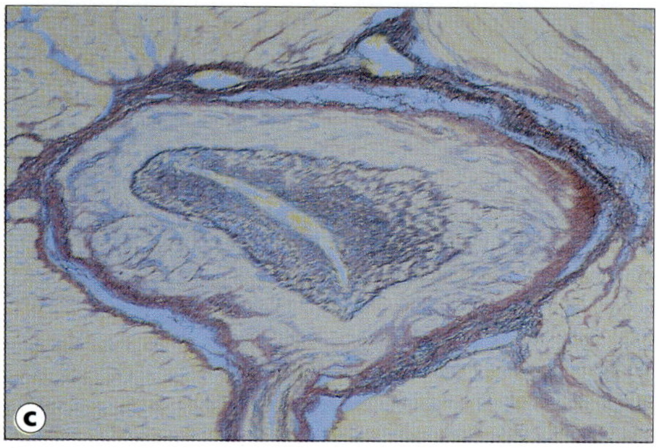

11.1 Pathology of congenital canine subaortic stenosis. **(a)** Opened left ventricular cavity demonstrates the subaortic ring (arrow) and severe left ventricular concentric hypertrophy. Note the proximity of the subaortic membrane to the anterior (i.e. septal or cranioventral) mitral leaflet. **(b)** Heart from another dog, cut to demonstrate the left ventricular outlet and the extent of the subaortic ridge which is very wide and is complete in this case. **(c)** Obstruction of ventricular outlow leads to sclerosis of intramural coronary arteries as a result of intimal fibroelastic thickening. This is a reaction to increased systolic transmural tension which is seen frequently in aortic stenosis (EVG stain).

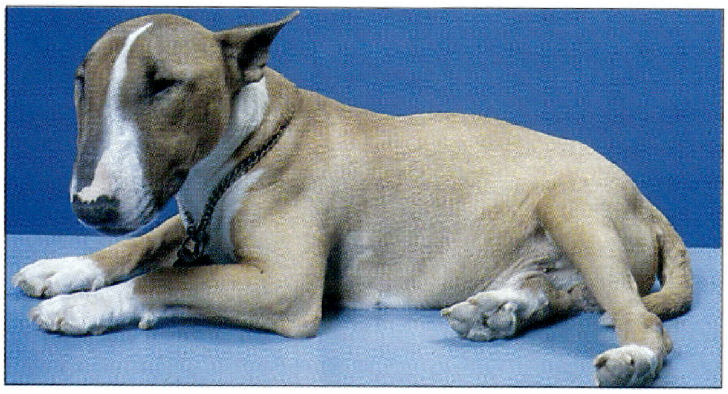

11.2 Dog (from **11.1a**) with severe subaortic stenosis. The dog was affected by exertional syncope and eventually developed dyspnoea owing to left-sided congestive heart failure.

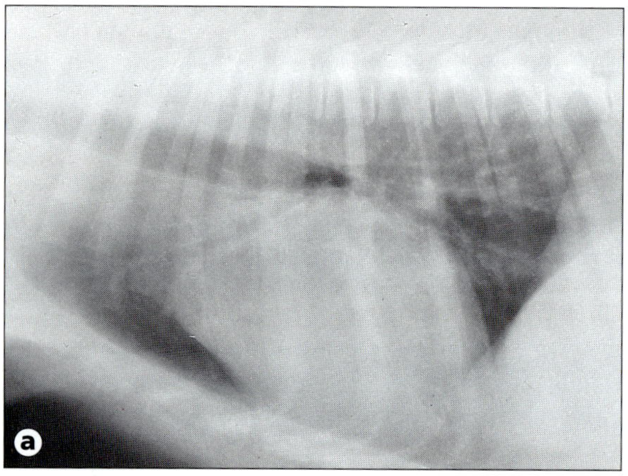

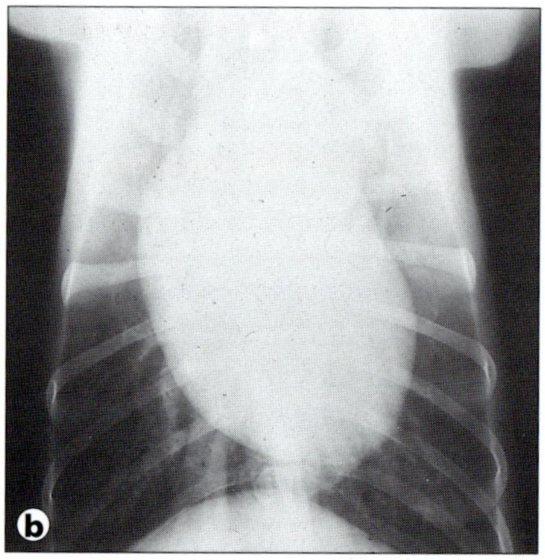

11.3 a and **b** Radiographs from two dogs with subaortic stenosis. In each case, the ascending aorta has been dilated due to post-stenotic turbulence leading to a widening of the cranial mediastinum.

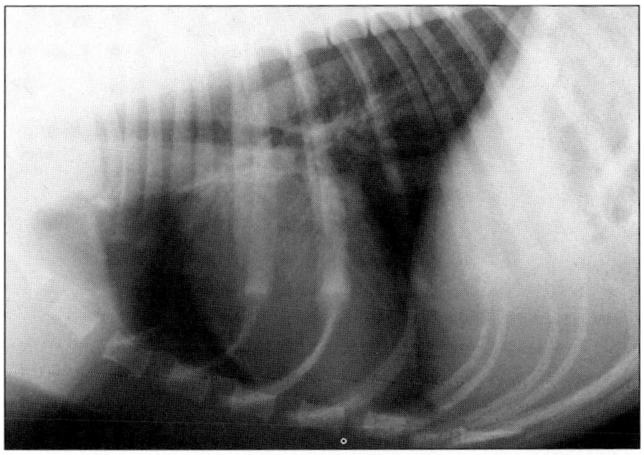

11.4 Lateral radiograph of a boxer with moderate aortic stenosis. Note the lack of identifiable cardiac enlargement or vascular changes – most enlargement will be concentric left ventricular hypertrophy, to which radiographs are relatively insensitive.

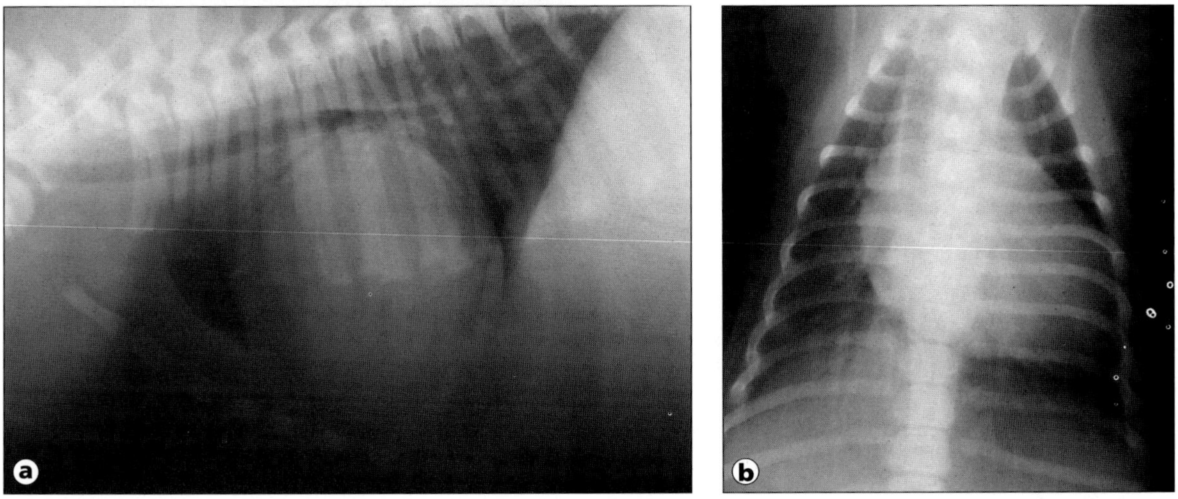

11.5 a and **b** Radiographs of a Labrador retriever puppy with aortic stenosis and mitral regurgitation, showing a very tall cardiac outline on the lateral film with straightening of the caudal border of the heart and loss of caudal waist, all indicating left atrial enlargement. The displacement of the apex to the left on the dorsoventral view is probably of no significance. On both views there is marked pulmonary vascular congestion and mild oedema, a pattern not usually seen with solitary aortic stenosis, but probably due to the associated mitral regurgitation in this case.

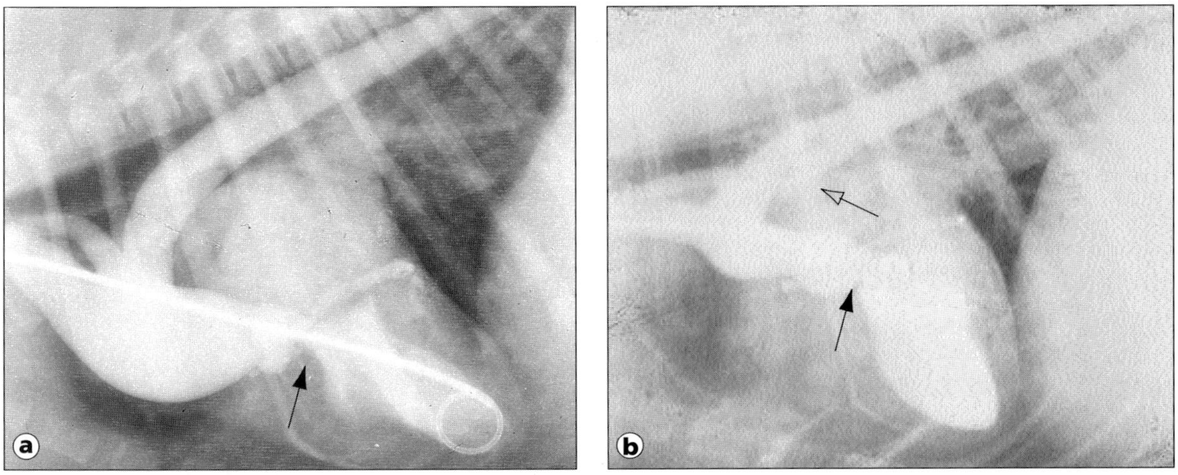

11.6 Angiocardiograms from two dogs with subaortic stenosis. (**a**) Left ventricular injection demonstrating a relatively long segment of subvalvular stenosis (arrow) and severe post-stenotic dilatation of the ascending aorta. (**b**) Discrete subvalvular stenosis (solid arrow). There is also opacification of a ductus arteriosus that had previously been ligated (open arrow).

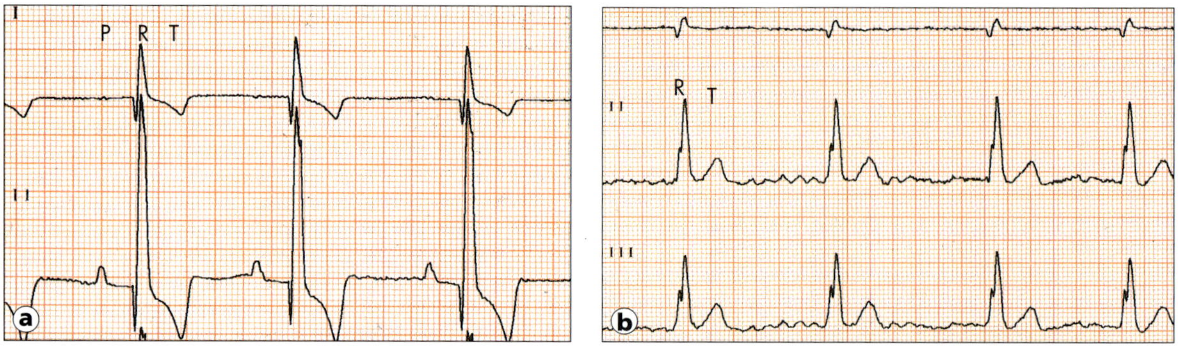

11.7 Electrocardiograms from dogs with subaortic stenosis. (**a**) ECG compatible with ventricular hypertrophy, demonstrating a normal frontal axis, increased amplitude, QRS complexes, minor intraventricular conduction disturbance (notched R waves), and secondary ST-segment changes. (50mm/sec; 10 mm/mV.) (**b**) A 6-lead ECG demonstrating atrial fibrillation and left ventricular conduction disturbance compatible with left bundle branch block (50 mm/sec; 10 mm/mV).

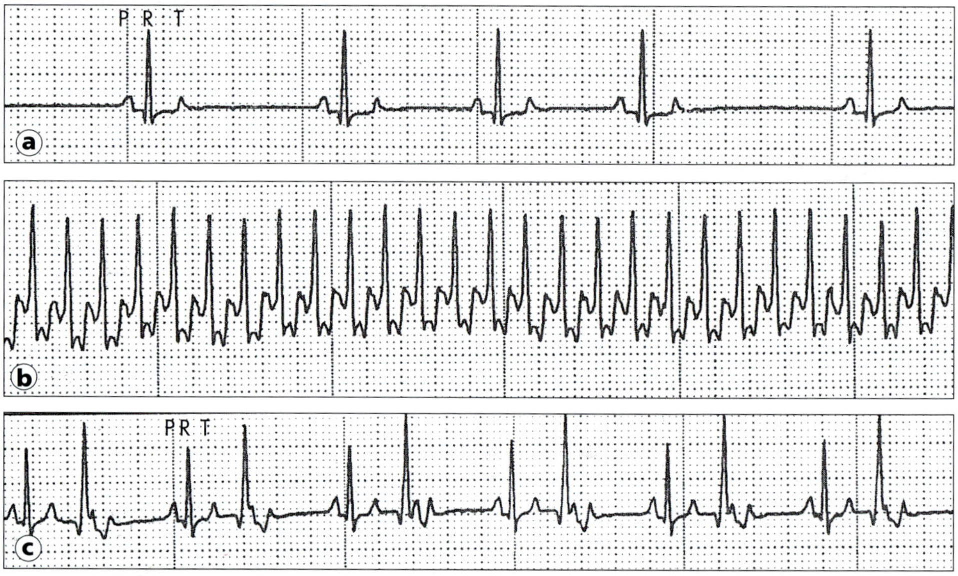

11.8 Ambulatory, Holter (tape recorded) ECGs obtained from a dog with severe subaortic stenosis. (**a**) Sinus arrhythmia with minimal ST-segment depression while standing. (**b**) Marked sinus tachycardia with severe ST-segment depression during exercise. These findings suggest significant subendocardial ischaemia and myocardial oxygen imbalance. (**c**) Bigeminal ventricular premature beats.

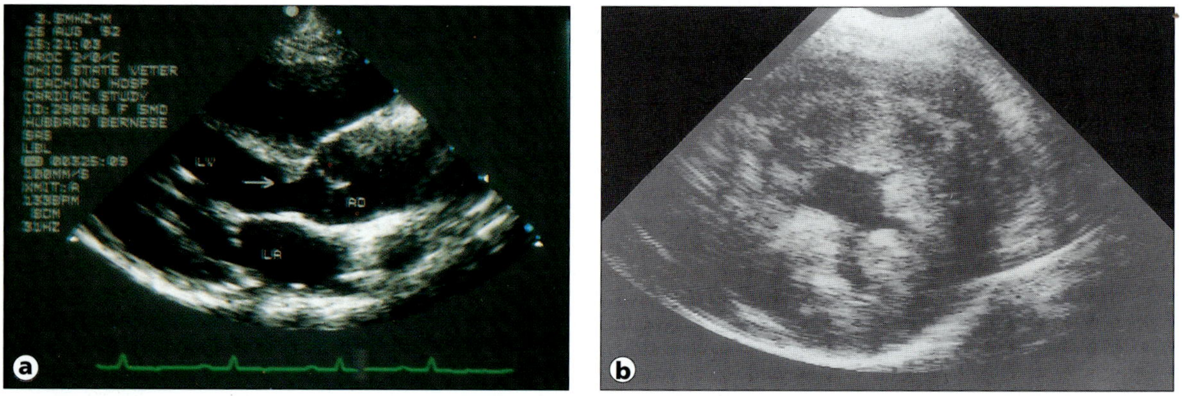

11.9 (**a**) Echocardiogram demonstrating a well-defined subaortic ridge (arrow) in a dog with subaortic stenosis. There is also obvious post-stenotic dilatation of the aorta (courtesy of Dr Linda B. Lehmkuhl). (**b**) Short-axis image of the left ventricle from a dog with subaortic stenosis demonstrating marked increase in echogenicity along the subendocardium. This finding is usually related to endocardial fibrosis which is a consequence of poor coronary perfusion of the thickened ventricle and areas of myocardial ischaemia and microinfarction or ischaemia-induced fibrosis.

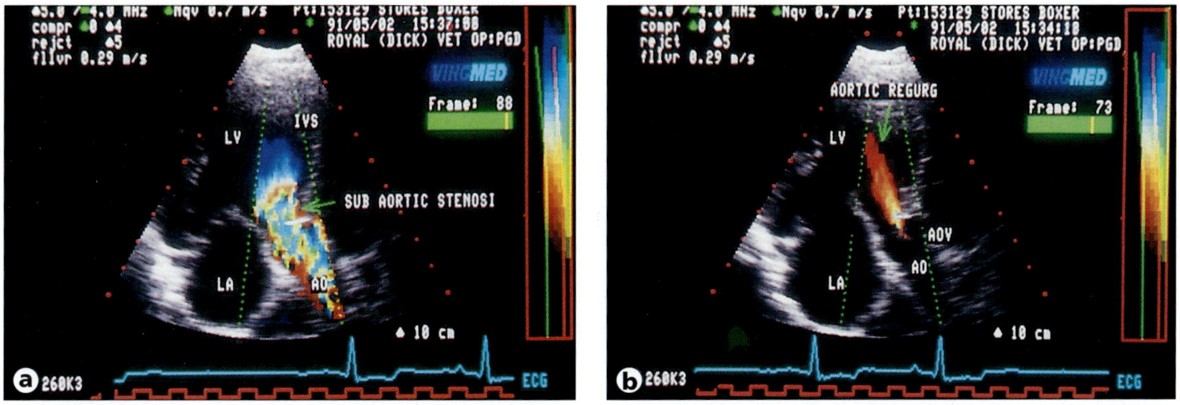

11.10 (**a**) Colour-flow Doppler recording from a boxer with subaortic stenosis. The obviously disturbed flow starts below the valve, at the stenosis, during systole. (**b**) Colour-flow Doppler recording from the same dog as in **a**, showing a jet of aortic regurgitation in diastole. Aortic regurgitation is common in subaortic stenosis.

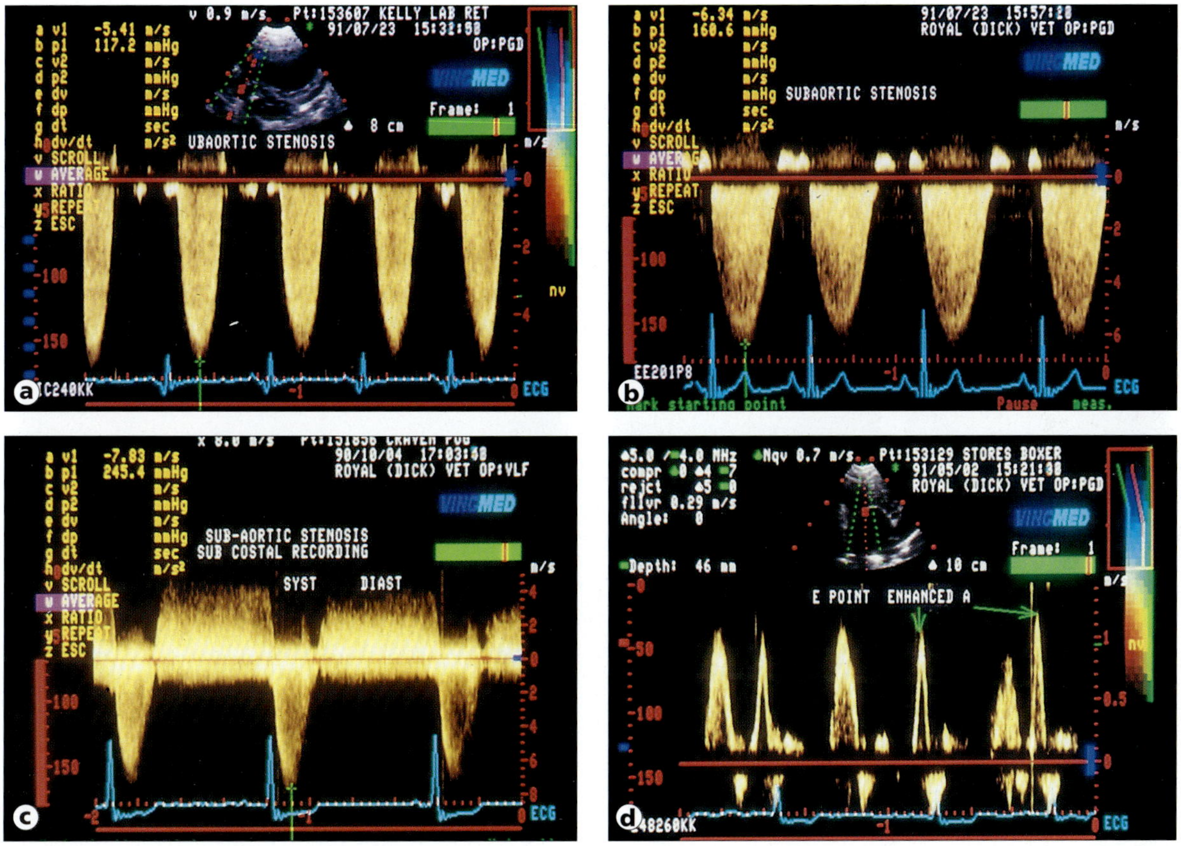

11.11 (**a**) HPRF pulsed-wave spectral Doppler recording from the dog in **11.5**, showing high-velocity disturbed flow, at 5.41 m/sec. This velocity represents a pressure gradient of approximately 117 mmHg (by the Bernoulli equation), indicating severe stenosis. (**b**) Continuous-wave spectral Doppler recording from the dog in **11.5** and **11.11**(**a**), showing mitral regurgitation of higher-than-normal velocity (6.34 m/sec), owing to elevated left ventricular systolic pressure. This recording also demonstrates that mitral regurgitation is of much longer duration than the aortic flow, accounting for a prolonged (pansystolic) murmur. (**c**) Continuous-wave spectral Doppler recording from a pug with subaortic stenosis, showing very high velocity aortic outflow (7.83 m/sec), together with aortic regurgitation (towards the transducer) in diastole. (**d**) Pulsed-wave spectral Doppler recording from the mitral valve of the boxer in **11.10**, with aortic stenosis. The A wave, representing ventricular inflow due to atrial contraction, is at an enhanced velocity (1 m/sec) owing to loss of compliance in the hypertrophied left ventricle.

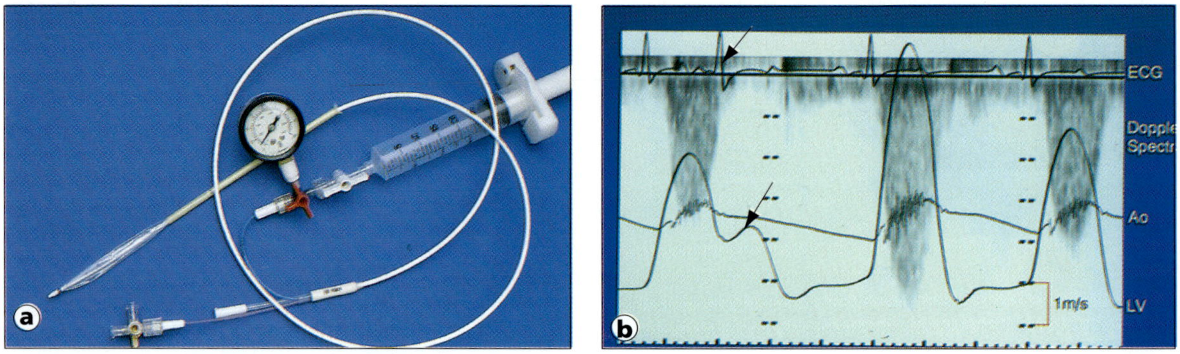

11.12 (**a**) A balloon catheter and inflation syringe with attached pressure manometer used to dilate a subaortic or valvular stenosis via cardiac catheterization. (**b**) Simultaneous pressure and Doppler recordings from a dog with subaortic stenosis. The pressure gradient (area between the left ventricular and aortic pressure curves in systole) varies owing to the presence of a ventricular premature beat (arrow) and post-extrasystolic potentiation. Note that the peak Doppler velocity varies directly with the gradient.

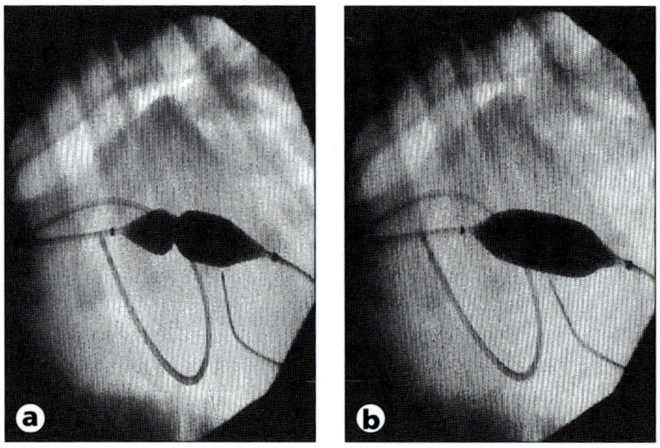

11.13 a and **b** Balloon catheter dilatation of a subaortic stenosis in a dog. (**a**) Initial inflation demonstrating the 'waist' of the stenosis. (**b**) Complete inflation of the balloon is evident and the waist is no longer present.

12. Aortic Regurgitation

Aortic regurgitation (AR, or aortic insufficiency) refers to incompetence of the aortic valve. This results in retrograde diastolic flow from the aorta into the left ventricle, increased left ventricular diastolic volume and pressure, and decreased aortic diastolic pressure. These haemodynamic effects are related to both the speed of onset and the magnitude of AR. The regurgitant volume in turn depends on the size of the regurgitant orifice (the lesion severity), the pressure difference between the aorta and left ventricle, and the duration of diastole. Trivial anatomic lesions, leading to mild AR, are well-tolerated both haemodynamically and clinically. Large regurgitant volumes predispose to significant ventricular volume overload, eccentric ventricular hypertrophy and eventually to left-sided congestive heart failure. Additionally, decreased aortic diastolic pressure may compromise coronary perfusion.

Aortic regurgitation in animals has three primary causes: congenital malformations, bacterial endocarditis and fibrous degeneration. Congenital subvalvular or valvular aortic stenosis is often associated with varying degrees of AR, and the condition can become more severe if endocarditis or progressive scarring develops, or as a result of balloon catheter dilatation of the stenosis. These disorders are most common in dogs, but congenital fenestrations of the aortic valve leaflets in horses have been reported. Ventricular septal defects in all species can be associated with AR because impaired support of the aortic root may allow an aortic leaflet to prolapse into the septal defect. Bacterial endocarditis may also injure the aortic valve, leading to AR (see Chapter 14). Degenerative linear thickening or beading of the aortic valve is a common finding in horses over 10 years of age, and this often leads to mild incompetence; infrequently, the AR becomes moderate-to-severe or is associated with concurrent mitral regurgitation. Affected horses may develop congestive heart failure, most notably when atrial fibrillation supervenes. AR has also been detected by Doppler echocardiography in old dogs and cats, though the lesion responsible is undetermined.

Clinical consequences of AR include a high-velocity regurgitant jet in the left ventricular outlet, and left ventricular eccentric hypertrophy. This flow disturbance is responsible for the holodiastolic murmur (with radiation to the right hemithorax) that is typical of AR, and which is best heard over the aortic valve area. The murmur in horses is remarkably variable, ranging from a soft, blowing decrescendo sound to a musical, cooing-dove, buzzing or vibratory event. The long duration of the typical murmur distinguishes this from a normal, brief, early diastolic murmur of ventricular filling. The cause of aortic regurgitation is best determined by combining clinical information with two-dimensional echocardiography.

Definitive documentation of the audible AR, and detection of subclinical regurgitation, can be made by angiocardiography (in small animals) or through Doppler echocardiography. Diastolic fluttering of the aortic valve, mitral valve or ventricular septum may be observed in individual cases with M-mode echocardiography. This vibration of adjacent structures is a result of the high-velocity jet.

The ECG and thoracic radiographs may demonstrate left ventricular hypertrophy in moderate-to-severe cases of volume overload. Serial radiographs or echocardiograms can be used to track the progression of disease. Abnormal coronary perfusion with myocardial ischaemia may precipitate ST–T segment changes in the ECG. Severe aortic regurgitation causes markedly elevated left ventricular end-diastolic pressure – an echocardiographic marker for this is premature closure of the mitral valve (before the QRS complex). Other consequences can include elevated left atrial pressure and pulmonary oedema.

Therapy for aortic regurgitation depends on the cause and severity of disease. The condition is rarely a serious issue in horses, as most will have passed their days of vigorous performance: mild AR is well tolerated and is not a contraindication to riding. In severe cases complicated by congestive heart failure, medical management is instituted with digitalis and diuretics (see Chapter 3). Arteriolar dilators are relatively contraindicated, as further lowering of aortic diastolic pressure can compromise coronary perfusion; however, with regular monitoring of blood pressure, angiotensin-converting enzyme inhibitors may be used at very low dosages. When AR is caused by bacterial endocarditis, appropriate antibiotic therapy should be considered, as discussed in Chapter 14.

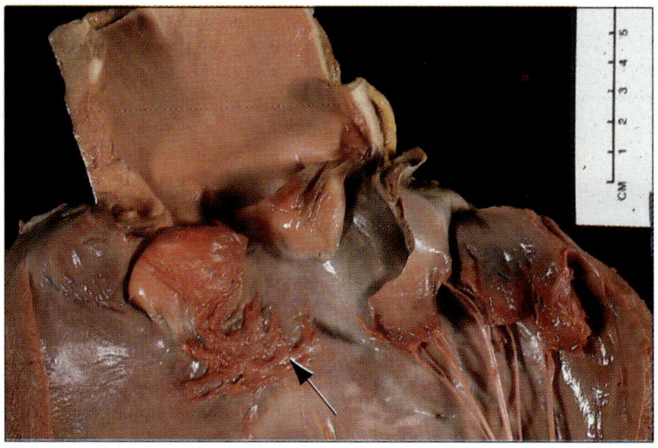

12.1 Aortic valve from a horse with chronic, degenerative aortic valve disease. Linear thickening of the valve is evident and a large jet lesion (arrow) can be observed in the segment of the left ventricular outflow tract that is shown.

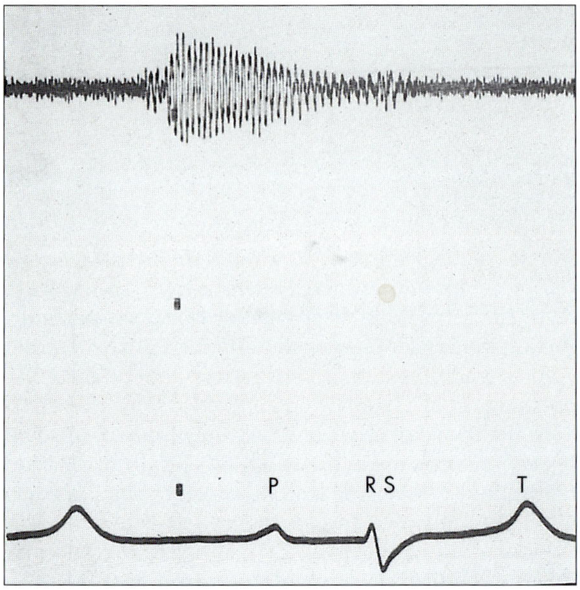

12.2 Typical decrescendo diastolic murmur of aortic regurgitation is demonstrated in this phonocardiogram (see also Chapter 3).

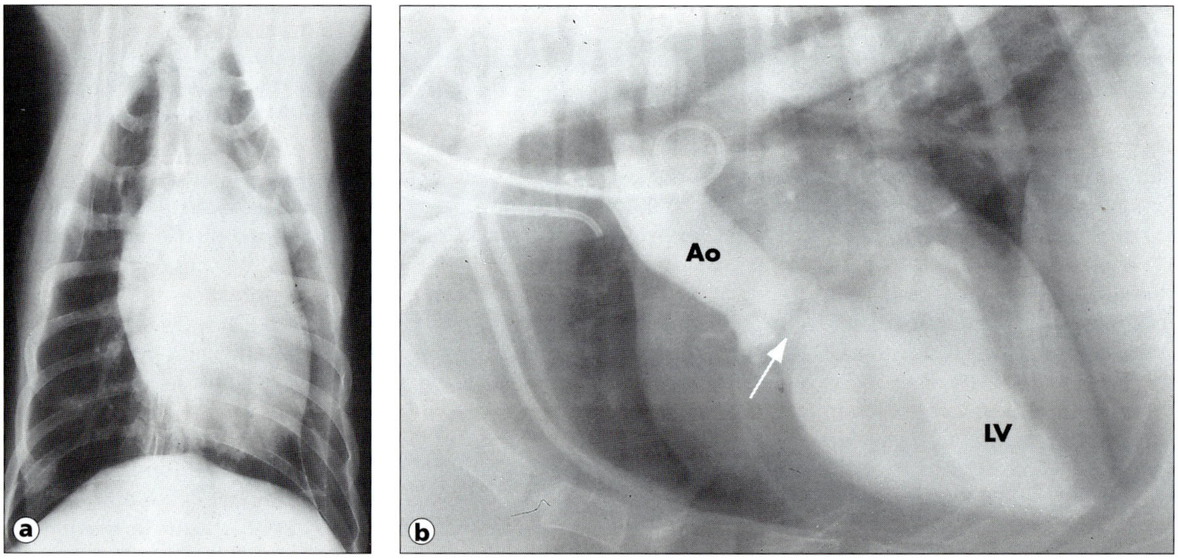

12.3 (**a**) Ventrodorsal radiograph showing left ventricular dilatation in a dog with aortic insufficiency secondary to bacterial endocarditis. (**b**) Angiogram obtained from a dog with congenital subaortic stenosis and secondary bacterial endocarditis of the aortic valve. After injection of contrast medium into the ascending aorta (Ao), the medium regurgitates into the left ventricle (LV) – which has hypertrophy of the papillary muscles. The aortic valve is very irregular owing to the vegetation (arrow).

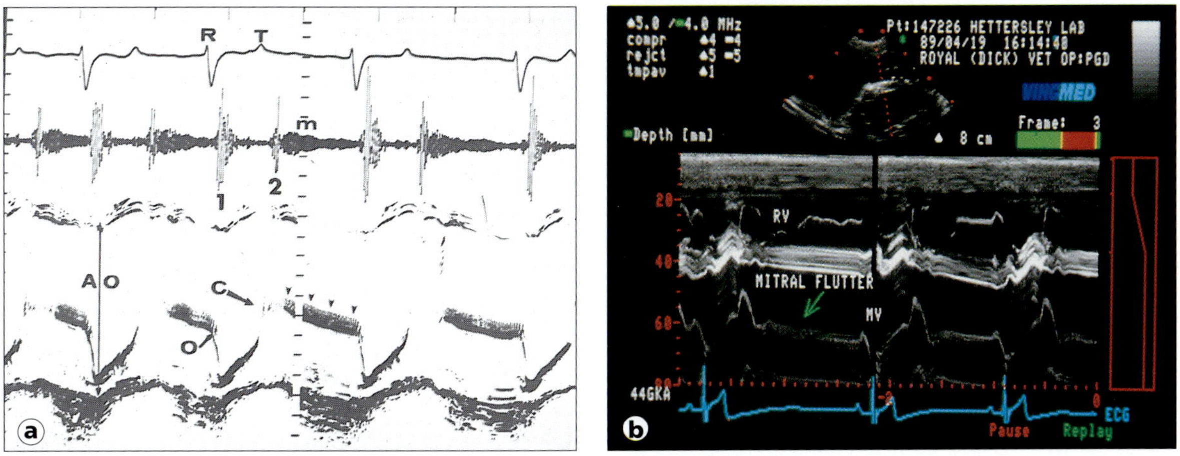

12.4 (**a**) M-mode echocardiogram of the aortic root and aortic valve and phonocardiogram from a horse with aortic insufficiency. A diastolic murmur (m) is evident and coincides with high-frequency vibrations on the imaged aortic valve leaflet. (**b**) M-mode echocardiogram from the mitral valve of a Labrador retriever with pulmonic stenosis, showing diastolic fluttering of the anterior mitral valve leaflet when struck by the jet of incidental aortic regurgitation. There is also right ventricular enlargement, and paradoxical septal motion, due to right ventricular overload.

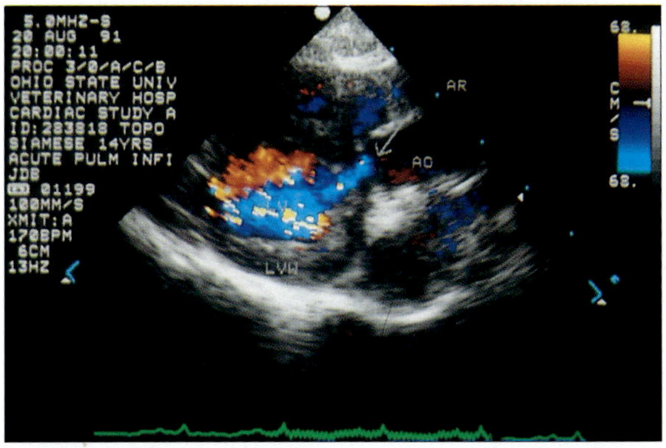

12.5 Colour-flow Doppler echocardiogram of aortic regurgitation (blue jet) in a cat receiving immunosuppressive therapy with suspected acute bacterial endocarditis of the aortic valve.

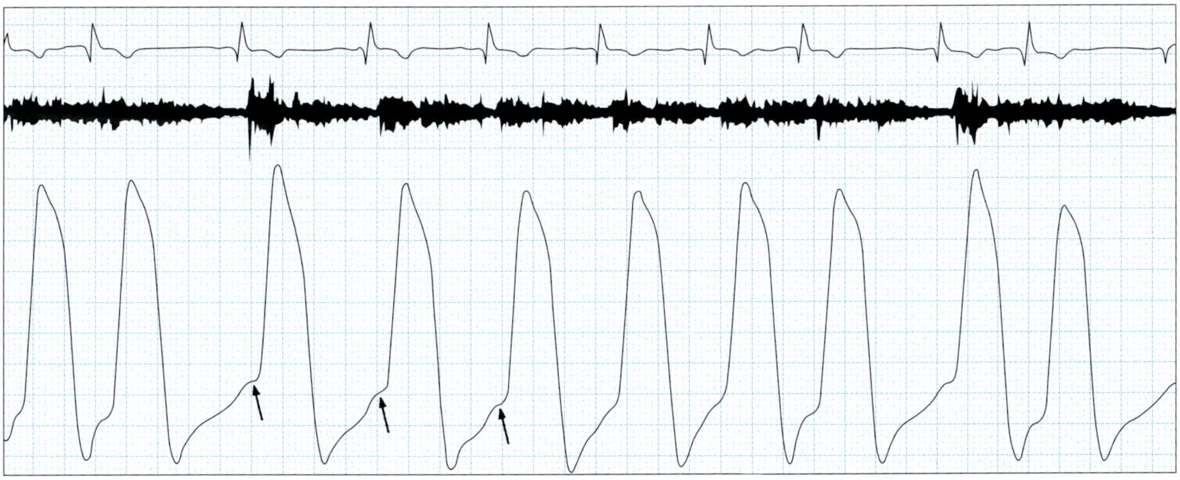

12.6 Simultaneous recording of ECG, phonocardiogram and left ventricular pressure, showing elevated left ventricular diastolic pressure and diastolic murmur of aortic insufficiency in a dog with bacterial endocarditis related to subaortic stenosis. The end-diastolic pressure (arrows) is approximately 40 mmHg. A systolic murmur is also recorded on the phonocardiogram.

13. Pulmonic Stenosis

Pulmonic stenosis (PS) is a congenital valve malformation characterized by a variety of morphologic lesions, which may include combinations of: hypoplasia of the valve, thickening of the valve leaflets, incomplete commissural separation of the leaflets and asymmetric valve leaflets. Infrequently, supravalvular stenosis is observed, but dysplastic pulmonary valves will often be associated with marked fibrous thickening at the base of the valve. Infundibular or valvular PS is a component of the tetralogy of Fallot which is discussed in Chapter 15.

The pathophysiology of PS and its effects on the right side of the heart are very similar to those previously described for the left side of the heart with subaortic stenosis (see Chapter 11). In this case, the hypertrophy involves the right ventricle, and post-stenotic dilatation is found in the main pulmonary artery. Infundibular muscular hypertrophy is of clinical significance as it adds a second level of dynamic obstruction that must be addressed by the cardiologist before selecting balloon catheter dilatation or surgery for treatment. Tricuspid valve malfunction often develops in severe PS, a consequence of concurrent malformation or hypertrophy of the papillary muscles (see Chapter 10).

This condition is found most frequently in certain breeds of dog, particularly beagles, boxers, chihuahuas, English bulldogs, schnauzers and all forms of terriers. It is clearly heritable in most of these breeds, probably as a polygenic trait. PS is encountered rarely in cats and foals. Signs of PS are variable and are summarized in Appendix A3, *Congenital Heart Disease in Animals*. In mild obstruction, dogs can be clinically normal, with only a left-sided systolic murmur to indicate the problem. Severe cases manifest exercise intolerance, syncope and often right-sided cardiac failure. The latter is particularly likely if there is concurrent tricuspid regurgitation, when abnormal jugular pulses or distension may be observed.

The murmur of PS is typically harsh and 'ejection' in character, usually best heard well forward (over the pulmonic valve), on the left side of the thorax. In virtually all cases, the murmur radiates dorsally to the thoracic wall. The ECG shows right ventricular hypertrophy in most cases and P-wave changes of right atrial enlargement may be observed. Thoracic radiographs show varying degrees of right ventricular enlargement; post-stenotic dilatation of the pulmonary artery can sometimes be seen, and the lungs often appear underperfused. Echocardiography demonstrates right ventricular hypertrophy and post-stenotic dilatation of the main pulmonary artery. The right atrium is often prominent. The stenotic lesion is not always well-demarcated, as clear imaging of the pulmonic valve can be difficult. Often the valve appears thick, and the systolic excursion is limited. Discrete subvalvular obstruction may also be noted, as well as generalized infundibular hypertrophy. As the disease progresses, dilatation of the right side of the heart becomes evident. Confirmation of the diagnosis requires either cardiac catheterization or Doppler echocardiography (see Chapters 6 and 7). Either technique permits measurement of the pressure gradient, which is useful in assessing prognosis.

The natural history of severe PS (non-anesthetized Doppler gradient > 100–125 mmHg) is that of sudden death or heart failure. Severe cases of PS can be partially relieved by balloon valvuloplasty or by surgery in many dogs. There are numerous factors to consider in treating this condition, and the patient should be referred to a cardiologist. Should right-sided CHF supervene, the medical management is similar to that described for pure tricuspid valve regurgitation in Chapter 10.

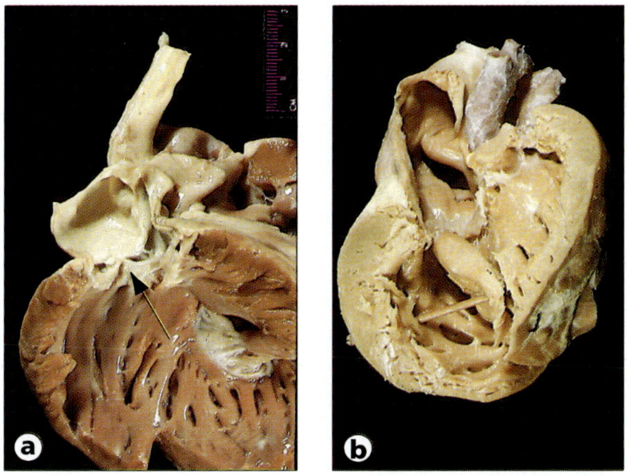

13.1 Pathology of pulmonic stenosis in dogs. (**a**) Opened right ventricular outflow tract demonstrates thickened, dysplastic valve (arrow), right ventricular hypertrophy, and post-stenotic dilatation of the main pulmonary artery. (**b**) Ventral view of open right atrium and ventricle demonstrating right atrial dilatation and hypertrophy, and marked right ventricular and papillary muscle hypertrophy. A hypoplastic pulmonary artery orifice is also evident.

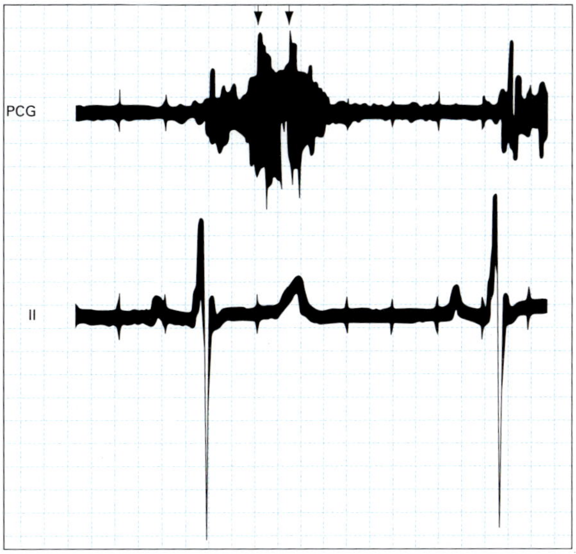

13.2 Phonocardiogram (PCG) from a dog with pulmonic stenosis demonstrating a typical ejection murmur (arrows).

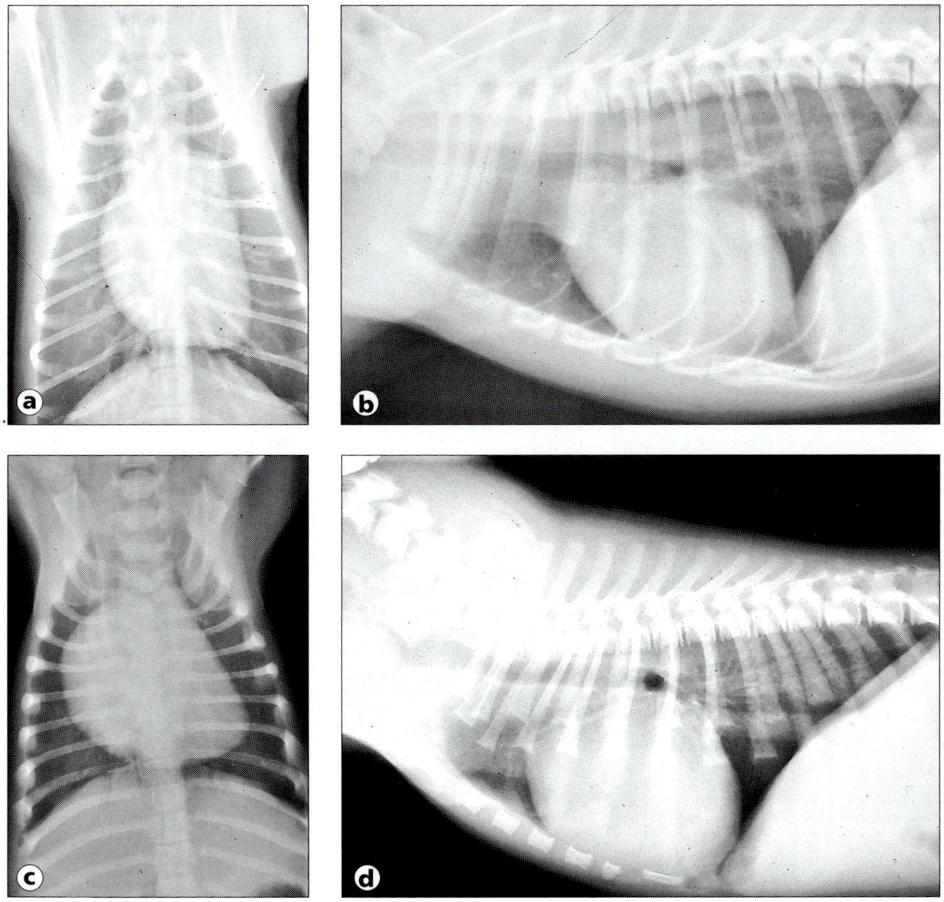

13.3 (**a** and **b**) Thoracic radiographs obtained from a dog with pulmonic stenosis. There is mild right ventricular enlargement and a prominent main pulmonary artery (post-stenotic dilatation – arrow). (**c** and **d**) Right ventricular enlargement and pulmonary undercirculation in a dog with pulmonic stenosis and patent foramen ovale. This combination causes right-to-left shunting and pulmonary under-perfusion.

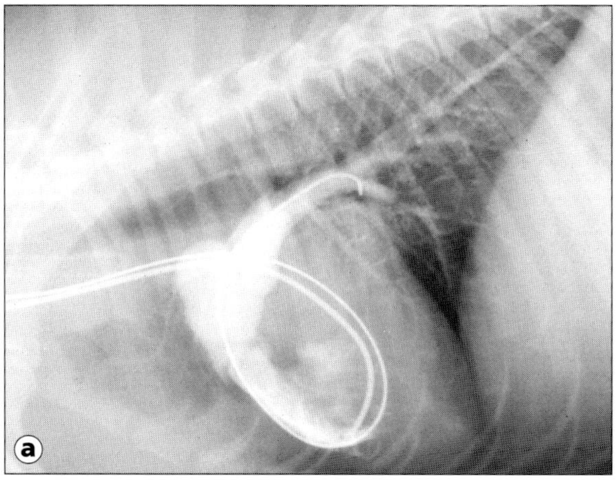

13.4 (**a**) Right ventricular angiogram of a 7-month-old miniature schnauzer with pulmonic stenosis. There is right ventricular hypertrophy with a narrowed ventricular chamber; there is also post-stenotic dilatation. A catheter guide-wire has been passed though the ventricle into the right main pulmonary artery prior to balloon vavuloplasty. (**b**) The stenotic valve (arrow) and post-stenotic dilatation of the pulmonary artery and lobar artery are evident.
(**c**) Valvular PS and subvalvular dynamic obstruction caused by muscular hypertrophy secondary to valvular obstruction.
(**d**) Right ventricular angiogram from a cat with pulmonic stenosis. Note the severe right ventricular hypertrophy and marked post-stenotic dilatation of the pulmonary artery.
(**e**) Pulmonic stenosis related to an anomalous coronary artery. Such cases should not be treated by balloon valvuloplasty.

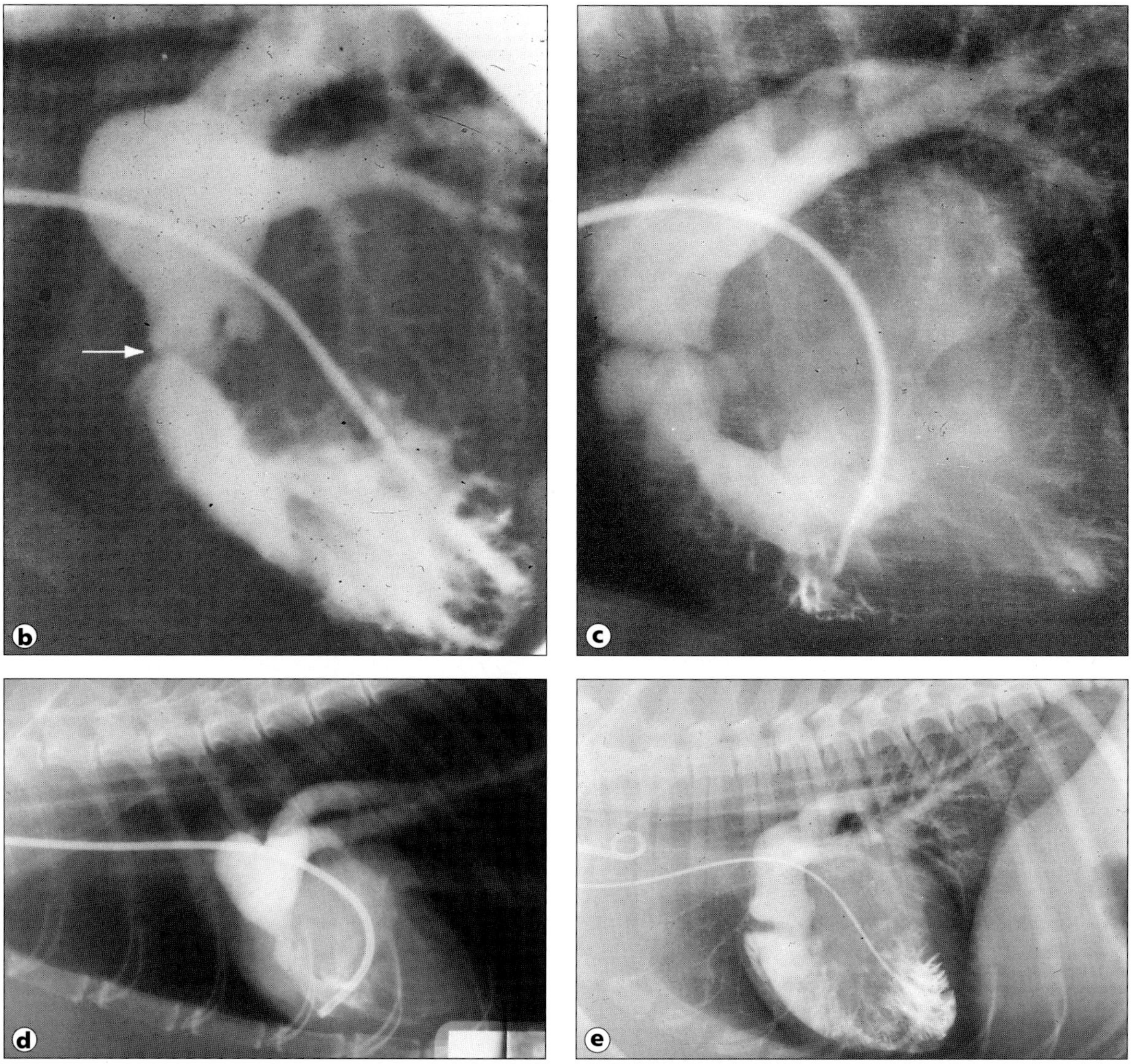

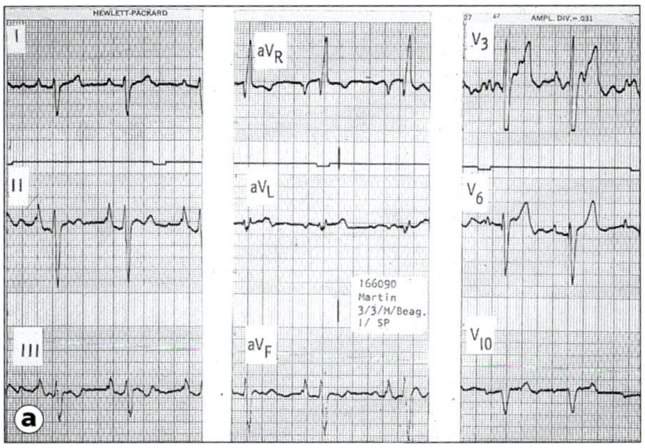

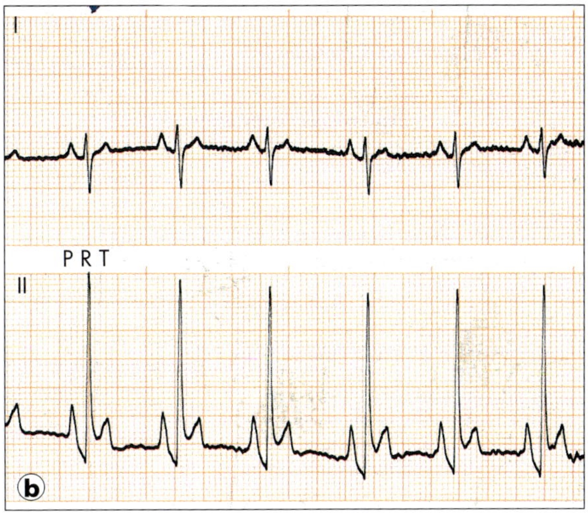

13.5 (**a**) ECG from a dog with pulmonic stenosis. Prominent P waves (right atrial enlargement) and right-axis deviation with prominent S waves in leads I, II, aV_F, and V_3 (indicating right ventricular hypertrophy) are evident.
(**b**) ECG (leads I and II) from a one-year-old golden retriever with pulmonic stenosis and tricuspid regurgitation. Note the P pulmonale (0.6 mV) in lead II representing marked right atrial enlargement, and the S wave in lead I. This dog has marked right atrial ventricular dilatation due to tricuspid regurgitation, and the ECG findings are not typical of most cases of simple pulmonic stenosis.

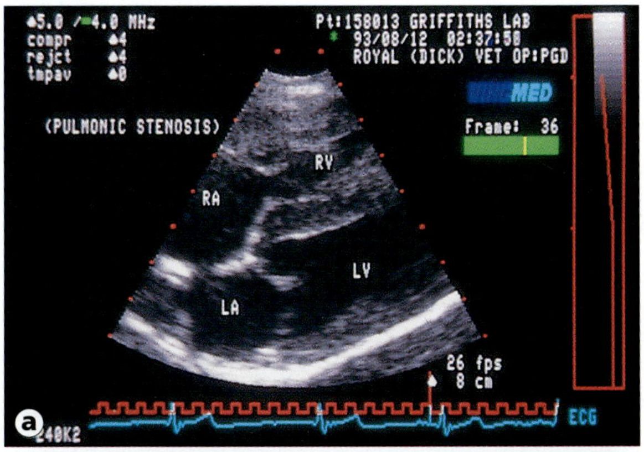

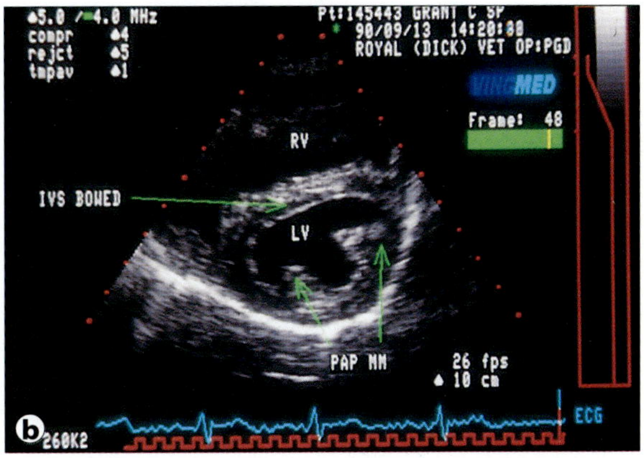

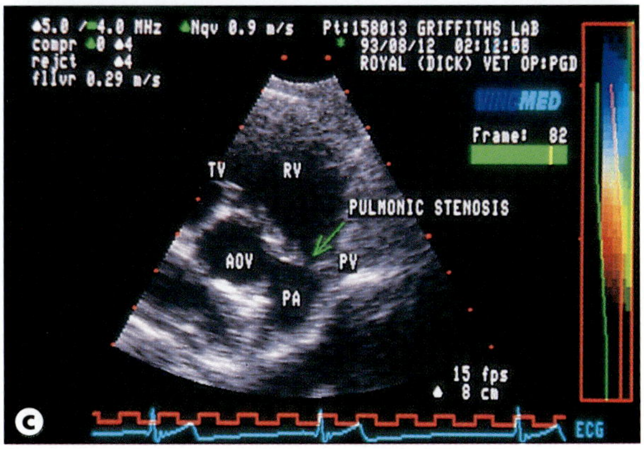

13.6 (**a**) Right, paracostal, long-axis, 4-chambered view of the heart of a Labrador retriever with pulmonic stenosis. There is marked right ventricular hypertrophy and moderate right atrial dilatation. (**b**) Short-axis view of the heart of a cocker spaniel with pulmonic stenosis, showing flattening of the interventricular septum due to elevated right ventricular pressure. (**c**) Short-axis view of the pulmonic valve of the dog in **13.6a**. The pulmonic valve is noticeably thickened.

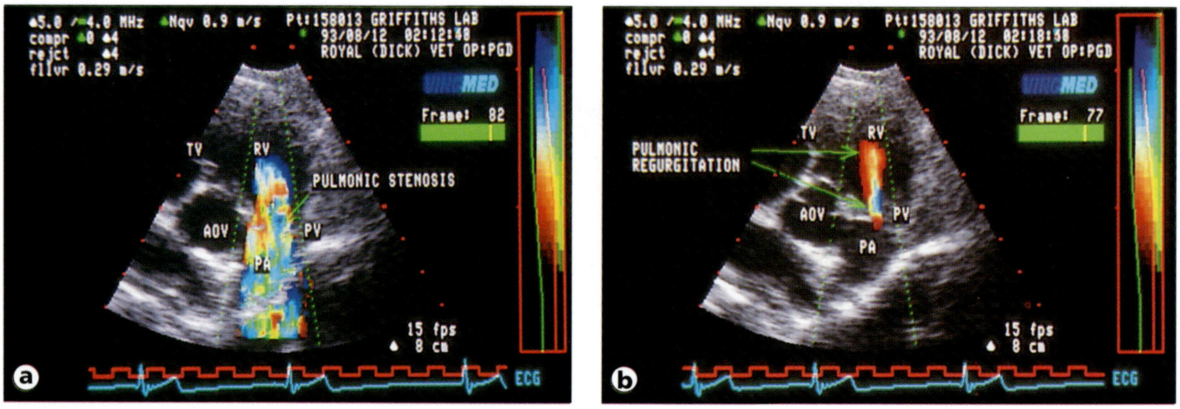

13.7 (**a**) Colour-flow Doppler recording from the pulmonary outflow of the dog in **13.6(c)** showing severely disturbed flow. (**b**) Colour-flow Doppler recording from the pulmonary outflow of the dog in **13.6(b)** showing pulmonic regurgitation.

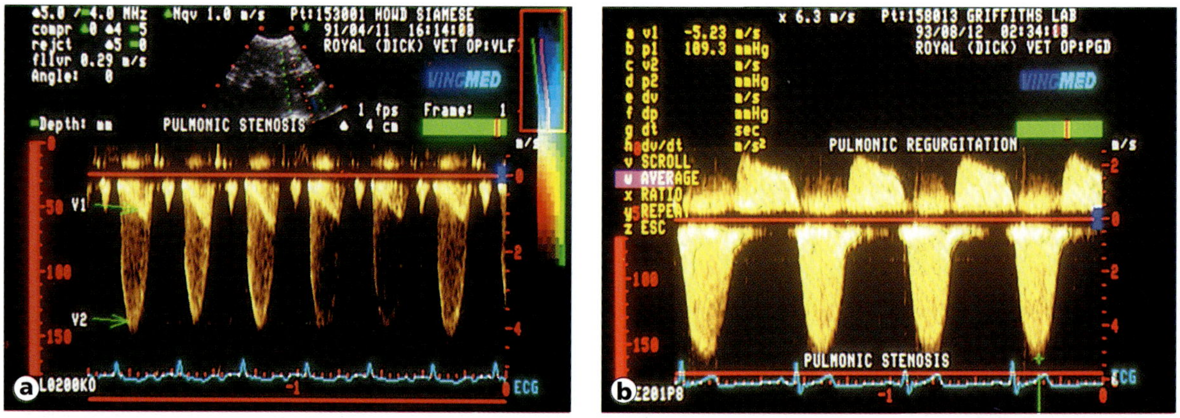

13.8 (**a**) HPRF pulsed-wave spectral Doppler recording from the pulmonary artery of a Siamese cat with pulmonic stenosis, showing disturbed (turbulent) flow, at high maximal velocity (4 m/sec) beyond the valve (V2). Flow of normal velocity (about 1 m/sec) at the outflow tract can also be seen in this recording (V2). With HPRF, the flow is sampled at multiple points down the line of the cursor. (Courtesy of Miss V. Luis Fuentes.) (**b**) Continuous-wave Doppler recording from the pulmonic valve of the dog in **13.6(a)**, **13.6(c)**, **13.7(a)** and **13.7(b)**, showing the increased velocity of outflow (5.23 m/sec) due to stenosis, and a diastolic pulmonary regurgitation. Diastolic regurgitation is common in pulmonic stenosis.

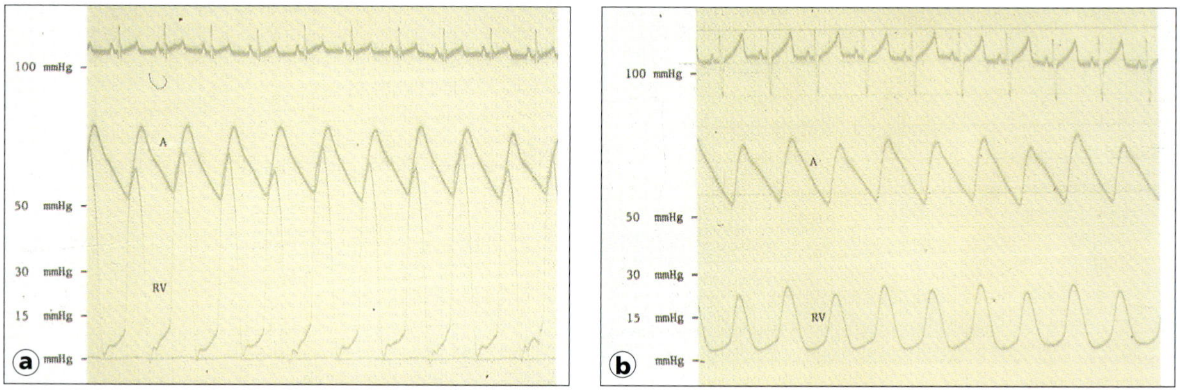

13.9 Aortic and right ventricular pressures recorded before (**a**) and after (**b**) therapeutic balloon valvuloplasty in a dog with congenital pulmonic stenosis. Normal right ventricular systolic pressure is approximately 16–20% of the aortic pressure.

14.

Bacterial Endocarditis

Bacterial endocarditis (BE) is a bacterial infection of the lining of the heart valves or, rarely, the mural endocardium. All domesticated species are affected by BE, though both the offending microorganisms and the affected valves vary.

Generally, endocarditis is assumed to be initiated by bacteraemia. Microorganisms can enter the blood through a break in a barrier which may normally harbour bacteria (skin, gut, mouth, urogenital tract or respiratory epithelium), from foci of infected tissues (e.g. abscess, osteomyelitis, prostatitis), or by introduction from medical or surgical procedures such as intravenous cannulation or dental prophylaxis. Bacteria of sufficient virulence, or those agglutinated by host antibody, may invade, ulcerate and colonize a valve surface. Abnormal haemodynamic conditions, with subaortic stenosis being most notable, predispose to endocarditis by altering normal valve endothelium and directing bacteria onto the valve surface at high velocity. Although diseased valves are thought to be more susceptible to bacterial endocarditis, it is noteworthy that dogs with endocardiosis and mitral regurgitation rarely develop BE. (There is also no compelling evidence for the 'association' between valvular heart disease and oral cavity disease in dogs.) Once bacteria penetrate the endothelium and expose collagen, platelets aggregate and there is local accumulation of fibrin. Subacute or chronic vegetations, which resemble thrombi, form on the valve surface. These are typically yellowish-red to grey and are covered by a thin layer of clotted blood. Deformation of the valve usually results in *valvular insufficiency*. Exuberant vegetations may also produce valve stenosis, but this is far less common.

There are well-recognized but unexplained species differences in valve predilection to BE: the mitral and aortic valves of the dog and cat, the tricuspid and pulmonic valves of the cow and other ruminants, and either left-sided or right-sided (less common) cardiac valves of the horse. The frequency of infection by specific bacteria also varies between species and is probably related to the environment and portal of entry. General guidelines include: dogs – streptococci, staphylococci, corynebacteria and *Erysipelothrix*; cats – streptococci and staphylococci; horses – streptococci; cattle – *Actinobacillus* (*Corynebacterium*) *pyogenes*; pigs – streptococci and *Erysipelothrix*. Gram -negative BE occurs with increasing frequency in hospitalized patients. This is probably related to the preponderance of antibiotic-resistant nosocomial infections. Other microorganisms (e.g. fungi) rarely cause endocarditis. Immunosuppressive drug therapy and injudicious use of antibiotics may predispose to infection.

The clinical signs of bacterial endocarditis are explained readily by appreciating the pathophysiological effects (**14.2**). Intermittent bacteraemia causes persistent or recurrent malaise, shivering and fever. Brain abscesses, splenitis, osteomyelitis, arthritis, nephritis and other remote infections may result from BE. It can be difficult in advanced cases to distinguish primary infection (portal of entry) from embolic infection. Emboli, either septic or 'bland' (aseptic) are shed from the vegetation, leading to embolic infection or thromboemboli. Potential lesions include myocardial infarction and myocarditis; renal infarction, suppuration, or glomerulonephritis; cerebral infarction, meningitis or encephalitis; bone infarcts and osteomyelitis; vascular obstruction including aortic–iliac occlusion; splenic infarcts; and intestinal ischaemia. Thus, endocarditis should be considered in any animal with signs of thromboembolism (though pulmonary embolism from BE is uncommon in dogs and cats owing to the low incidence of right-sided BE) and clinical signs can be varied. Immune complexes formed in response to the infection may contribute to morbidity. These complexes can be filtered and trapped in joints, kidneys or meninges, attract complement and leucocytes, and produce inflammation in these tissues. The clinical signs of fever with sterile polyarthritis or polymyositis can be easily confused with primary immune-mediated disorders, prompting injudicious therapy with corticosteroids.

A variety of cardiac manifestations are possible with BE, including: valvular incompetence or stenosis; coronary arterial occlusion by thromboemboli (with consequent myocardial infarction); myocarditis; myocardial abscess; pericarditis; or arrhythmia (**14.2**). Arrhythmias may be related to myocarditis, 'toxaemia', or extension of aortic root abscesses into the conduction system causing AV block. Congestive heart failure may develop if valvular injury is severe. Other possible clinical signs of BE include vasculitis, small vessel thromboses, haemorrhages and disseminated coagulopathy.

The clinical features of BE have essentially been described above. The history may suggest previous or concurrent wound or infection, or perhaps a recent diagnostic or therapeutic procedure or treatment that could predispose to bacteraemia. Persistent or recurrent fever is a hallmark and should always alert the clinician to the possibility of BE, particularly if the fever is responsive to antibiotic therapy. A high level of suspicion is essential to diagnose BE, and this should always be considered in the differential diagnosis of immune-mediated disorders such as polyarthritis. A cardiac murmur, particularly a 'new' or changing murmur, is characteristic of BE.

Laboratory tests can contribute to the diagnosis. Haematology may demonstrate mild anaemia, leukocytosis with neutrophilia and monocytosis, or red cell fragments, vasculitis or disseminated intravascular coagulopathy. Serum biochemical abnormalities such as elevated fibrin degradation products and azotaemia reflect organ injury from infection, thrombosis, infarction, or poor perfusion from heart failure. Tests of autoimmune responses (LE preparation, antinuclear antibody) can be positive in patients with BE and this can be misleading. Urinalysis may demonstrate haematuria, proteinuria, pyuria or casts, should embolic nephritis or glomerulitis be present. Culture of the urine may be revealing, but it cannot be assumed that organisms cultured from urine are also responsible for the cardiac infection. Cerebrospinal fluid and joint-fluid cytology and culture may provide evidence for either septic or immune-mediated inflammation. The laboratory test of choice is blood culture, with preferably two or more samples taken 30–60 minutes apart. Sufficient blood (5–10 ml) must be taken and transferred into special broth media tubes (usual blood:media ratio of 1:10). Successive cultures positive for the same microorganism, and obtained from an animal with compatible clinical signs, are diagnostic of BE.

Additional investigations may substantiate the diagnosis and indicate the degree of cardiac injury. Radiography may indicate cardiomegaly, valve calcification, congestive cardiac failure or (rarely) embolic pneumonia. Angiocardiography documents valvular insufficiency and may outline the vegetation, but this technique can dislodge thrombi and has been supplanted by echocardiography. Electrocardiography in BE gives variable results, but may indicate chamber enlargement or document an arrhythmia. AV block may suggest aortic valve involvement with a perivalvular inflammation affecting the AV junction. The echocardiographic study is useful, especially for prognosis. Routine two-dimensional or M-mode echocardiography may demonstrate a vegetation and signs of haemodynamic overload (cardiomegaly); however, the echo cannot reliably differentiate mitral BE from mitral endocardiosis in older dogs, nor can it reliably identify small vegetations or acute ulcerative endocarditis. Doppler studies can document valvular regurgitation or stenosis. Identification of a large vegetation by two-dimensional echocardiography carries a poor prognosis since substantial valvular dysfunction usually persists even following successful antibiotic therapy. The natural history of such cases parallels those described in the previous chapters detailing valvular heart diseases.

The principles of treatment of BE include the administration of bactericidal drugs that penetrate fibrin, reference to blood or other cultures for ultimate antibiotic selection, and long-term antibiotic therapy. Since bacteria are sequestered within the vegetation, normal defence and healing processes (e.g. granulation) are impeded. The antibiotic should be capable of penetrating fibrin, thus excluding from consideration most sulphonamide drugs. Long-term therapy (4–8 weeks) may be needed to ensure sterilization of the vegetation. Ideally, intravenous therapy should be used to obtain the highest possible plasma concentrations. Antibiotic therapy should be guided by blood cultures whenever possible. It is appropriate to delay therapy for 2–4 hours while blood cultures are obtained, unless the patient is demonstrating signs of septic shock. Empirical therapy for BE often includes the following drugs:

- Penicillins (high doses) which are safe and useful for streptococcal infections.
- Aminoglycosides combined with a synthetic penicillin or cephalosporin provide wider antimicrobial coverage. Use of these drugs requires good patient hydration and careful monitoring for nephrotoxicity.
- A patient with renal failure may be treated with a newer generation cephalosporin (e.g. moxalactam) instead of an aminoglycoside. Rifampin may be used in horses.

Should congestive heart failure develop, treatment is similar to that outlined in Chapter 3 (see also specific valvular lesions). Prophylactic antibiotic therapy should be used if the animal undergoes any procedure that may cause bacteraemia, though the general subject of prophylactic therapy of BE is unresolved and no firm recommendations can be made.

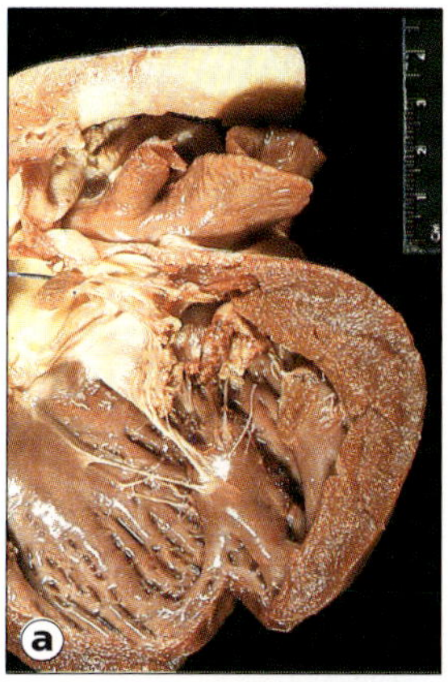

14.1 Pathology of bacterial endocarditis. (**a**) Proliferative vegetation on the mitral valve of a dog. (**b**) Mitral valve endocarditis in a colt. (**c**) Large tricuspid valve vegetation in a horse viewed from the dorsal perspective. Compare the lesion to the normal valves. (**d**) Chronic suppurative endocarditis of the tricuspid valve due to *Actinobacillus (Corynebacterium) pyogenes* in a Friesian cow. (**e**) Small aortic valve vegetation on the aortic valve of a horse. A jet lesion of aortic insufficiency is evident below the valve (arrow). (**f**) Large pulmonary valve vegetation is evident in this specimen from a cow. (**g**) Histologic section of an infective heart valve demonstrating fibrin and cellular deposition in the valve (×16).

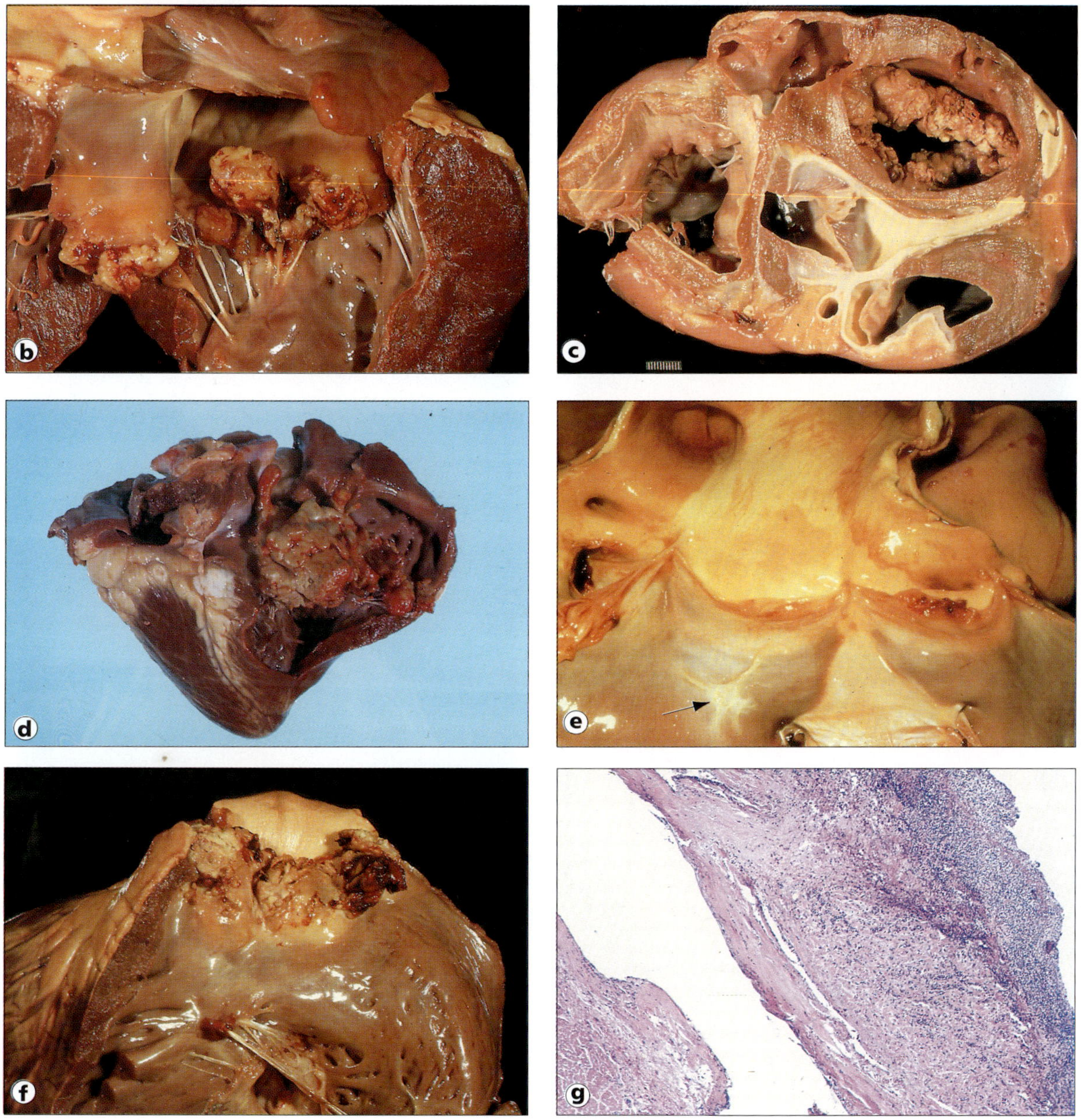

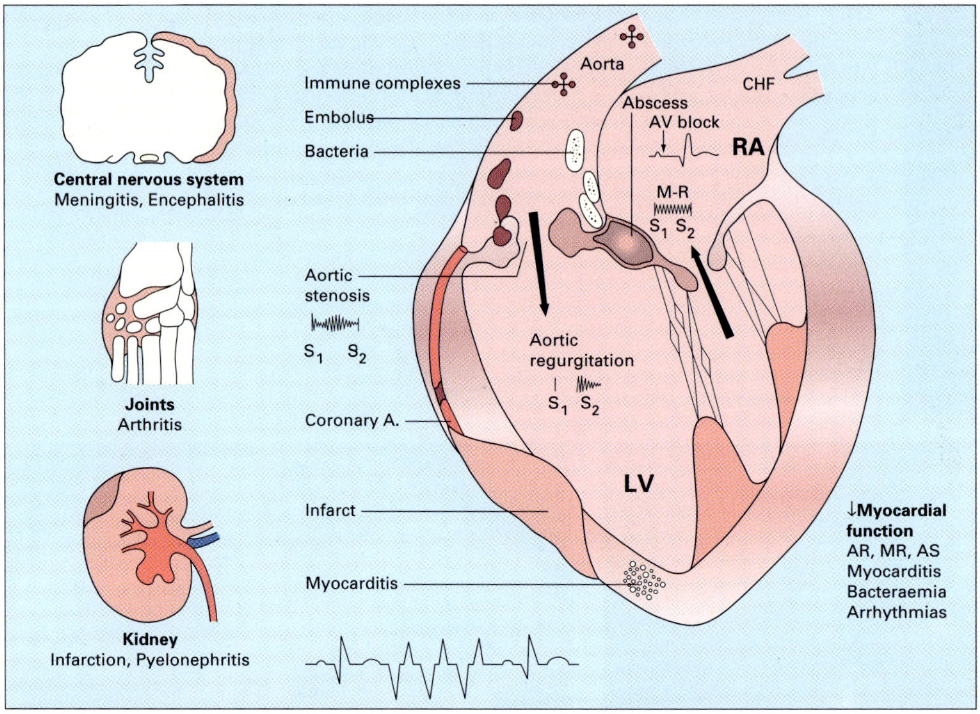

14.2 Pathophysiology of bacterial endocarditis (see text for details).

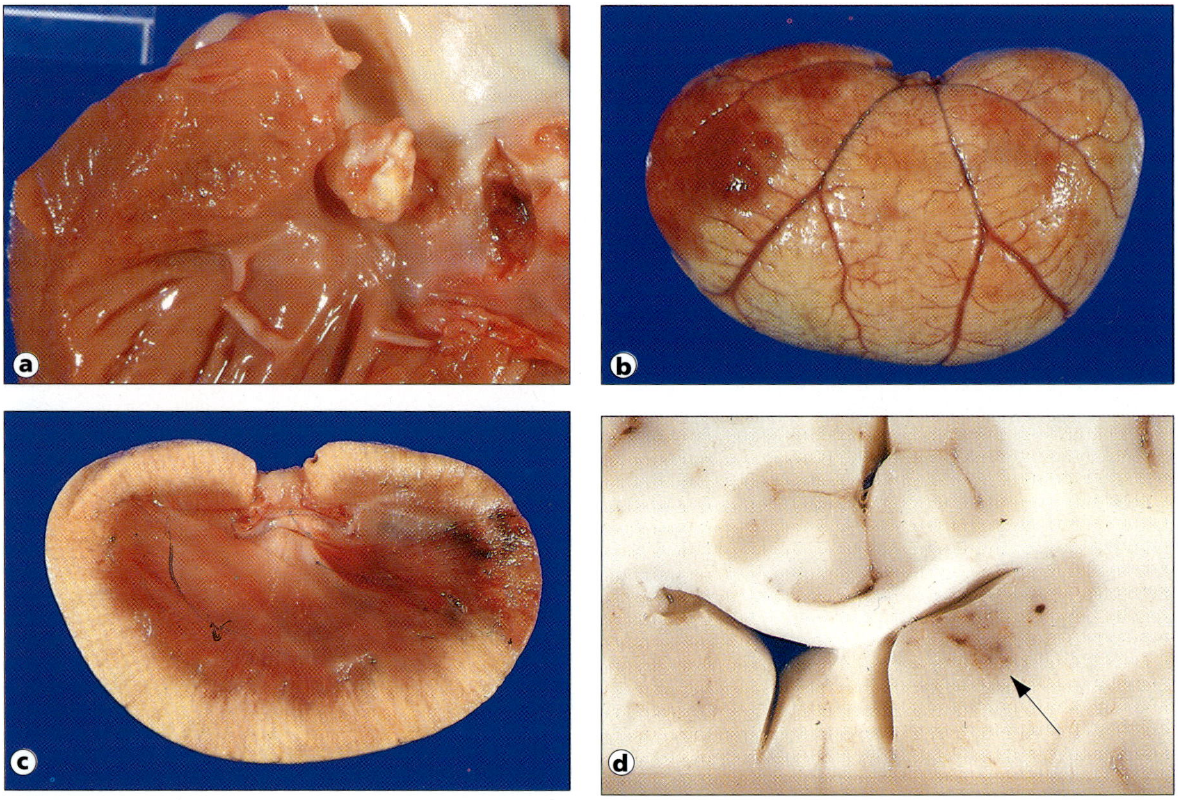

14.3 (**a**) Aortic endocarditis in a 4-year-old female Burmese cat. A valve cusp is obscured by a large, firmly adherent mass of thrombus. Aortic valve endocarditis is often complicated by thromboembolism and renal infarction. (**b**) Thromboembolic infarction of the kidney in a cat with vavular endocarditis. (**c**) Cut surface of the kidney from the same cat as in (**b**). (**d**) Brain infarction (arrow) in a 7-year-old Dalmatian dog with valvular endocarditis.

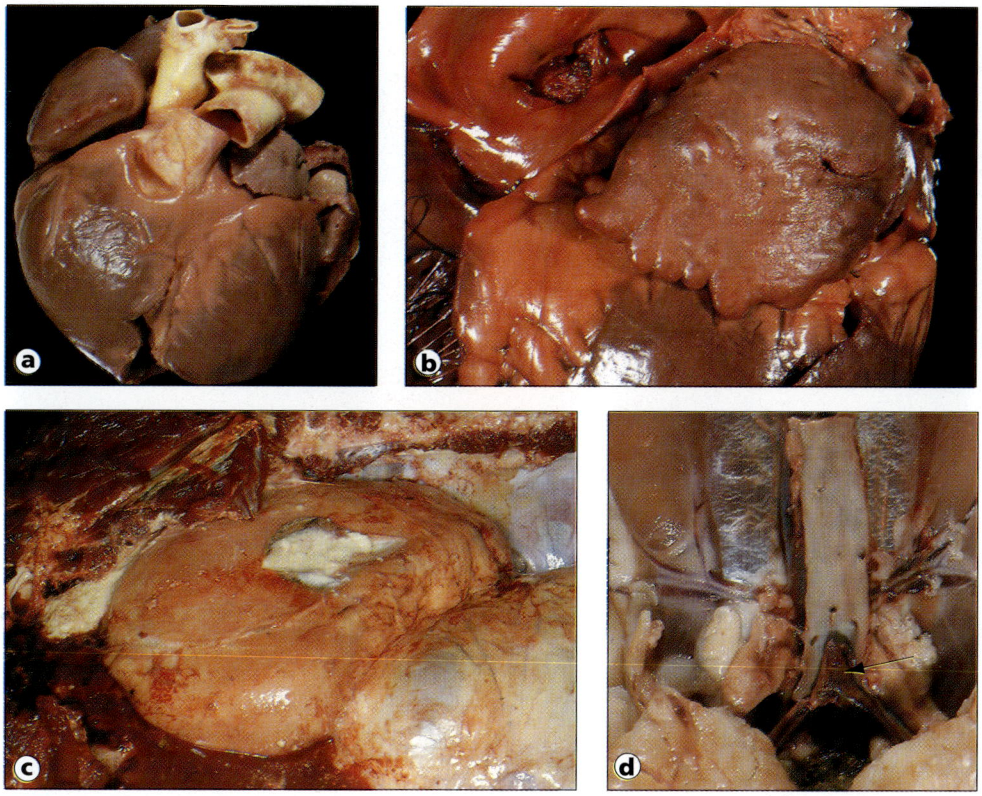

14.4 (**a**) Enlarged right atrium in a yearling with tricuspid valve endocarditis and congestive heart failure. (**b**) Grossly dilated left atrium and auricular appendage in a horse with acute mitral valve endocarditis. (**c**) Pulmonary abscess in a horse with right-sided endocarditis and embolic infection of the lung. (**d**) Aortic thrombosis ('saddle thrombus' – arrow) in a cat with bacterial endocarditis.

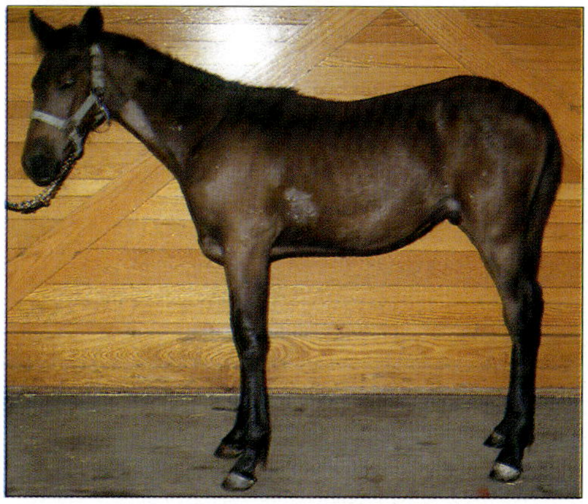

14.5 Yearling with endocarditis (see **14.1c**) showing poor condition and subcutaneous, ventral oedema secondary to right-sided cardiac failure.

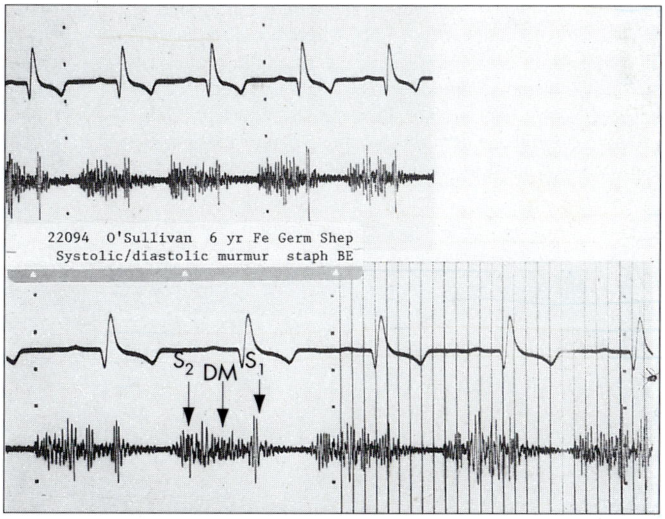

14.6 Phonocardiogram of aortic regurgitation in a dog with aortic valve endocarditis. The finding of this diastolic murmur (DM) in a dog with a fever strongly suggests infection of the aortic valve in this species. (S_1 – first heart sound; S_2 – second heart sound.)

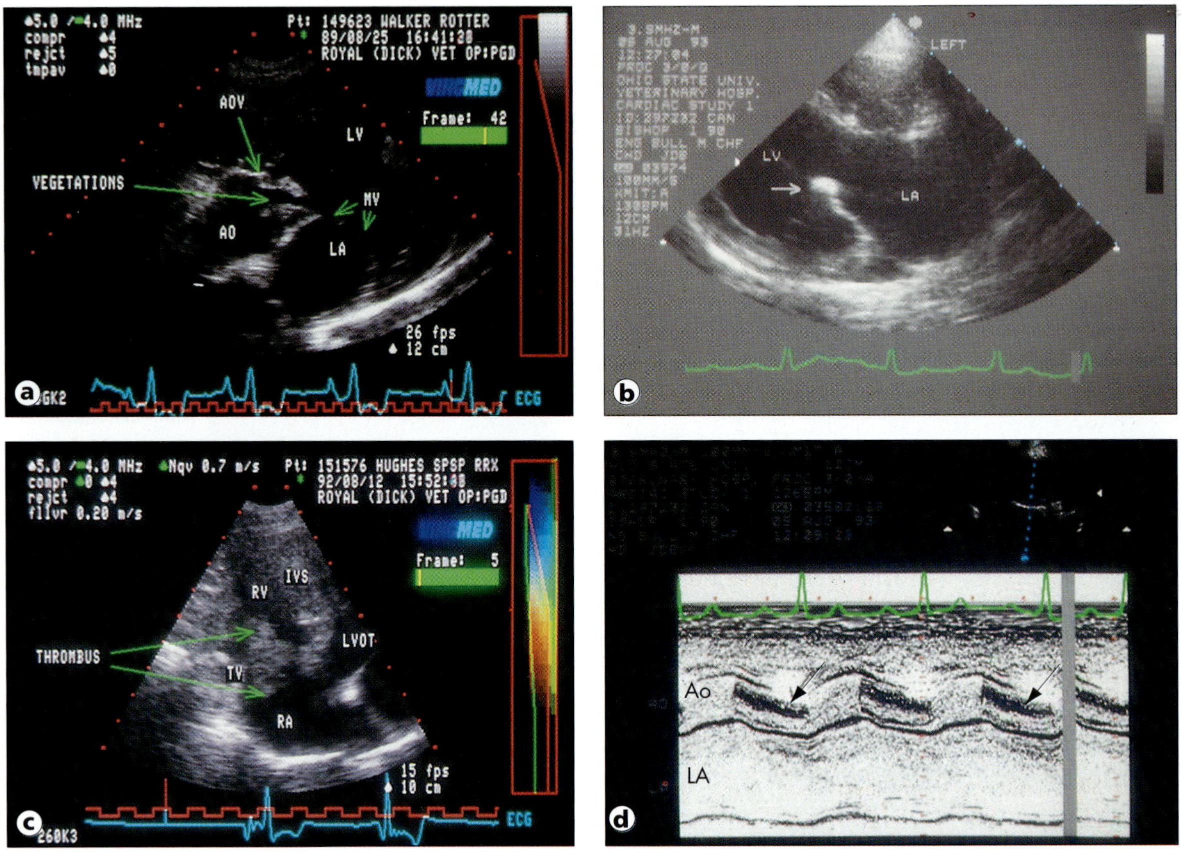

14.7 (**a**) Two-dimensional echocardiogram of the aortic valve of a Rottweiler with bacterial endocarditis, showing vegetations of the aortic valve. (**b**) Mitral valve vegetation (arrow) evident as a hyperechoic valve cusp in an English bulldog with bacterial endocarditis of the left heart valves and congestive heart failure. Both the left atrium and left ventricle are dilated. (**c**) Left apical two-dimensional image of the heart of a springer spaniel, showing a thrombus attached to the tricuspid valve. This was associated with a cardiac pacing lead. Bacterial endocarditis was confirmed at necropsy. (**d**) M-mode echocardiogram of an aortic valve demonstrating bacterial endocarditis in a dog (arrow). The typical pattern of movement during the cardiac cycle is evident. The vegetation is most evident in diastole (arrow) when the valve is closed. The left atrium (LA) is dilated.

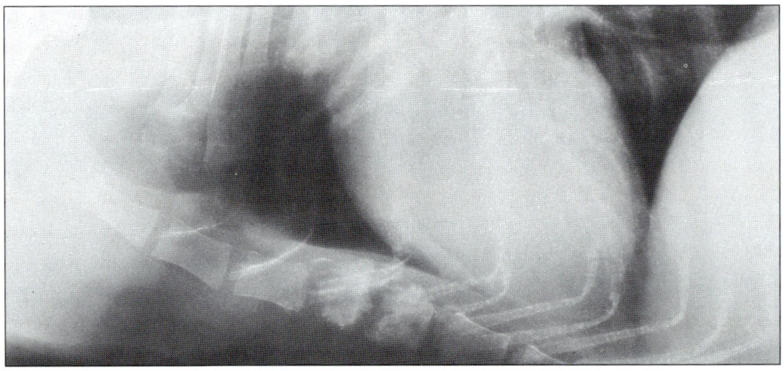

14.8 Osteomyelitis of the sternum in a golden retriever with bacterial endocarditis. A proliferative and destructive lesion is evident typical of embolic infection. The original source of this staphylococcal infection was an infected surgical wound from which the same bacteria was isolated. Blood cultures were also positive.

15. Defects of the Cardiac Septa

Congenital myocardial malformations most commonly involve defects in the cardiac septa. Malformations usually occur in specific areas of the atrial and ventricular septa. Often, septal defects are isolated, but they may be associated with valve malformations.

ATRIAL SEPTAL DEFECT

An atrial septal defect (ASD) usually results from a failure of closure of the fetal ostium primum or ostium secundum. Following birth, blood will shunt through the lesion along the path of least resistance. This is invariably from the left to the right side of the heart unless there is another reason for elevated right-sided pressures such as pulmonic or tricuspid valve malformation or pulmonary hypertension. A patent foramen ovale is similar in effect, although this would close if there were not another defect maintaining patency of the fetal orifice. Any persistent elevation in right atrial pressure (e.g. from severe pulmonic stenosis) may prevent the foramen ovale from sealing and thereby provide an avenue for right-to-left shunting, as occurs normally in the fetus. Severe dilatation of the left atrium (e.g. with mitral stenosis) may also stretch the foramen ovale sufficiently to prevent anatomic closure following birth. In cats, an ASD is often part of a complex endocardial cushion defect, combined with a ventricular septal defect and an atrioventricular valve malformation (usually a common or bridging septal leaflet).

In itself, an ASD causes few specific signs. Any murmur is due to increased flow across the pulmonic valve, and radiographic and electrocardiographic findings are mainly those of right-sided cardiac enlargement. The colour of mucous membranes is normal unless there is another lesion promoting right-to-left shunting, in which case cyanosis may occur. The pulmonary artery is dilated in this condition due to high flow volume and turbulence, and pulmonary overcirculation may be detected by radiography. The definitive diagnosis is usually made following referral to a specialist. Either cardiac catheterization or preferably two-dimensional echocardiography with Doppler studies is used to establish the diagnosis. Salient clinical features are summarized in Appendix A3, *Congenital Heart Disease in Animals,* and clinical examples are found in this chapter.

VENTRICULAR SEPTAL DEFECT

The ventricular septal defect (VSD) appears to be the most common congenital malformation across all animal species, although other defects are more common in dogs. Many breeds of cattle and cats are affected with ventricular septal defects, and the English bulldog and Arabian horse breeds are clearly predisposed. A VSD is at times found in association with pulmonic stenosis, pulmonary atresia, truncus arteriosus and double-outlet right ventricle. Often in these cases, the defect is partially straddled by the aortic root ('overriding'), as with the tetralogy of Fallot. An isolated VSD is most commonly located dorsally within the septum, and there are elaborate and inconsistent methods of classifying the defect, based on location relative to the right-sided valves or ventricular septum. The most common form of VSD in animals is found between the subaortic septum on the left and the perimembranous or inlet, right ventricular septum, adjacent to or just below the septal tricuspid cusp on the right. In ruminants, the defect often has a subpulmonic location, just ventral to the pulmonic valve in the outlet portion of the ventricular septum. The septal defect permits left-to-right shunting of blood unless there is a mechanism to reverse the shunt as previously described for an ASD.

The pathophysiologic and clinical effects are variable according to the size and location of the defect and associated malformations. Very often, animals have a small defect ('restrictive' VSD), with maintenance of the normal left-to-right pressure gradient between the ventricles, and with little clinical dysfunction. This is typical of most cases that survive for more than 6 months. As described in Chapter 12, an aortic valve leaflet can prolapse into the defect, leading to concurrent aortic regurgitation. Left-to-right shunting may lead to considerable volume overload of the pulmonary circulation, left atrium and left ventricle with a large VSD. The right ventricle is variably affected, because the location of most defects causes the right ventricle to serve as a conduit for flow during systole. In general, larger defects are associated with more right-sided enlargement, though there are exceptions.

A VSD is recognized initially by cardiac auscultation, except when it is associated with complex congenital heart disease, in which case cyanosis may be a presenting sign. In nearly all cases there is a harsh, holosystolic murmur, audible maximally over the ventral right thorax, often near the sternum. In animals with subpulmonic defects (typically cattle), the murmur is most intense near the pulmonary valve area at the left cranial thorax. In severely affected cases, if ventricular pressures have equilibrated, the murmur may be either soft or loud. Murmurs of relative pulmonic stenosis or aortic regurgitation may be audible with VSD.

ECG findings are variable and related to the degree and type of volume overload, although a common feature is an intraventricular conduction disturbance affecting the Q wave in leads II and aVF. Pulmonary overcirculation is the most common sign seen radiographically. Radiography and echocardiography show left atrial and ventricular dilatation with varying degrees of right-sided and main pulmonary artery enlargement. The diagnosis is confirmed by cardiac catheterization or by two-dimensional echocardiography with Doppler studies. Defects of less than 35% of the diameter of the aorta and associated with high-velocity shunting (> 4 m/sec) have a reasonable likelihood of being restrictive and well-tolerated despite the appearance of cardiomegaly. The salient clinical features of an isolated VSD are summarized in Appendix A3, *Congenital Heart Disease in Animals*.

The natural history of the large, isolated VSD is early death from left-sided or biventricular congestive heart failure, or hypoxaemia and cyanosis from the development of pulmonary vascular disease with pulmonary hypertension and reversal of the shunt (Eisenmenger's physiology). The natural history of a small-to-moderate isolated defect may include spontaneous closure of the lesion, tolerance of the defect despite volume overload, and cardiomegaly, exercise intolerance or late onset of heart failure. Accurate assessment and management requires consultation with an experienced cardiac specialist.

COMBINATION WITH OTHER DEFECTS

A large VSD is often encountered with other congenital heart defects. Among the most common of these is the tetralogy of Fallot – this combines pulmonic stenosis (often subvalvular), unrestrictive VSD, right ventricular hypertrophy and over-riding aorta. Tetralogy of Fallot is a serious disorder, causing right-to-left shunting (which leads to chronic hypoxaemia), and therefore recurrent bouts of exercise intolerance, weakness or collapse. Polycythaemia commonly results from the arterial hypoxaemia. Cyanosis is usual, this being the commonest cause of cyanotic heart disease in young animals (see Appendix A3, *Congenital Heart Disease in Animals*). Thoracic radiographs show undercirculation of the lungs, and right ventricular prominence. The ECG usually demonstrates right ventricular hypertrophy. The diagnosis is readily made by two-dimensional echocardiography, with Doppler studies or contrast echocardiography to demonstrate right-to-left shunting. Angiocardiography and cardiac catheterization can be used to make the diagnosis, but these are rarely needed if careful echocardiographic studies are undertaken. The management of this condition includes phlebotomy to reduce the packed cell volume to 62–65%. Palliative surgery by an experienced thoracic surgeon can improve pulmonary flow.

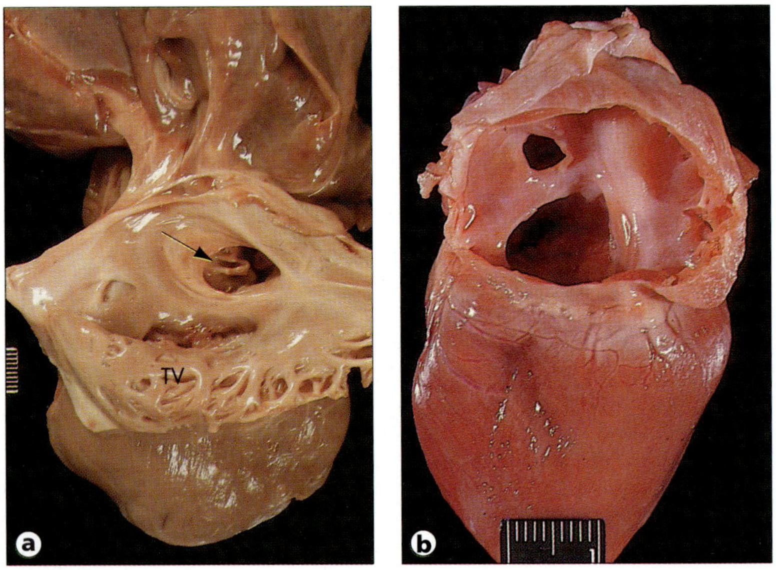

15.1 (**a**) Atrial septal defect in a ruminant (goat). The lesion is typical of an ostium secundum defect and is located in the fossa ovale (arrow). The orifice of the coronary sinus is evident to the left and the tricuspid valve (TV) is also observed. (**b**) Ostium primum (large) and ostium secundum (smaller) septal defects in a cat. Shunting will occur across these defects.

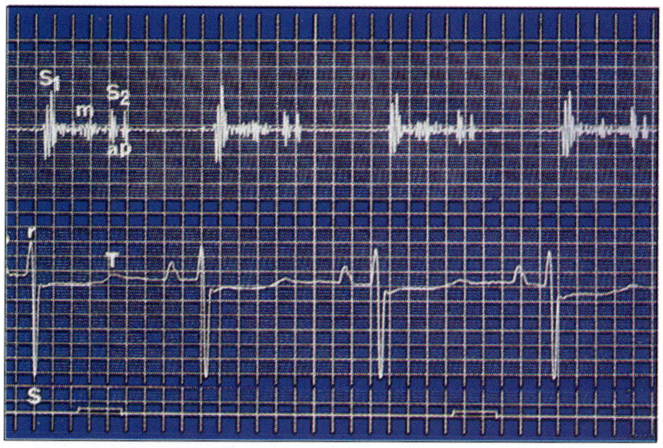

15.2 Phonocardiogram of relative pulmonic stenosis in a dog with atrial septal defect. The second heart sound (S_2) is also split. (Courtesy of Drs David Smetzer and Robert L. Hamlin.)

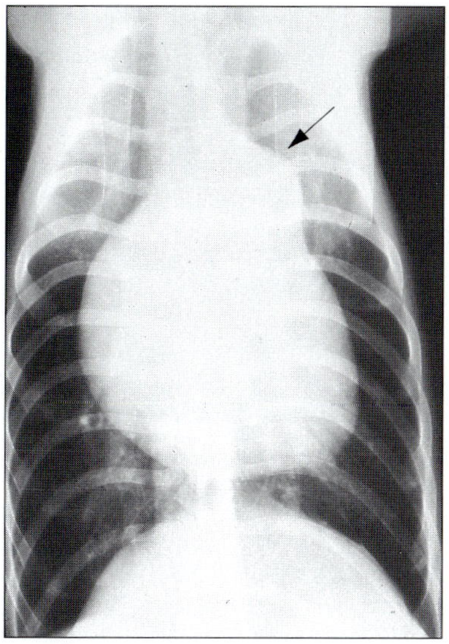

15.3 Dorsoventral radiograph of a young dog with Eisenmenger's syndrome and right-to-left shunting. The dog had a large VSD, and ASD, a PDA, and severe pulmonary vascular disease. There is a prominent pulmonary artery dilatation (arrow) and right ventricular enlargement.

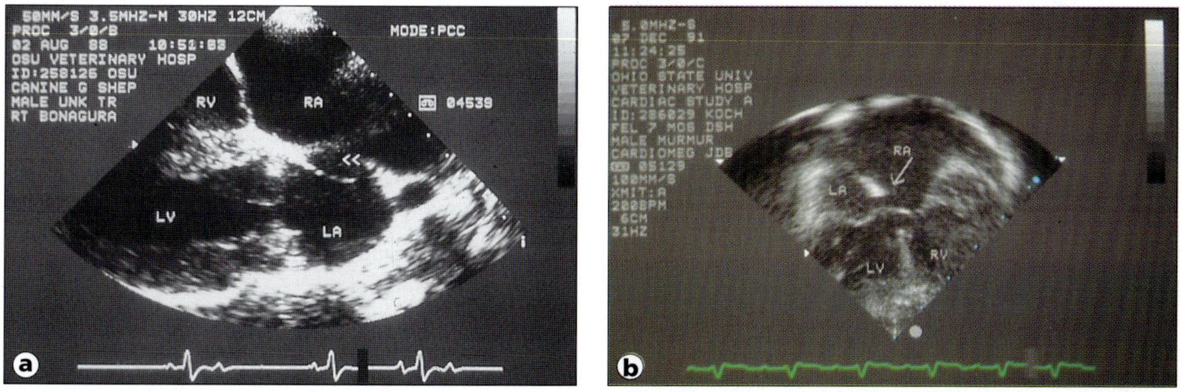

15.4 **(a)** Patent foramen ovales (arrow heads) in a dog with tricuspid dysplasia and volume overload of the right atrium and right ventricle. Right-to-left shunting occurred across this defect. **(b)** Primum atrial septal defect (arrow) and inlet ventricular septal defect in a cat with an endocardial cushion defect. The septal leaflet of the atrioventricular valves has a common attachment to the dorsal ventricular septum.

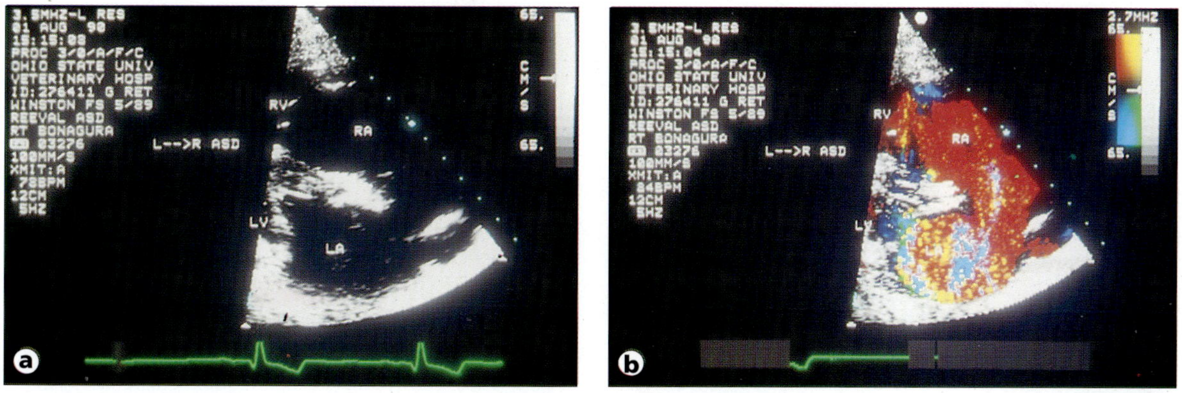

15.5 Atrial septal defect in a golden retriever. **(a)** Large secundum atrial septal defect. **(b)** Colour-flow Doppler: flow across the defect (left to right) is shown coded in red.

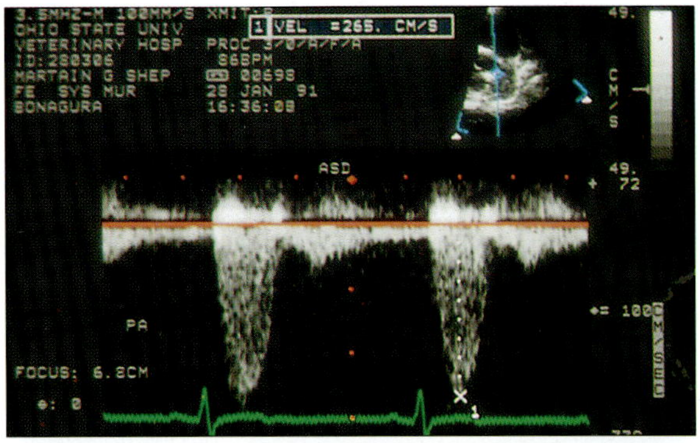

15.6 Continuous-wave Doppler recording of increased pulmonary artery velocity in a dog with atrial septal defect. The pulmonic valve was normal. The increased volume of flow, across a normal valve, leads to increased velocity (relative stenosis) and a murmur similar to that recorded in **15.2**.

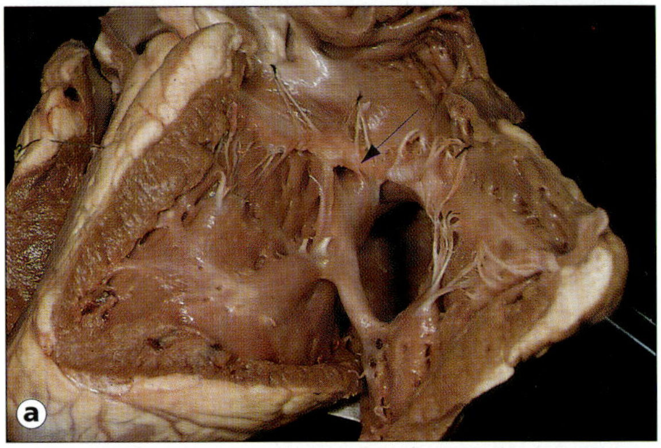

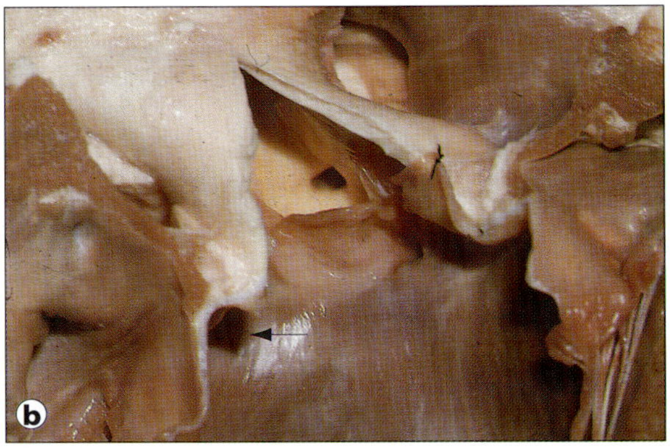

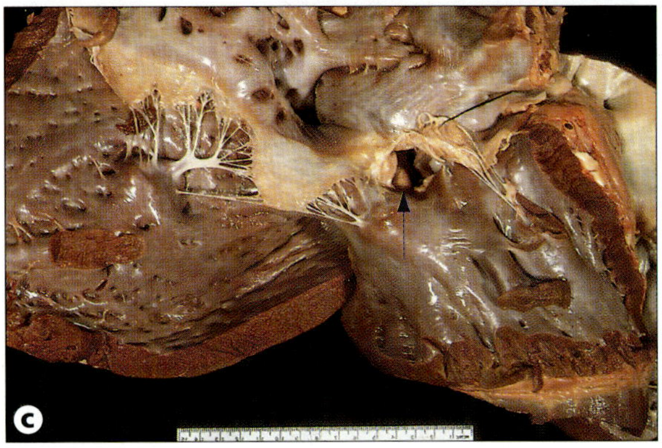

15.7 Ventricular septal defects in a calf and a foal. (**a** and **b**) The right ventricular and subaortic location of a perimembranous VSD in a calf. The VSD are indicated by arrows. The opening of a coronary artery is also evident in **b**. (**c**) Right ventricular position of a VSD (arrow) in a horse. The dorsal, subaortic locations of these defects and the close proximity to the tricuspid valve are typical features of VSD in animals.

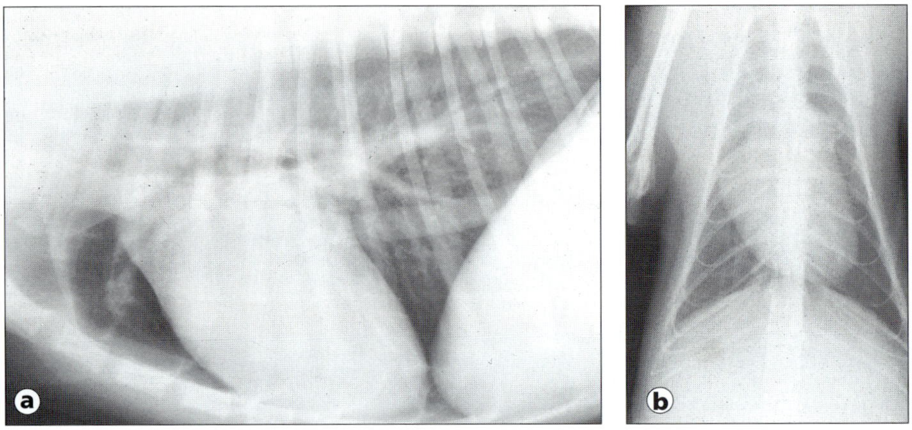

15.8 (**a**) Radiograph of a young Irish setter with a ventricular septal defect. Pulmonary overcirculation and mild left atrial enlargement are evident. (**b**) Radiograph of a 1-year-old West Highland white terrier with a ventricular septal defect, showing a rounded cardiac silhouette on the right, indicating right ventricular enlargement. There is also enlargement of the pulmonary arteries and evidence of pulmonary overload.

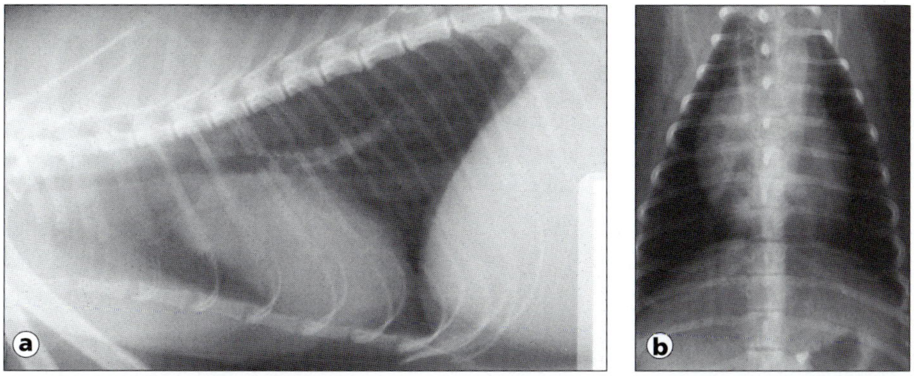

15.9 (**a** and **b**) Radiographs of a Devon rex cat with a ventricular septal defect showing generalized cardiac enlargement, affecting notably the right ventricle, together with a marked pulmonary artery dilatation and evidence of pulmonary overperfusion.

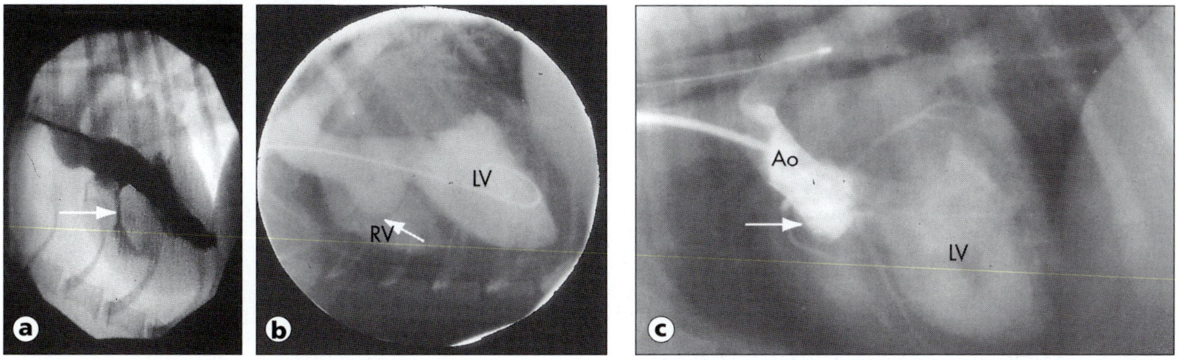

15.10 (**a**) Angiocardiogram demonstrating a small ventricular septal defect in a dog. Note that the jet (arrow) originates dorsally along the septum. (**b**) Left-to-right shunting and prolapse of an aortic valve leaflet (arrow) into a ventricular septal defect in a dog. (**c**) Angiogram demonstrating aortic regurgitation in a dog with VSD. The aortic valve had prolapsed into the VSD (arrow), partially occluding the defect, but leading to valvular incompetence.

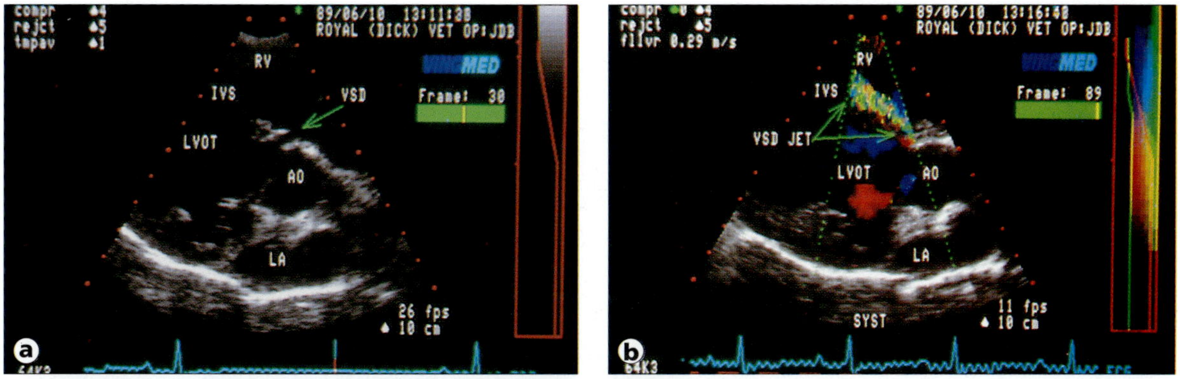

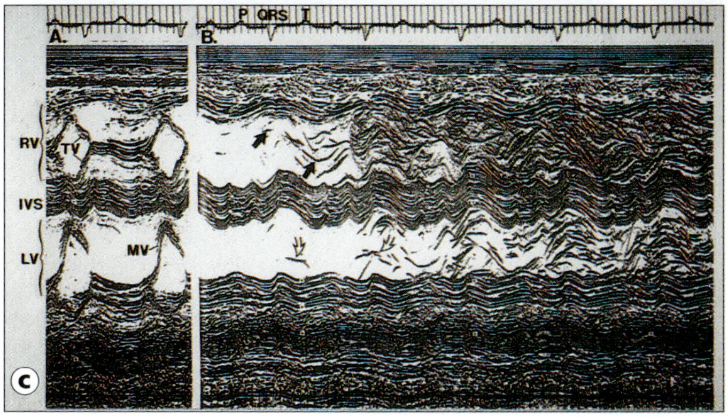

15.11 (**a**) Two-dimensional echocardiogram of a border collie with a small ventricular septal defect in the upper septum. (**b**) Colour-flow Doppler recording from the dog in (**a**), showing a small jet of disturbed flow into the right ventricle during systole. (**c**) Contrast M-mode echocardiogram from a calf with a ventricular septal defect and truncus arteriosus. A right-to-left shunt is evident as echocontrast opacifies the right and then the left ventricle. (TV – tricuspid valve; MV – mitral valve.)

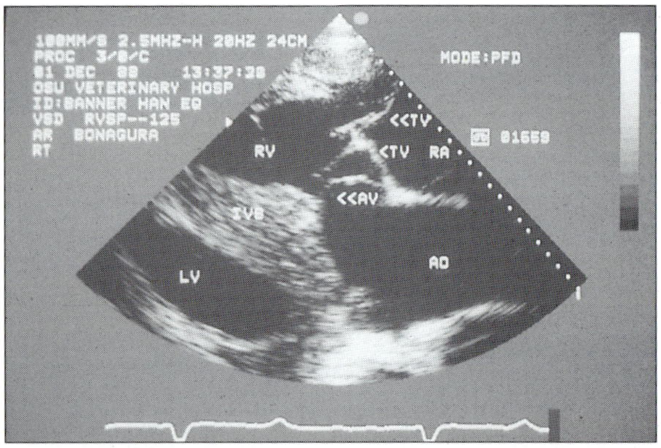

15.12 Angled image of an equine heart that shows malalignment of the aortic root with over-riding of the aorta across a ventricular septal defect. An aortic valve (AV) leaflet has prolapsed into the right ventricle just below the septal tricuspid valve (TV) leaflet.

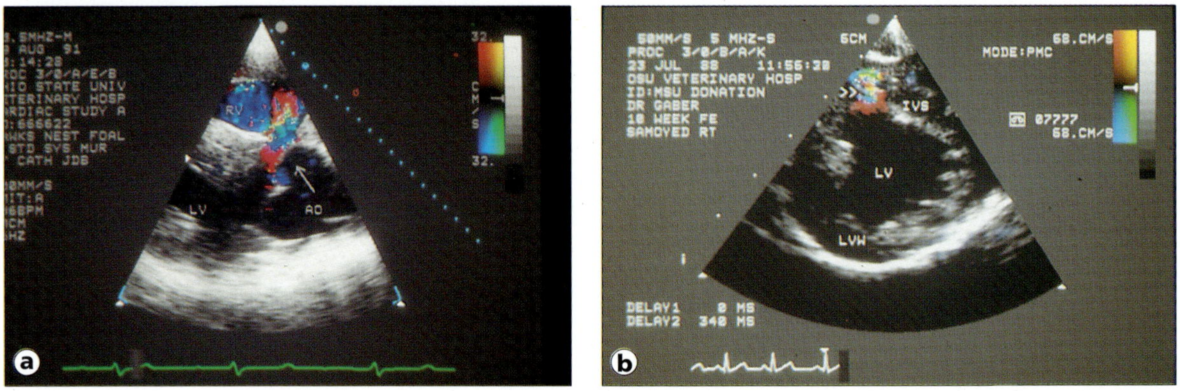

15.13 Colour-flow studies from ventricular septal defects that demonstrate left-to-right shunting. (**a**) Paramembranous VSD in a horse with flow across the defect (red, then turbulent). (**b**) An unusual muscular ventricular septal defect in a dog. The lesion is observed in a short axis image plane.

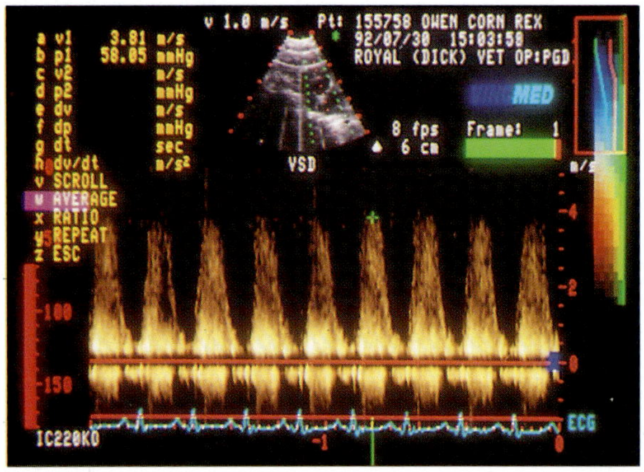

15.14 HPRF pulsed-wave spectral Doppler recording from a Cornish rex cat with a ventricular septal defect. The disturbed flow occupies much of the cardiac cycle, at a maximum velocity of 3.81 m/sec. This suggests a restrictive lesion.

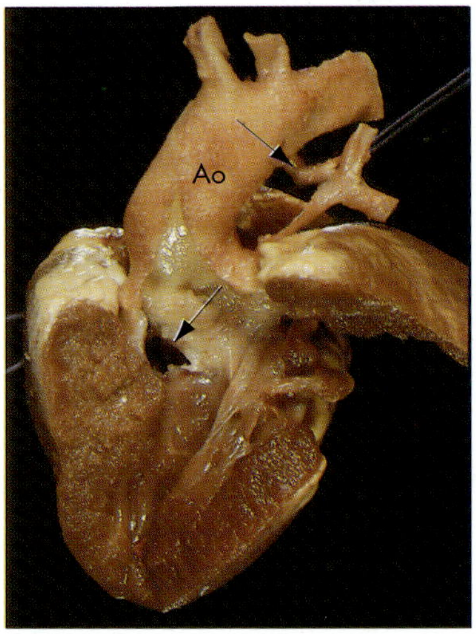

15.15 Tetralogy of Fallot with pulmonary atresia (pseudotruncus arteriosus) in a cat. The left ventricle has been opened to demonstrate the large, unrestrictive VSD (arrow), dilated ascending aorta (Ao), hypoplastic main pulmonary artery connecting to small left and right pulmonary arteries and a ductus arteriosus (arrow). Pulmonary perfusion in this situation depends on flow through the ductus or bronchial artery collateral vessels.

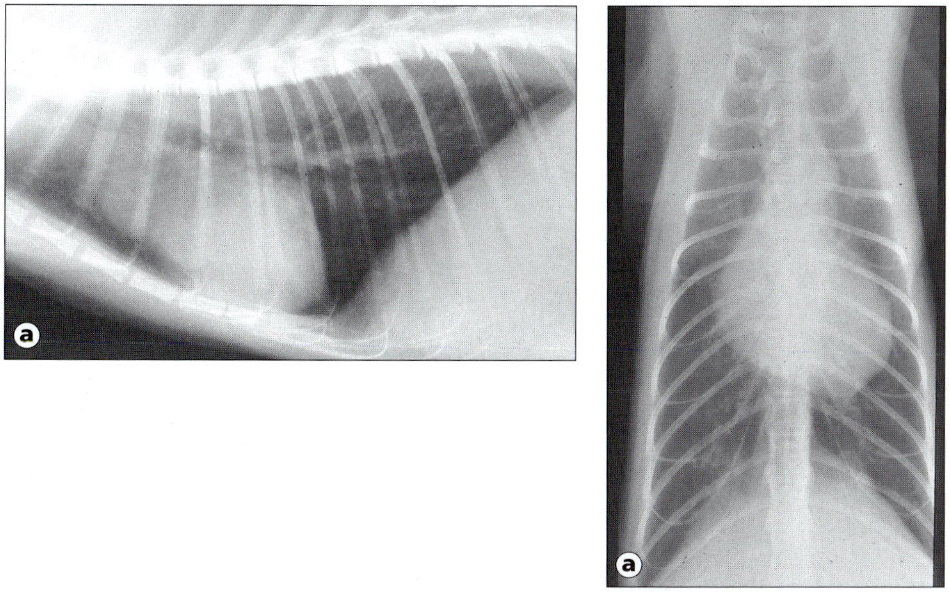

15.16 (**a** and **b**) Radiographs from the cat in **15.15**. (**a**) The dilated aorta is evident in the cranial mediastinum and pulmonary circulation is diminished. The ventrodorsal view (**b**) shows rounding of the heart compatible with right ventricular hypertrophy.

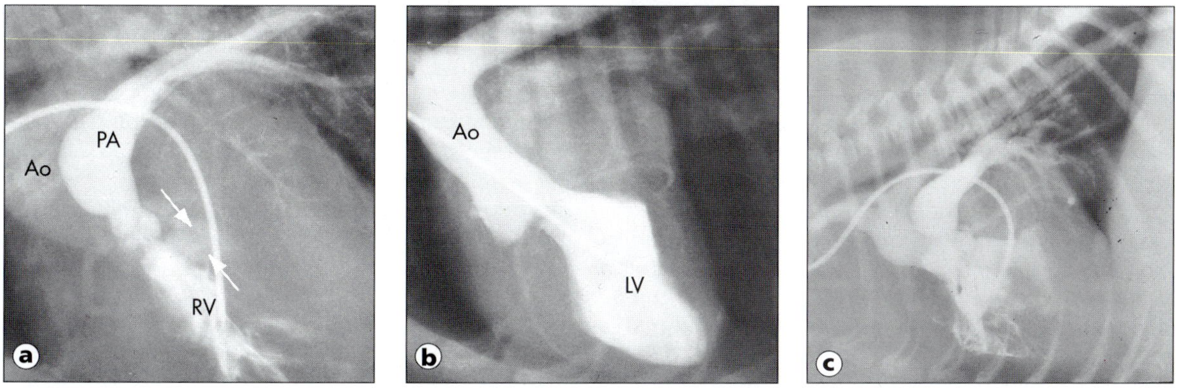

15.17 Angiography in canine tetralogy of Fallot. (**a**) Right ventricular injection demonstrates pulmonic stenosis and right-to-left shunting with opacification of the VSD (arrows) and the ascending aorta. (**b**) Left ventricular injection from the same dog shows over-riding of the aorta, straddling the VSD. (**c**) Right ventricular injection in a bulldog showing pulmonic stenosis and simultaneous opacification of the left ventricle and aorta.

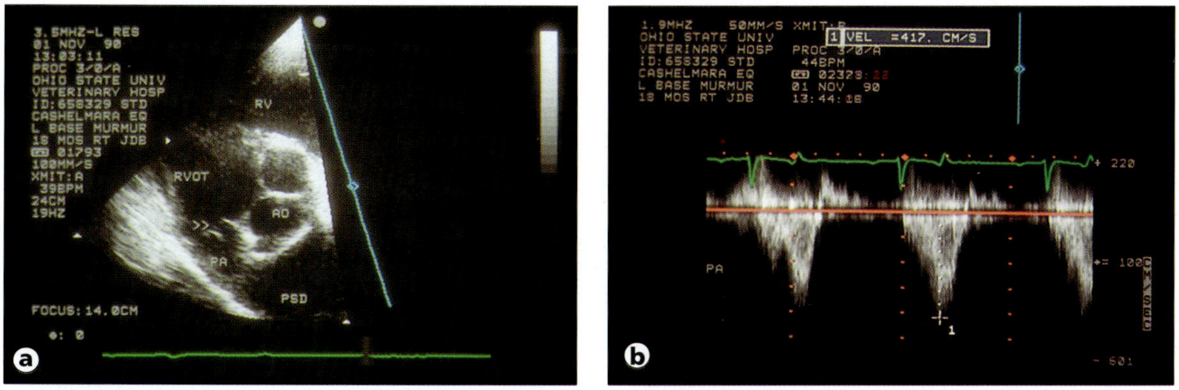

15.18 (**a**) Two-dimensional echocardiogram of tetralogy of Fallot in a filly. A large VSD is evident between the aortic root and the right ventricular outlet. The pulmonary valve is hypoplastic and stenotic (arrow heads). There is post-stenotic dilatation (PSD) of the main pulmonary artery. (**b**) Continuous-wave Doppler recording across the outflow tract demonstrates a high-velocity jet (almost 4.2 m/sec) of pulmonic stenosis.

16.

Dilated Cardiomyopathy

Idiopathic dilated cardiomyopathy (DCM) leads to heart failure in almost all species, most notably the dog, where it ranks second among causes of congestive heart failure (CHF). Dilated (previously called 'congestive') cardiomyopathy is characterized by a reduced myocardial contractility. Lesions observed at necropsy are nonspecific, but include generalized cardiac chamber dilatation and a 'flabby' appearance to the myocardium that cannot be explained by co-existing congenital heart defect, valvular lesion or coronary artery disease. Microscopic findings are also nonspecific, and are consistent with an underlying myocyte biochemical disorder; they include eccentric hypertrophy, focal endocardial fibrosis, muscle cell degeneration and necrosis, and separation of cells by oedematous extracellular ground substance or connective tissue. Ventricular dilatation (and fibrosis) also contribute to varying degrees of diastolic dysfunction and elevated ventricular end-diastolic pressure. Stretching of the valve annulus often causes mild-to-moderate mitral or tricuspid regurgitation. When moderate-to-severe loss of ventricular systolic function occurs, problems include exercise intolerance, atrial fibrillation and CHF (Chapters 1 and 3). Dilated cardiomyopathy often precipitates sudden death, probably from cardiac asystole or ventricular dysrhythmias.

The myopathic process may be the end-result of diverse disorders that affect myocardial cell function, including deficiencies of metabolic substrates or essential factors (taurine in cats, cocker spaniels and small breed dogs, L-carnitine in some dogs, selenium in horses and cattle), myocarditis associated with necrosis of myocytes (e.g. following parvovirus infection), severe global myocardial ischaemia (e.g. chronic ventricular tachyarrhythmia) or toxic injury to myocytes (e.g. doxorubicin administration in dogs and monensin ingestion in horses). The condition occurs most frequently in dogs, and is seen sporadically in cats, horses cattle, and ferrets. The larger canine varieties are most often affected, and a genetic predisposition is found in many breeds. Various spaniel breeds are also affected by DCM. Burmese and Abyssinian cats are predisposed, particularly if their diet is marginal in taurine. Furthermore, DCM is prevalent in some herds of Holstein–Friesian cattle.

Clinical signs of dilated cardiomyopathy (regardless of the affected species) are very similar. In contrast to chronic valvular heart disease, dogs affected by DCM are often relatively young, with many cases presenting between 2 and 5 years of age, though the range is very wide. Male dogs are affected more than females. Mild cases usually show few clinical signs, though a gallop sound, systolic murmur or arrhythmia may be detected during a routine examination. Symptomatic animals are usually presented for signs referable to progressive heart failure (see Chapters 1 and 3), including exercise intolerance, dyspnoea, coughing or fluid accumulation. Severe weight loss is often noted in giant canine breeds, though this is not a consistent finding. The pulse and left apical impulse are weak and may be irregular if an arrhythmia is evident. A gallop sound is the most consistent auscultatory finding, though soft heart sounds and apical systolic murmurs of mild-to-moderate intensity are often identified. Clinical signs typical of left-sided, biventricular or right-sided CHF are evident in advanced cases. Rapid, irregular, chaotic, variable-intensity heart sounds typify atrial fibrillation, which is the arrhythmia most commonly associated with DCM.

Advanced DCM is characterized by generalized cardiomegaly and radiographic signs of CHF (see Chapters 1 and 4). Echocardiography is the current clinical 'gold standard' for diagnosis of DCM and the cardinal findings are ventricular and atrial dilatation with depressed myocardial systolic function (fractional shortening $< 25\%$, and usually $< 15\%$ in symptomatic dogs). Doppler studies often demonstrate mitral regurgitation or tricuspid regurgitation, as well as the decreased aortic ejection velocity typical of myocardial failure. The ECG usually, but not always, shows abnormalities which may include signs of cardiomegaly or myocardial disease (see Chapter 5), persistent sinus tachycardia, atrial premature complexes, atrial tachycardia, atrial flutter or fibrillation, ventricular premature complexes, or ventricular tachycardia. Ventricular arrhythmias are especially common in boxers, and it is emphasized that ventricular arrhythmias in boxers, English bulldogs and some other breeds may be related to DCM or may represent the cardinal manifestation of a primary *arrhythmogenic cardiomyopathy* (e.g. so-called 'boxer myocarditis') which sometimes progresses to DCM. Routine haematology in DCM is usually normal, unless altered by heart failure, therapy for heart failure, or concurrent disease. Prerenal azotaemia, which is generally mild, occurs in about 25–30% of cases and may influence the dosage of digoxin (which is eliminated by the kidneys). Mild hypoproteinaemia is relatively common when there is ascites. Low plasma taurine concentration can be demonstrated in many affected cats and some cocker spaniels and small dogs with DCM. Low plasma or myocardial L-carnitine concentrations can be measured in some dogs with DCM, but these tests are not widely available .

Therapy for canine dilated cardiomyopathy involves the following principles: treatment of CHF; identification and control of significant cardiac arrhythmias; treatment of the underlying disorder, if known. The emergency treatment of severe CHF accompanied by cardiogenic shock (oedema with hypotension) is occasionally needed, and should include a 24–72 hour infusion of dobutamine or dopamine until the patient is stable. Thoracocentesis, intravenous furosemide, oxygen, and judicious vasodilator therapy (with blood pressure monitoring) are often required to control critical CHF. Once stable, home care for affected dogs or cats includes digoxin, diuretics, an angiotensin-converting enzyme inhibitor and dietary sodium restriction as outlined in Chapter 1. Atrial fibrillation is managed by controlling the fast ventricular rate with digoxin, and subsequently adding either a beta blocker or diltiazem (see Chapter 23 for details). Ventricular tachycardia is controlled with suitable antiarrhythmic drugs, typically procainamide, mexiletine or tocainide (see Chapter 23). Should plasma concentrations of taurine be low, a taurine supplement (feline dosage: 250 mg b.i.d.–t.i.d.; canine dosage: 500 mg b.i.d.–t.i.d.) should be prescribed, and the diet re-examined. Some cardiologists recommend empirical therapy with L-carnitine (50 mg/kg/day) for dogs with DCM; however, the cost:benefit ratio of supplementation has not been evaluated critically.

The prognosis of DCM with CHF, atrial fibrillation or recurrent ventricular tachycardia is guarded. With excellent home care and regular veterinary attention, most dogs live for 6–12 months following the initial onset of CHF or syncope. Experience with Doberman pinschers is most unfavourable, and those presented in cardiogenic shock, even when stabilized, often die within 3–6 months. Some breeds (e.g. the Irish wolfhound, Saint Bernard, Great Dane, and cocker spaniel) seem to stabilize after 1–2 months of therapy, and often live a good-quality life for 1 year or more. While the echocardiographic shortening fraction is diagnostic, it is not prognostic unless obvious improvement follows dietary supplementation; this is most often observed in cats and cocker spaniels with taurine-deficient DCM. The presence of recurrent ventricular arrhythmias increases the possibility of sudden death, even when CHF is well-controlled.

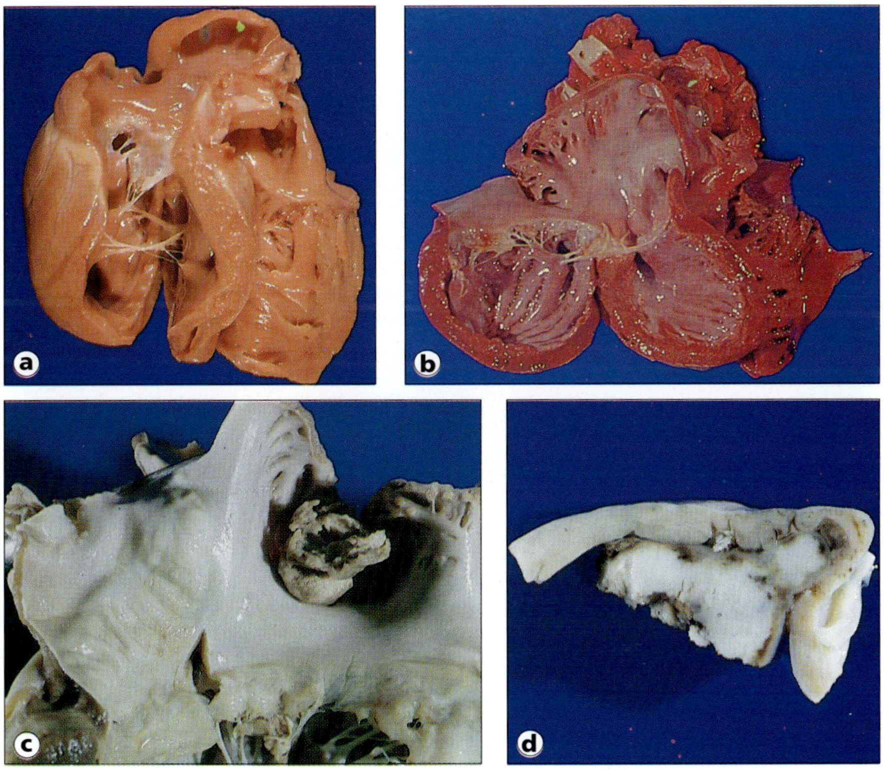

16.1 (**a**) Dilated cardiomyopathy in an 18-year-old female cat. The heart shows generalized chamber dilatation. (**b**) Dilated cardiomyopathy in a 6-year-old Irish wolfhound. There is massive generalized dilatation of the cardiac chambers, with secondary dilatation and incompetence of atrioventricular valves. (**c**) Atrial thrombosis in an 8-year-old Great Dane dog with atrial fibrillation. There is a thrombus firmly attached to the endocardium of the left auricular appendage. (**d**) In the same dog as **c**, thromboembolism has caused left ventricular myocardial infarction as a result of occlusion of the coronary arterial supply to the inner myocardium. Thromboembolism is more common in cats.

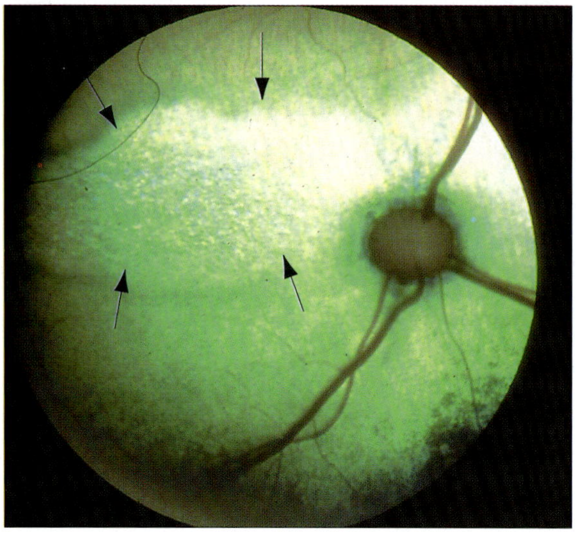

16.2 Retinal degeneration (arrows) in a cat with taurine-deficiency-related DCM. (Courtesy of Dr David Wilkie.)

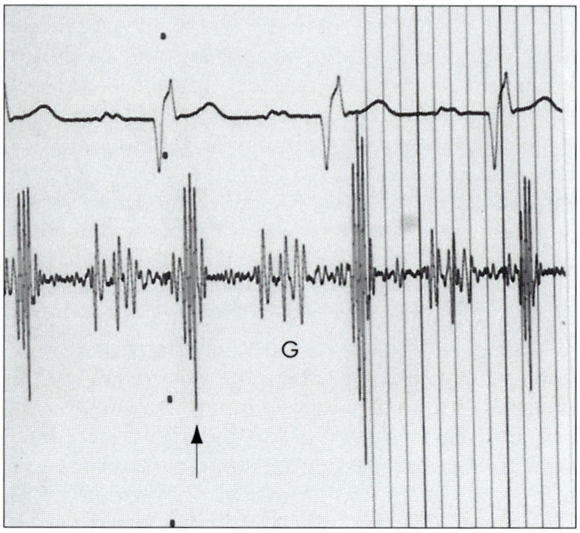

16.3 Phonocardiogram from a dog with DCM. The first sound is evident at the apex (arrow) as well as an S_3 and S_4 gallop (a summation gallop – G). The second sound is not recorded at this position (see also Chapters 3 and 5).

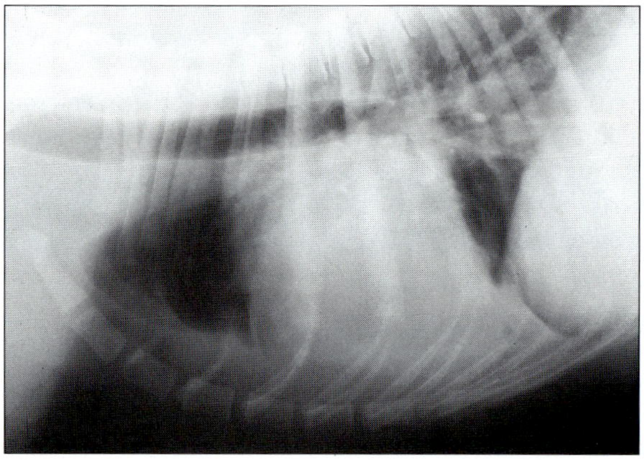

16.4 Lateral thoracic radiograph from an Old English sheepdog with DCM, showing pleural effusion which partly occludes the cardiac silhouette. There is also mild generalized cardiomegaly, with elevation of the caudal trachea, straightening of the caudal border of the heart, and pulmonary vascular congestion.

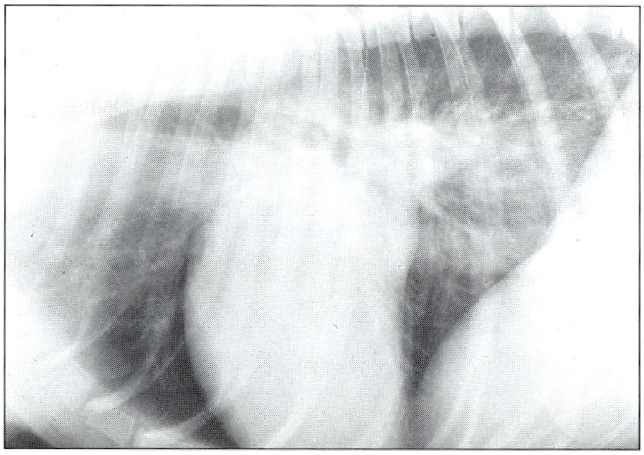

16.5 Lateral radiograph of a Doberman pinscher with dilated cardiomyopathy. Dogs of this breed with DCM often show much less cardiac enlargement than shown by other breeds. Most enlargement is typically seen in the left atrium, as in this view. There is also some pulmonary oedema and enlargement of the caudal vena cava.

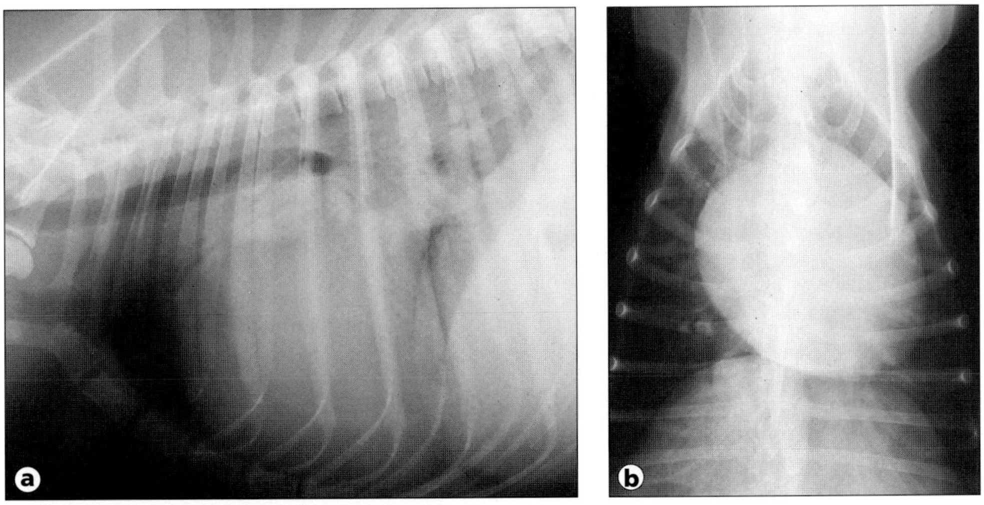

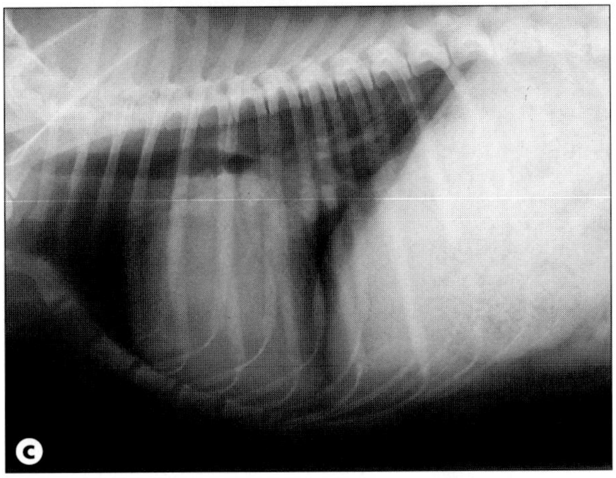

16.6 (**a** and **b**) Radiographs from a cocker spaniel with DCM, showing generalized cardiomegaly with marked left atrial enlargement. There is also pulmonary alveolar oedema that affects particularly the dorsocaudal lung fields. (**c**) Lateral radiograph from the same dog, 2 weeks later, showing a marked reduction in cardiac size and obvious improvement in pulmonary patterns. This radical improvement with routine therapy for congestive cardiac failure in DCM has been seen in a several cocker spaniels.

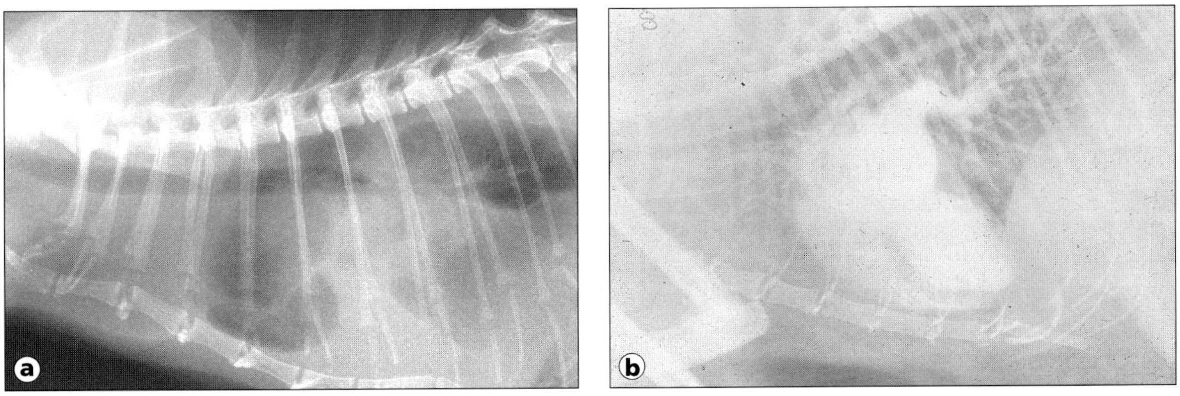

16.7 (**a**) Lateral radiograph of a cat with dilated cardiomyopathy and congestive heart failure. Pleural effusions mask the heart and diaphragm. The trachea is elevated – a finding that may indicate cardiomegaly or a large pleural effusion.
(**b**) Nonselective angiocardiogram from a cat with dilated cardiomyopathy demonstrating a dilated left atrium and left ventricle.

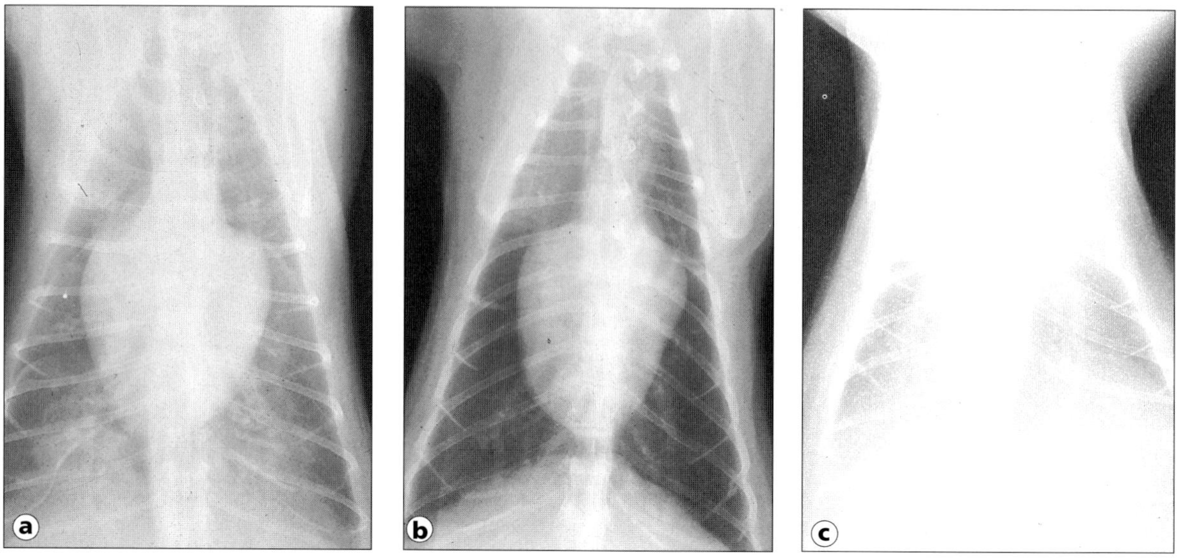

16.8 (**a**) Radiograph of a cat with DCM and alveolar pattern of pulmonary oedema caused by congestive heart failure. Note the 'valentine' shaped heart that is more usually attributed to hypertrophic conditions in cats. This demonstrates the lack of specificity of cardiomegaly patterns in cats with heart disease. (**b**) Following therapy, the lung parenchyma is normal, though the left ventricular elongation and left auricular enlargement are still evident. (**c**) Many months later, there is further decompensation; the same cat has a large pleural effusion that has responded poorly to medical therapy.

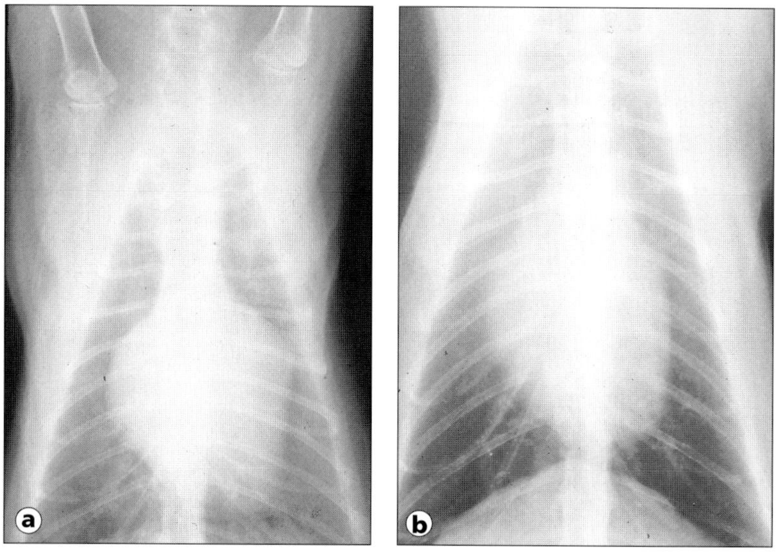

16.9 Radiographs from a cat with taurine-response DCM, before (**a**) and after (**b**) 5 months of taurine supplementation. The heart disease was largely reversible in this case.

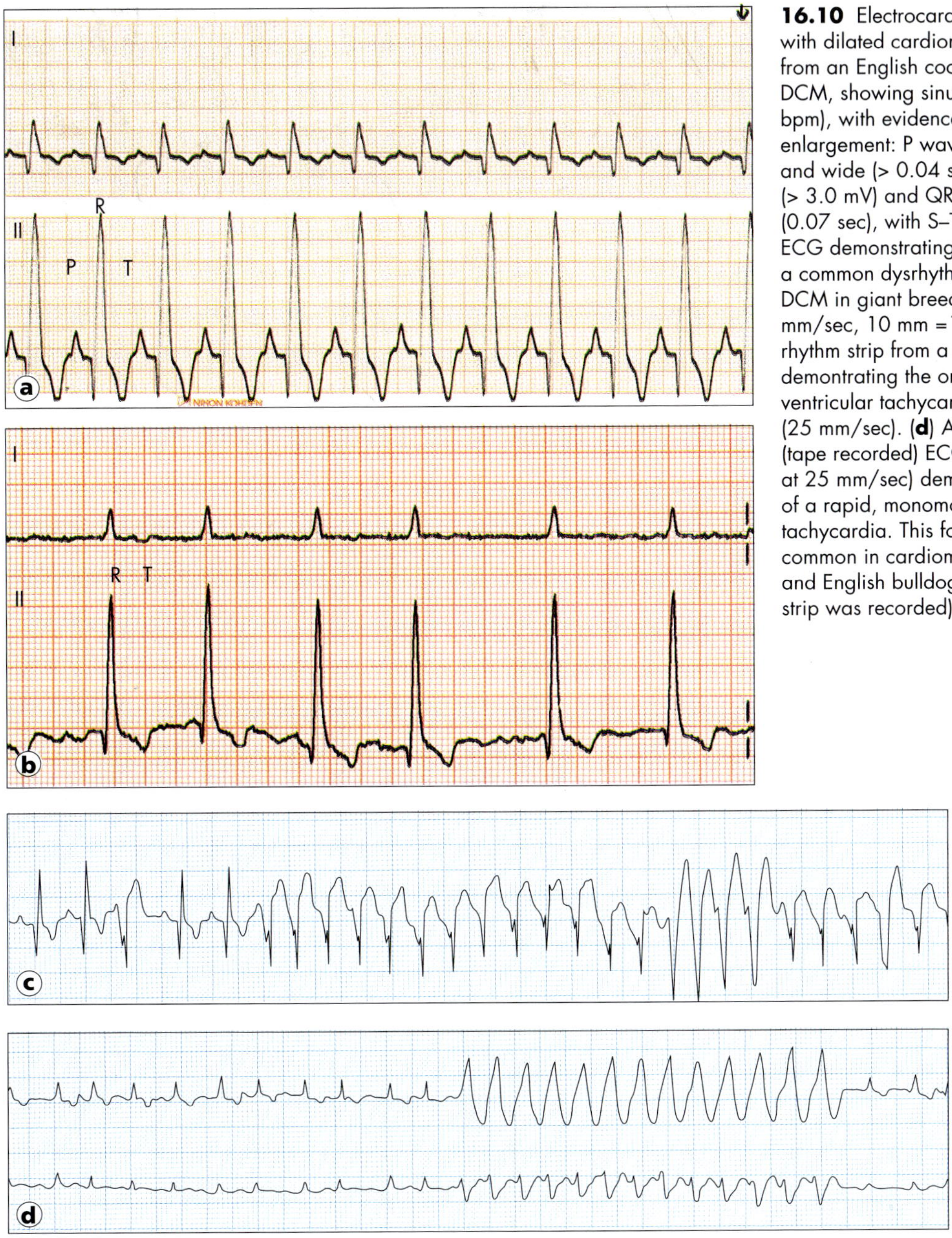

16.10 Electrocardiograms from dogs with dilated cardiomyopathy. (**a**) ECG from an English cocker spaniel with DCM, showing sinus tachycardia (200 bpm), with evidence of marked cardiac enlargement: P wave is tall (0.6 mV) and wide (> 0.04 sec); R wave is tall (> 3.0 mV) and QRS is prolonged (0.07 sec), with S–T coving. (**b**) An ECG demonstrating atrial fibrillation – a common dysrhythmia associated with DCM in giant breeds of dog (50 mm/sec, 10 mm =1 mV). (**c**) Lead II rhythm strip from a Doberman pinscher demontrating the onset of polymorphic ventricular tachycardia at a rapid rate (25 mm/sec). (**d**) Ambulatory Holter (tape recorded) ECG record (recorded at 25 mm/sec) demonstrating the onset of a rapid, monomorphic ventricular tachycardia. This form of arrhythmia is common in cardiomyopathies of boxers and English bulldogs (from which the strip was recorded).

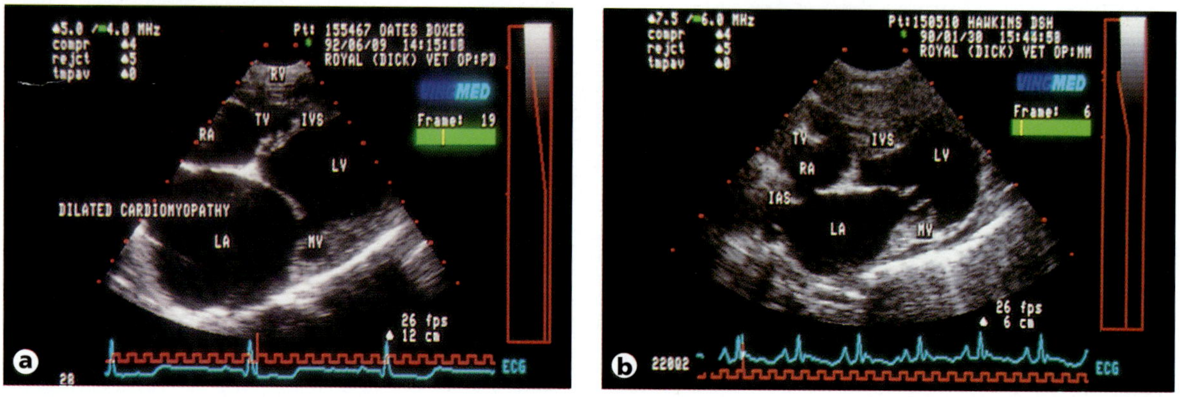

16.11 (**a**) Two-dimensional echocardiogram from a boxer dog with DCM, showing marked dilatation of the left side of the heart. (**b**) Two-dimensional echocardiogram from a domestic, short-haired cat with DCM, showing dilatation of the left side of the heart and the right atrium. (Courtesy of Mr Mike Martin.)

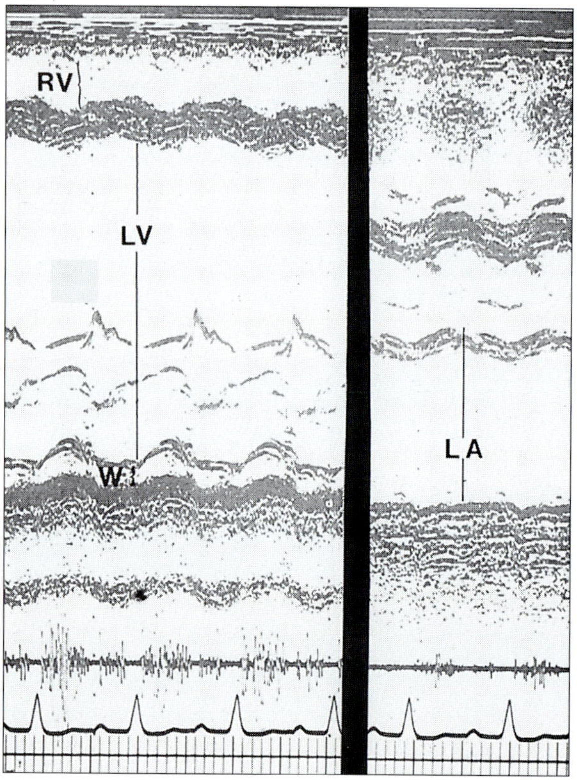

16.12 M-mode echocardiogram from a dog with DCM. The left ventricle is markedly dilated and the septum and free wall contract feebly, leading to a very low ejection fraction. The dilatation and low transmitral flow account for the poor opening of the mitral valve.

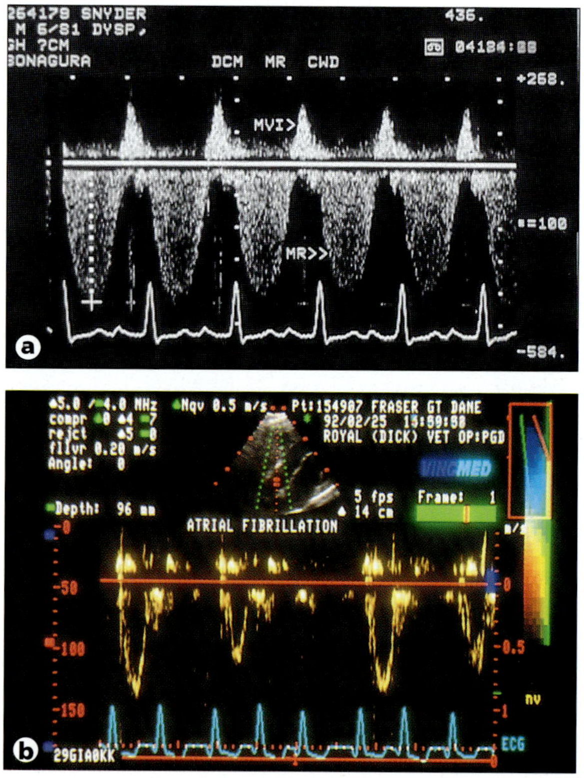

16.13 (**a**) Continuous-wave Doppler study from a dog with mitral regurgitation (MR) secondary to DCM. A high-velocity regurgitant jet is recorded below the zero baseline during systole. (**b**) Pulsed-wave spectral Doppler recording from the aorta of a Great Dane with DCM and atrial fibrillation, showing large variations and absent flow signals, related to variable preload. This is typical of animals with this disorder, and it accounts for the varying pulse and pulse deficit that is often present. Additionally, the maximum velocity of flow is reduced, the pre-ejection period is prolonged, and the ejection time is reduced – all typical features of loss of left ventricular systolic function in DCM.

17. Hypertrophic Cardiomyopathy

Hypertrophic cardiomyopathy (HCM) is a condition characterized by left ventricular hypertrophy that is unexplained by other causes. This disorder, which is common in cats, probably involves a genetic predisposition to abnormal myocardial protein synthesis. The resultant left ventricular hypertrophy (LVH) may be diffuse or segmental, with various patterns recognized echocardiographically and at necropsy. In the most common cases, the hypertrophy involves the free wall, papillary muscles and ventricular septum, and the ventricular lumen is normal-to-reduced in size. Intramural coronary arterial sclerosis is also evident at necropsy, and this may be important in limiting oxygen delivery to the hypertrophied myocardium. Cases of HCM have also been recognized sporadically in dogs, most notably in Boston bull terriers. Left ventricular hypertrophy can also be caused by a number of other diseases from which HCM must be differentiated, including feline hyperthyroidism, congenital aortic stenosis, systemic arterial hypertension and growth hormone excess (acromegaly).

Cats with HCM mainly have concentric hypertrophy, which reduces left ventricular distensibility. Diastolic function is further weakened by myocardial fibrosis, impaired relaxation (an active, energy-dependant process) and myocardial ischaemia. Higher than normal pulmonary venous and left atrial pressures are required to fill the left ventricle, predisposing the cat to pulmonary oedema. Stress-induced tachycardia can adversely affect myocardial oxygen balance, and may be responsible for sudden development of left-sided heart failure. Cats with hypertrophic cardiomyopathy may also be affected by abnormal systolic function. Mitral regurgitation, often related to systolic anterior motion of the mitral valve, is very common in HCM. Dynamic LV outflow tract obstruction may also occur, and can be demonstrated by Doppler as high-velocity, turbulent ejection through the outflow tract. Left atrial dilatation is common in cats; it is explained by the noncompliant left ventricle, mitral regurgitation and the elevated venous pressures that usually develop with this condition. Abnormal thrombogenesis often leads to left atrial thrombi which may dislodge to cause systemic thromboembolism.

Cases of HCM may be identified in asymptomatic cats of any age (even under one year old) during the course of a routine health examination; males and some breeds (e.g. Maine coon cats) are predisposed. A gallop sound, often with a systolic murmur over the left apical sternal border, is the most typical finding. Most clinically affected cats are presented with tachypnoea and dyspnoea caused by congestive heart failure or for signs of aortic thromboembolism (see Chapter 21). Congestive heart failure may be precipitated in compensated cases by stress, fever, moderate-to-severe anaemia, thyrotoxicosis, anaesthesia or fluid therapy.

Diagnostic studies can further characterize the clinical condition and rule out other causes of LVH. Radiographs usually demonstrate cardiomegaly (elongation) and left atrial/auricular enlargement (most evident on the VD view). Abnormal lung densities compatible with pulmonary oedema or a bilateral pleural effusion may be present. Prominent pulmonary vascular patterns may indicate pulmonary hypertension secondary to elevated left ventricular diastolic pressure. The ECG is often, but not always, abnormal, demonstrating various combinations of: atrial enlargement, LVH, left anterior fascicular block (see Chapter 5), atrial premature complexes or atrial fibrillation. Hypertrophic cardiomyopathy is characterized by echocardiography as increased left ventricular wall thickness (> 5.5 mm in cats), normal-to-decreased intraluminal size, normal or increased systolic shortening (in chronic cases, systolic function may deteriorate), possible ventricular septal hypertrophy obstructing the LV outlet, and left atrial enlargement. Two-dimensional echocardiographic studies often identify regional septal LV hypertrophy that is not evident in the left ventricular free wall, and over-reliance on one echocardiographic measurement is not advised. Most cats with clinically significant LVH have left atrial enlargement as well. Since similar echocardiographic findings can be encountered in congenital subaortic stenosis, systemic hypertension, or with hyperthyroidism, these conditions must be excluded for a definitive diagnosis. Doppler studies usually demonstrate mitral regurgitation and subtle-to-marked increases in flow velocity across the left ventricular outflow tract.

The management of life-threatening heart failure in cats with HCM includes rest, oxygen (40–50%) and sedation if necessary (acepromazine – 0.05–0.1 mg/kg, subcutaneously, unless hypothermia is severe).

Furosemide (2–4 mg/kg IV or IM) is given as an initial dose to ensure diuresis; the dosage is subsequently reduced to 1–2 mg/kg every 12 hours for the first 24–48 hours of therapy. Thoracocentesis is performed if there is a large pleural effusion. Nitroglycerine ointment may be given when there is florid pulmonary oedema (Appendix A2). Following diuresis, judicious fluid therapy may be needed if the cat will not drink or if azotaemia ensues.

Long-term medical management of feline HCM involves prescribing either a beta blocker (propranolol or atenolol) or a calcium-channel blocker (diltiazem) to prevent bouts of pulmonary oedema. Beta blockers block adverse sympathomimetic effects, prevent tachycardia and maximize ventricular filling time. Beta blockade is also helpful for reducing left ventricular outflow obstruction if significant gradients have been proven by Doppler studies. The dosage of the beta blocker should be titrated to obtain a resting heart rate of less than 150 bpm. The use of a calcium-channel blocker – diltiazem – is increasingly popular for chronic management of HCM and is usually preferred when cats have CHF or moderate-to-severe LVH demonstrated by echocardiography. Diltiazem may decrease the heart rate (less effectively than a beta blocker), improve ventricular relaxation, increase myocardial perfusion (since the drug is a coronary vasodilator) and lead to regression of hypertrophy. Further treatment is needed in cats with congestive heart failure. Furosemide is continued in cats that have experienced pulmonary oedema; however, the dosage often may be gradually reduced to a relatively low level (0.5 mg/kg once or twice daily), and increased as needed should fluid retention become more severe (up to 4 mg/kg t.i.d.). Adequacy of dosage is best determined by monitoring respiratory rate and thoracic radiographs. Renal function and serum potassium should be monitored regularly. Enalapril (0.25–0.5 mg/kg q12–24h) can be administered for refractory pulmonary oedema or pleural effusion. Nitroglycerine may also be used at home, particularly if the cat has episodes of dyspnoea or if the owner has trouble medicating their pet. Cats with atrial fibrillation can be managed with a beta blocker (or diltiazem) if necessary, with digoxin to control the ventricular rate. Dietary sodium restriction and aspirin (20–25 mg/kg two or three times weekly) or warfarin (Coumadin, 0.5 mg daily with careful monitoring of clotting times) are often prescribed in an attempt to prevent thromboemboli. The survival varies from weeks to years: thromboembolism and unresponsive CHF are poor prognostic factors.

Management of canine cases of HCM is difficult. Firstly, systemic hypertension should be excluded as the cause of LVH since this condition is managed differently (see Chapter 21). Beta blockers and diuretics have been used for management of canine cases, using suitable canine dosages (see Appendix A2). In contrast to the cat, sudden death is common in HCM in the dog, and it is advisable to monitor the heart with a 24 hour Holter ECG. Most cases should be evaluated by a cardiologist.

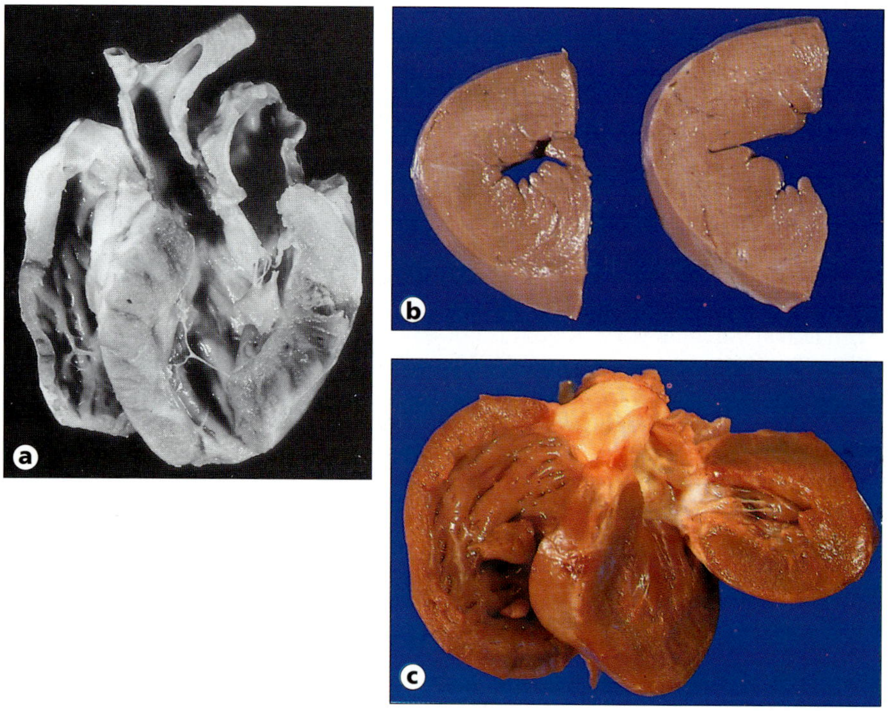

17.1 (**a**) Hypertrophic cardiomyopathy in a cat. (**b**) Hypertrophic cardiomyopathy in a 7-year-old Boston terrier that died unexpectedly, shortly after general anaesthesia. There is massive concentric hypertrophy of the left ventricular myocardium. This impinges on the ventricular lumen, compromising stroke volume. Under stress, dogs with such hearts may die suddenly. (**c**) Hypertrophic cardiomyopathy in an 18-month-old cairn bitch. The heart is enlarged (48.75 g) because of hypertrophy of all chambers. The relative heart weight (13.38 g/kg) is considerably greater than the normal range in dogs (6.6 +/– 0.3 g/kg) (Liu, Maron and Tilley, 1979).

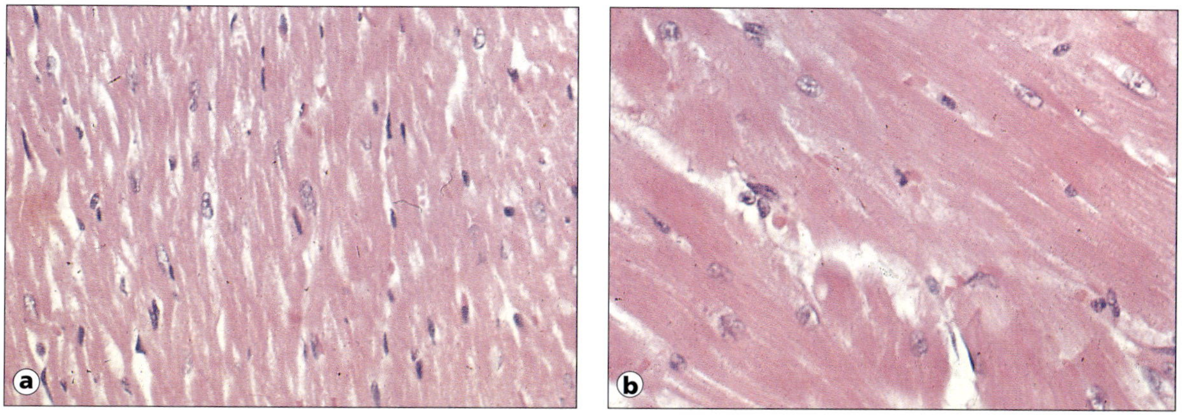

17.2 Photomicrograph of normal left ventricular myocardium (**a**) together with the hypertrophied fibres (**b**) from the heart in **17.1b**.

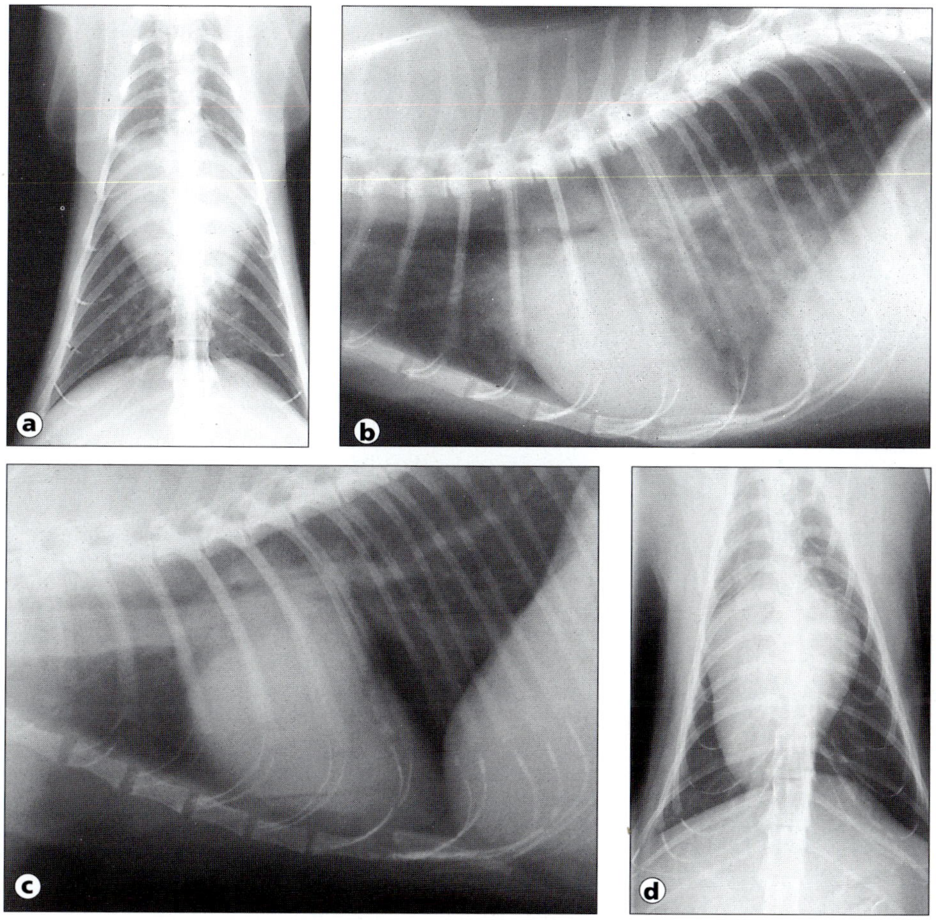

17.3
(**a**) Ventrodorsal radiograph demonstrating the classic 'valentine'-shaped heart of HCM. The elongated shadow indicates left ventricular hypertrophy while the large left auricle adds breadth across the heart. This finding is in no way pathognomonic for HCM. (**b**) Lateral radiograph of a cat with HCM and pulmonary oedema. Note the more dependent location of the alveolar infiltrate which is not uncommon in cats. The left ventricle is elongated. (**c** and **d**) Radiographs of a 7-year-old domestic short-haired cat with aortic thrombosis and hypertrophic cardiomyopathy showing gross cardiac enlargement, including both atria, and vascular overload, including the pulmonary vessels and caudal vena cava.

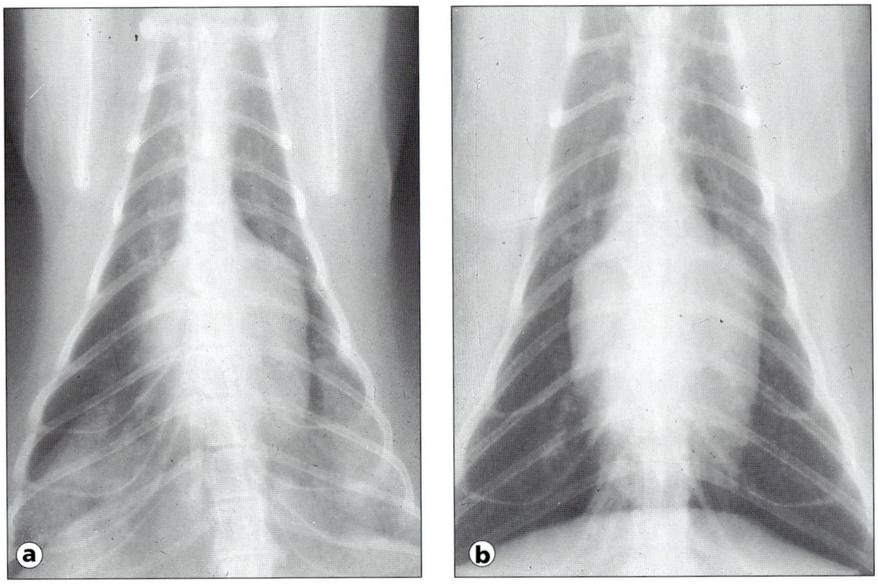

17.4 Radiographs of a cat with HCM before (**a**) and after (**b**) therapy for pulmonary oedema. The cat was treated with furosemide, nitroglycerine ointment and oxygen. There is also a slight decrease in cardiac size after therapy.

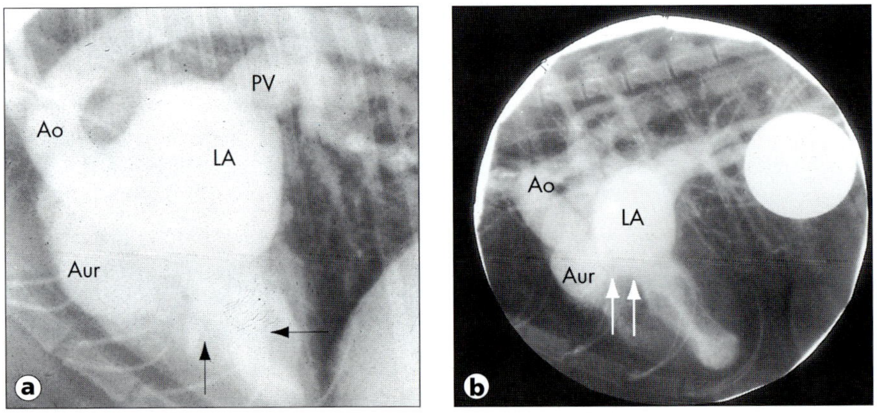

17.5 Nonselective angiograms of cats with HCM. (**a**) Distended, dilated pulmonary veins (PV), dilated left atrium (LA) and left auricle (Aur), and hypertrophied ventricle with prominent papillary muscles (arrows) are principal features. (**b**) Hypertrophic ventricle in systole demonstrating near complete obliteration of the midventricular cavity with outflow obstruction (arrows).

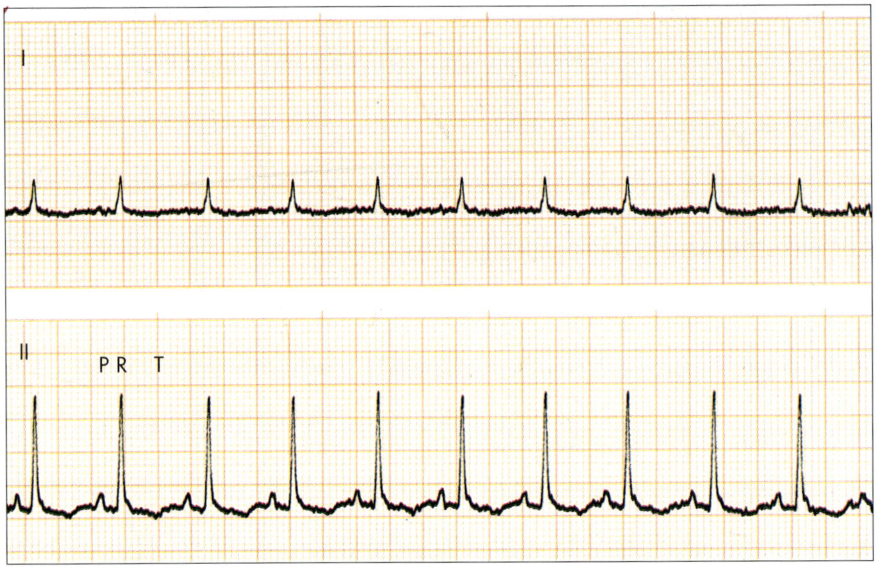

17.6 ECG of a 15-year-old short-haired domestic cat with hypertrophic cardiomyopathy, showing sinus tachycardia at a heart rate of about 240 bpm, and tall R waves in lead II (1.7 mV), consistent with left ventricular hypertrophy. (50 mm/sec; 100 mm/mV)

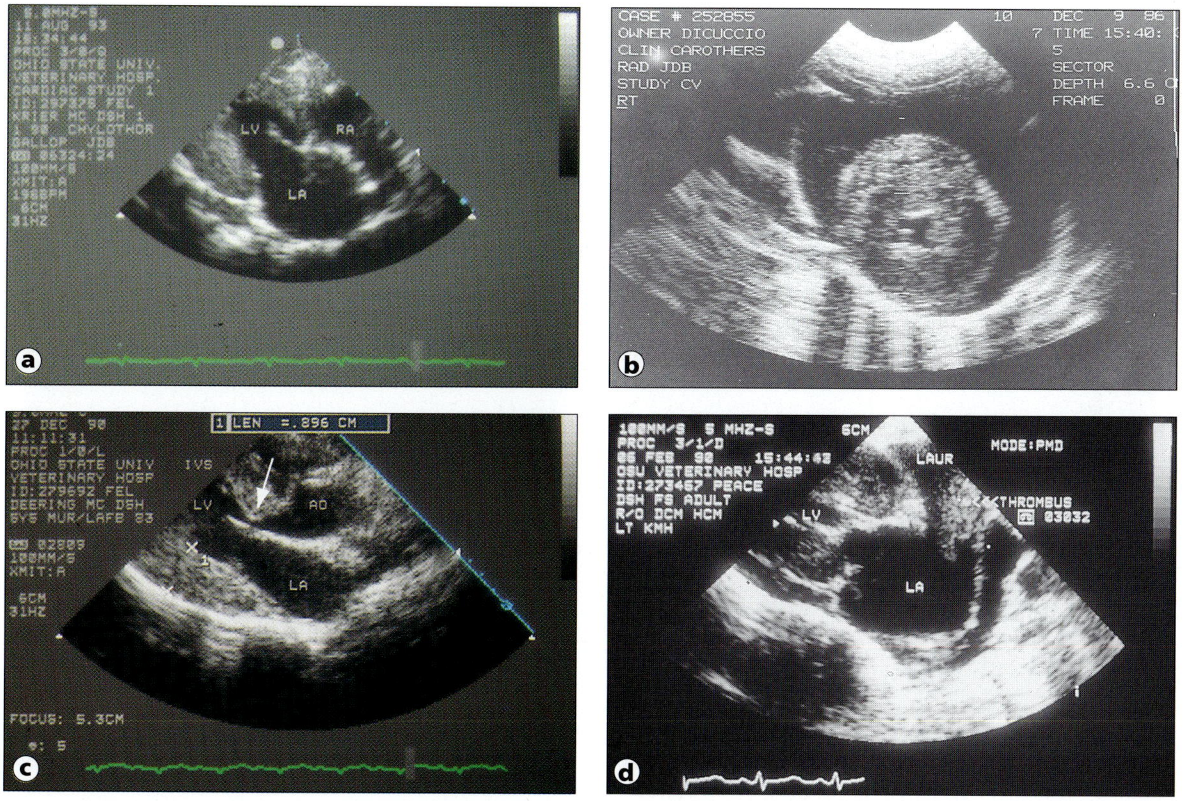

17.7 Echocardiograms from four cats with HCM. (**a**) Left atrial dilatation and asymmetric hypertrophy, with the free wall thicker than the septum. (**b**) Symmetric hypertrophy in the short-axis plane that is symmetrically involving the septum, free wall, and medial and lateral walls of the left ventricle. A pericardial effusion, related to congestive heart failure is also observed. (**c**) HCM involving the free wall and ventricular septum with a prominent dorsal septal bulge (arrow). (**d**) Left cranial dorsal placement of the transducer to evaluate the left auricle and the left atrium. There is a marked dilatation of the atrium and a mural thrombus is evident within the left auricle.

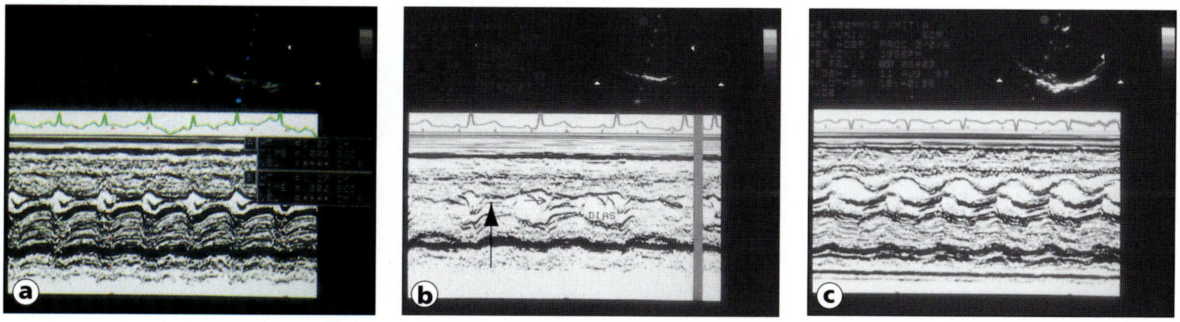

17.8 M-mode echocardiograms obtained from cats with HCM. (**a**) Severe hypertrophy of the free wall and septum in a young cat with HCM. (**b**) Mild HCM with systolic anterior motion of the mitral valve. The mitral septal contact (arrow) is indicative of a functional outflow obstruction – a potentially complicating factor in this disease. (**c**) M-mode study from the same cat as figure **17.7**(**a**). The free wall is markedly thicker than the septum, which is normal in thickness.

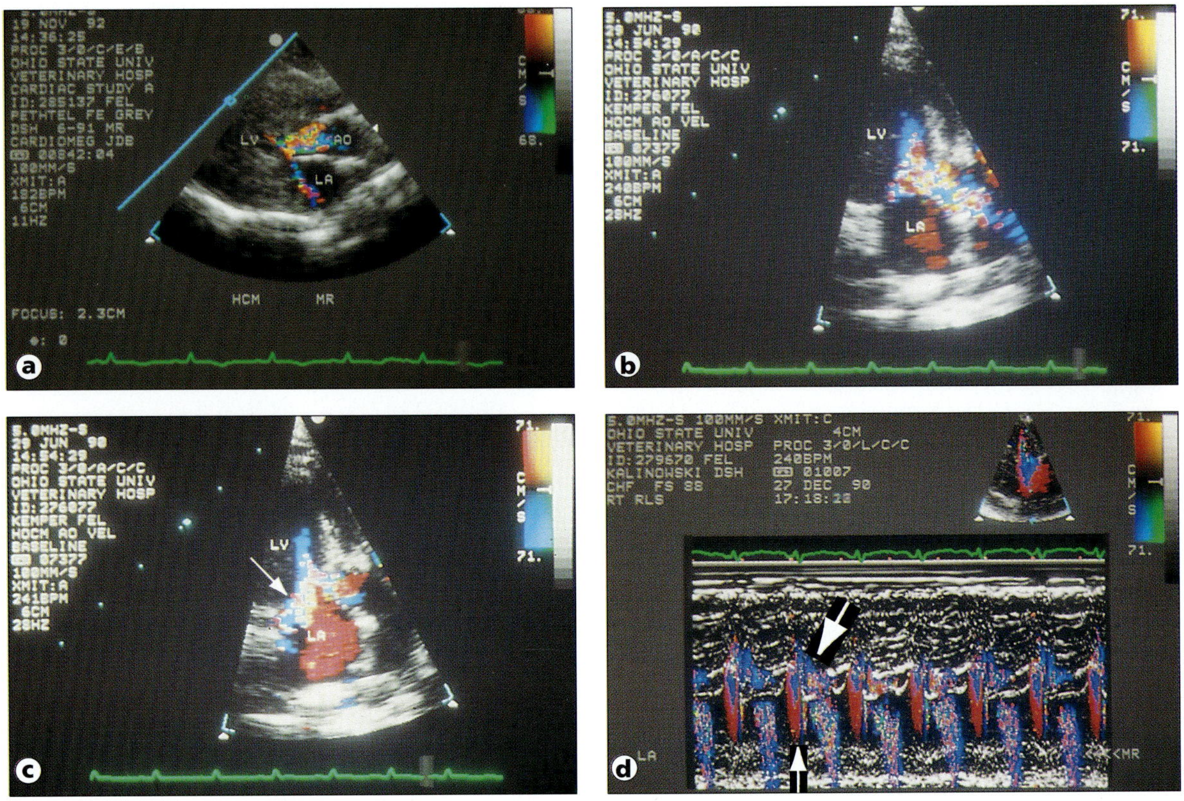

17.9 Doppler studies from cats with HCM. (**a**) Colour-flow study obtained from the right hemithorax that demonstrates a turbulent outlet jet and a mitral regurgitant jet. The apical left ventricular cavity is obliterated. (**b** and **c**) Early and late systolic frames from a cat with hypertrophic obstructive cardiomyopathy. Initial ejection into the aorta is followed by systolic anterior motion of the mitral valve which narrows the outflow tract and causes a jet of mitral regurgitation (arrow). The red flow pattern indicates normal venous return wells behind the mitral leaflets. (**d**) Colour M-mode Doppler demonstrating the timing of venous return (small arrow), ejection into the outflow tract (arrow) and mitral regurgitation. Mitral regurgitation begins after the onset of ejection.

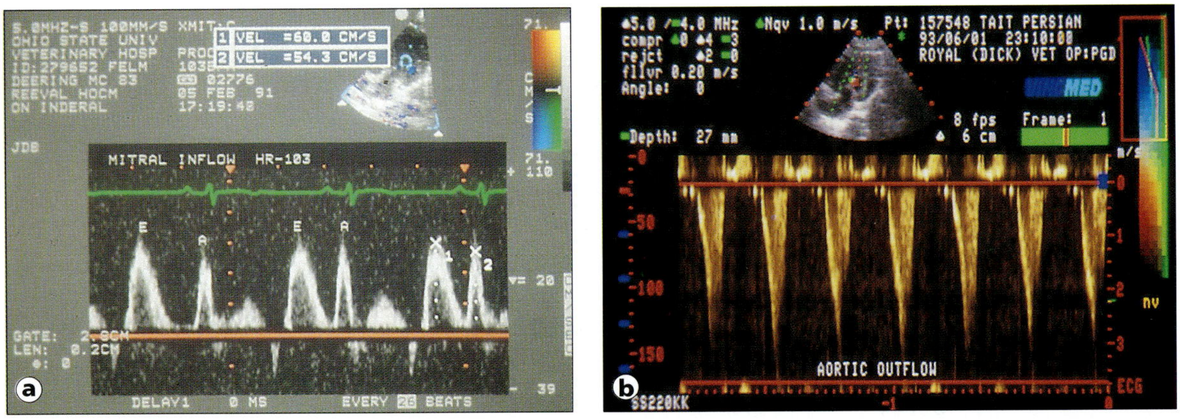

17.10 (**a**) Pulsed-wave spectral Doppler from the mitral inflow of a cat with HCM, showing an increase in the A wave (due to atrial contraction), and E–A reversal (owing to the decreased compliance of the left ventricle). (**b**) Pulsed-wave spectral Doppler recording from the aortic valve of a Persian cat with HCM. In this cat, there is excessive hypertrophy of the upper septum, causing outflow obstruction. This causes an increase in outflow velocity (to 3 m/sec) and disturbance in laminar flow.

18. Restrictive Cardiomyopathy

Careful investigation of cats with cardiac disease indicates that some primary myocardial disorders cannot be characterized as either hypertrophic or dilated forms of cardiomyopathy. These conditions have been termed *restrictive* or *intermediate cardiomyopathy* (RCM).

Various lesions have been observed in cats with clinical features of RCM: striking left or biatrial dilatation is typical; the left ventricle (LV) may be hypertrophied, dilated or normal in size; often there is regional thinning of the LV free wall or apex interspersed with focal or regional wall hypertrophy; prominent papillary muscle hypertrophy or fibrosis may be evident. Endomyocardial fibrosis of the LV is the characteristic diagnostic lesion and it may be patchy, multifocal or diffuse. Histologic lesions include endocardial thickening, endomyocardial fibrosis, myocardial interstitial fibrosis, myocyte hypertrophy, and focal myocytolysis and necrosis. While the pathogenesis of these lesions is undetermined, a prior bout of myocarditis is a possible cause. RCM in some cats seems to represent a late stage of hypertrophic cardiomyopathy complicated by myocardial failure or myocardial infarction. Extensive fibrosis also may occur in kittens with endocardial fibroelastosis; however, this condition is rare.

The pathophysiology of RCM in the cat probably involves aspects of both diastolic and systolic dysfunction of the left ventricle. These relate to stiffening of the ventricle from fibrosis, and to a decreased number or functional capacity of ventricular myocytes. LV fibrosis and marked left atrial dilation and fibrosis increase the resistance to right ventricular ejection, thereby leading to chronic pulmonary hypertension which can precipitate biventricular heart failure. Stasis of blood in a dilated left atrium undoubtedly predisposes affected cats to atrial thrombosis and systemic thromboembolism.

Cats affected with RCM are usually middle aged or older. Clinical signs are indistinguishable from those of hypertrophic cardiomyopathy in cats (see previous chapter). The ECG is frequently abnormal. Ventricular enlargement and myocardial disease can be manifested as any of the following abnormalities: widened QRS complexes (> 0.04 sec); increased amplitude R waves (> 0.9 mV) in leads II, aV_F, or III; intraventricular conduction disturbances including splintered R waves, right-axis deviation or left-bundle branch block; and ventricular extrasystoles. Atrial enlargement is supported by widened (> 0.035 sec) or tall (> 0.2 mV) P waves, atrial ectopic rhythms, or atrial fibrillation. The thoracic radiograph is characterized by marked left atrial dilatation and cardiac elongation that is typical of LV enlargement. Sometimes, generalized cardiomegaly is observed while other cats have a 'valentine'-shaped heart reminiscent of hypertrophic cardiomyopathy. Advanced cases often have radiographic evidence of pulmonary hypertension, pulmonary oedema or bilateral pleural effusions. Nonselective angiography (see Chapter 4) reveals marked left atrial dilatation and irregular filling defects of the left ventricular lumen. The most characteristic echocardiographic feature of RCM is marked left atrial or biatrial dilatation. LV shortening fraction is either normal or just mildly reduced (generally >25%) and the mitral opening (E point) to septal distance is minimally increased. However, marked regional wall dysfunction may be noted, most often affecting segments of the LV free wall. While the ventricle may be mildly dilated immediately ventral to the mitral valve, the left ventricular apex often appears hypertrophied and the papillary muscles appear thick or 'wooden'. Discrete thinned areas of ventricular scarring may be seen along with focal or diffuse, hyperechoic endocardial wall segments indicative of fibrosis. The right atrium and ventricle may be dilated in symptomatic cats, but are otherwise devoid of structural lesions. Doppler studies may indicate mild atrioventricular valve regurgitation. Clinical laboratory findings are not specific and most are attributable to heart failure, diuretic therapy, or thromboembolism. Plasma or whole-blood taurine should be measured, as decreased concentrations have been observed occasionally. Analysis of pleural effusates indicates either a transudate, modified transudate or chyle.

The immediate management of heart failure in cats with RCM is similar to that described in the previous chapter (see also Chapter 1). Diuretic therapy and thoracocentesis are crucial if advanced left-sided or biventricular failure is evident. Chronic therapy is centered on management of CHF and is identical to that described for dilated cardiomyopathy (see Chapter 16), including digoxin, furosemide, enalapril and a sodium-restricted diet. The daily furosemide dosage depends on the severity of fluid accumulation and must be adjusted to effect. Efficacy of diuretic therapy is monitored by respiratory rate, level of activity and chest radiography. Excessive diuretic or vasodilator therapy can be detected by periodic measurement of blood pressure, serum urea, creatinine and electrolytes. Mild azotaemia may be the necessary price of effective diuretic therapy in this disorder. The value of other treatments (e.g. diltiazem) in RCM is unresolved. Aspirin (1/4 of a 300 mg tablet, every 3 days) or warfarin (Coumadin, 0.5 mg daily with careful monitoring of clotting times) are often prescribed to inhibit thrombosis. Should progressive pleural effusion or ventricular tachycardia develop, the clinician should consider referring the cat to a cardiologist. Diltiazem or a beta blocker may be indicated in cases of RCM complicated by atrial fibrillation, as either drug can slow the rapid ventricular rate response to <200bpm (see Chapter 23). The long-term prognosis of RCM is guarded and quite variable. Unfortunately, relentless CHF, refractory pleural effusion or systemic thromboembolism offer formidable obstacles to long-term survival.

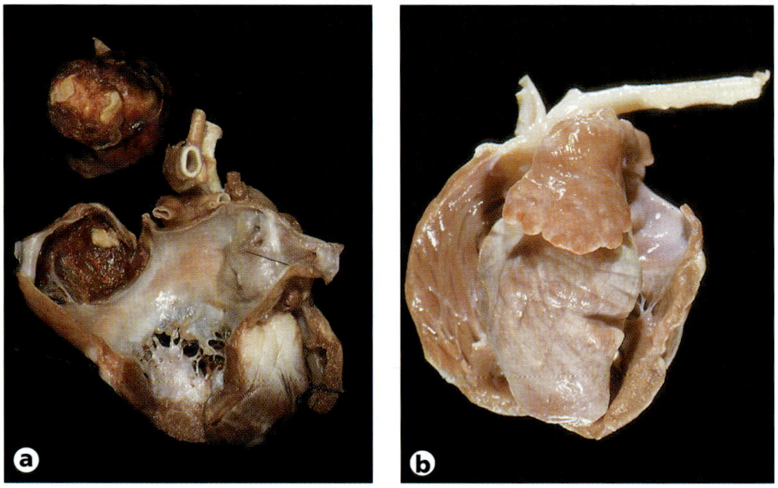

18.1 Pathology of feline restrictive cardiomyopathy (RCM). (**a**) Opened left auricle and ventricle viewed from above. A large ball thrombus has been removed from the left auricle. There is a dilated left auricle. The left ventricle has a large area of white discoloration that was found to be fibrous tissue. This is most evident in the papillary muscle. (**b**) Heart viewed from the left lateral perspective. The principal features in this cat are left auricular dilatation, focal areas of myocardial necrosis and fibrosis, and diffuse white discoloration of the ventricular muscle. Histological examination indicated severe, diffuse, myocardial fibrosis.

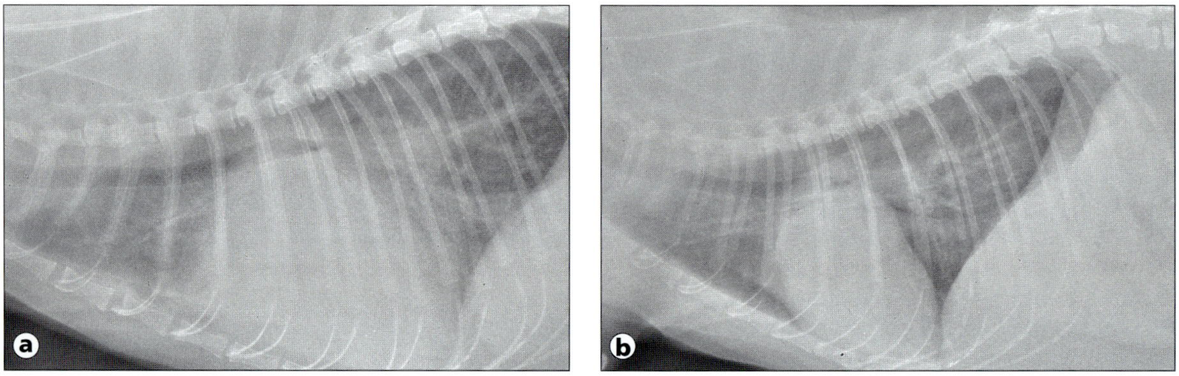

18.2 Lateral radiographs from a cat with RCM taken before (**a**) and after (**b**) therapy for heart failure. There is improvement but not complete resolution of the pulmonary infiltrates. The marked reduction in cardiac size is a consequence of diuresis and resolution of pericardial effusion. Pericardial effusion is a common sign of biventricular congestive heart failure in cats.

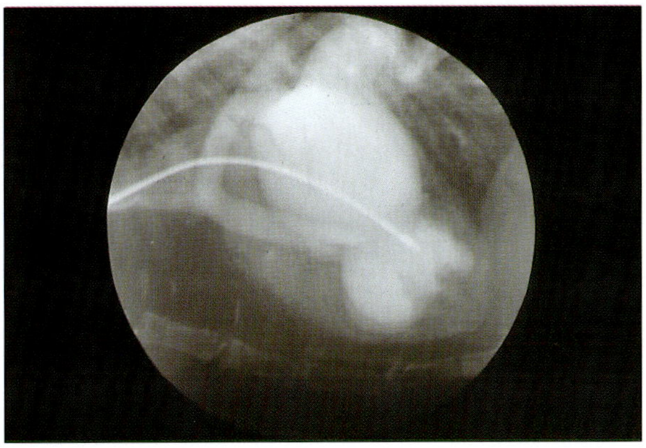

18.3 Nonselective angiogram from a cat with restrictive cardiomyopathy demonstrating a marked filling defect in the apical portion of the left ventricle, mild dilatation at the basilar left ventricle and severe left atrial dilatation.

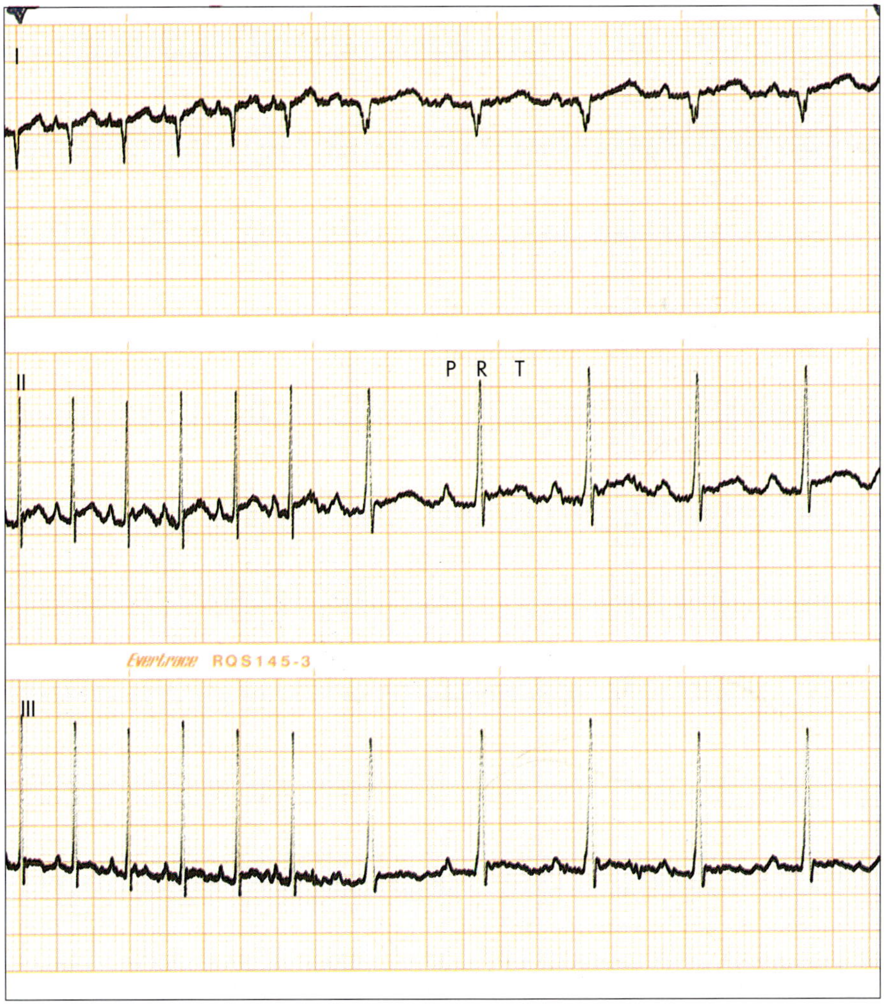

18.4 ECG recorded in leads I, II and III at 25 and 50 mm/sec from a 17-year-old short-haired domestic cat with restrictive cardiomyopathy, showing regular sinus rhythm at a heart rate of about 205 bpm. There is a right axis deviation, with a tall R wave in leads II and III (2.0 mV), consistent with biventricular enlargement.

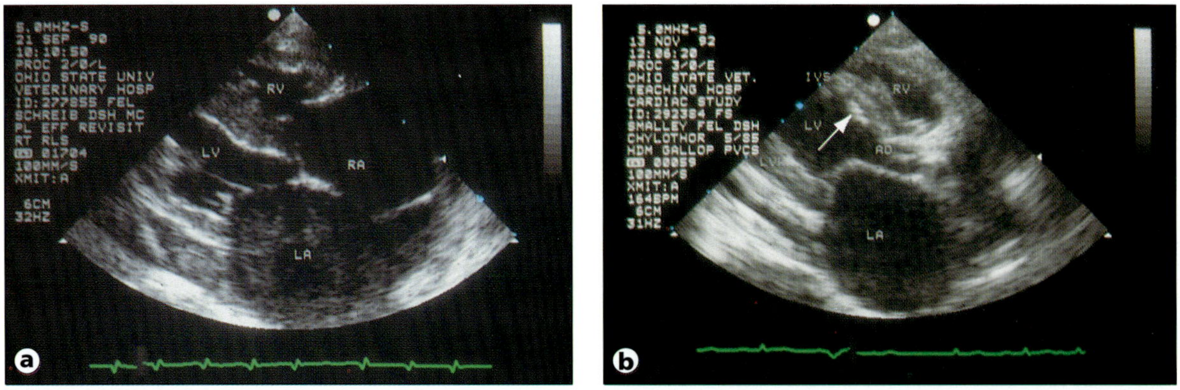

18.5 Two-dimensional echocardiograms from two cats with RCM. (**a**) Severe biatrial dilatation is evident in this frame. There is also a pleural effusion. (Courtesy of Dr Rebecca L. Stepien.) (**b**) Severe left atrial dilatation, mild left ventricular free wall hypertrophy, small pericardial effusion, and hyperechoic ventricular septal endocardium (arrow) from a cat with RCM.

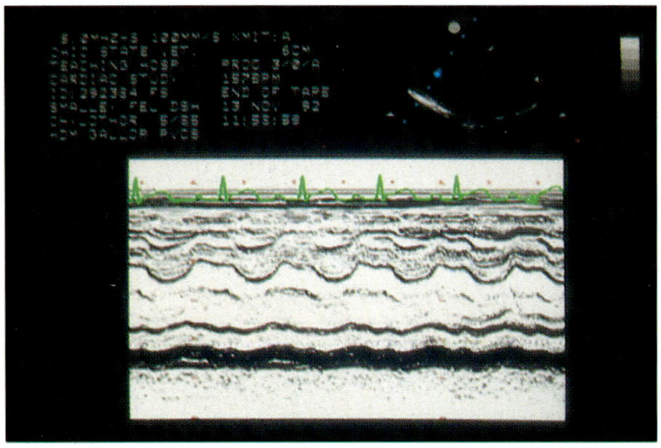

18.6 M-mode echocardiogram from a cat with RCM (same cat as in **18.5b**). There is marked regional dysfunction of the left ventricular free wall characterized by diminished thickening and contraction.

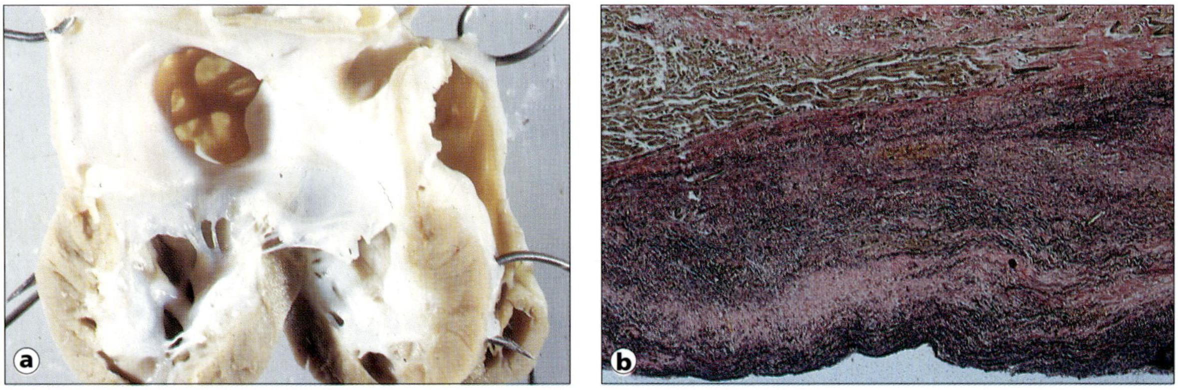

18.7 (**a**) Endocardial fibroelastosis in a 5-year-old male Siamese cat showing diffuse opacity of all chambers. (**b**) Photomicrograph from another cat with endocardial fibroelastosis, showing diffuse opaque endocardial pallor caused by collagen and elastic fibre deposition. This fibrosis has a constrictive effect on chamber filling and may encroach on conduction fibres, interfering with myocardial contraction.

19. Secondary Myocardial Diseases

In addition to the idiopathic cardiomyopathies described in the previous two chapters, a number of well-characterized agents and diseases can cause myocardial injury. Many of these disorders are multisystemic and the heart represents just one target organ; in other instances, cardiac disturbances are prominent. The myocardium can be affected by infectious or immune-mediated myocarditides or neoplasia, or injured by contusion, nutritional deficiency, genetic diseases, metabolic and endocrine disturbances or ischaemia (see Chapter 21). Should myocardial injury be widespread, a significant loss of contractility can lead to cardiac failure. Myocardial diseases can also predispose the heart to dysrhythmias, either by interfering with conduction or by acting as foci for re-entry or ectopic pacemaker activity. Cardiac-related tumours can obstruct blood flow, leading to ascites or oedema or they may bleed into the pericardial sac, causing cardiac tamponade (see Chapter 20). Consequently, cardiac manifestations of secondary myocardial disease are quite variable. Examples of these conditions are discussed in this chapter.

A myocardial disorder may be suspected when a dysrhythmia is detected by auscultation and confirmed by an ECG. Physical examination and blood pressure monitoring may demonstrate signs of inadequate circulatory function or even congestive heart failure. Thoracic radiographs usually show no specific changes, but merely reflect the state of myocardial contractility and circulatory function. However, with cardiac neoplasia, heart-base tumour or secondary pericardial effusion, radiographic changes are often observed. Echocardiography is valuable for the identification of myocardial dysfunction, or cardiac or pericardial neoplasia. Large myocardial infarcts and areas of myocardial degeneration, necrosis or cellular infiltration may be observed with high quality ultrasonography or other new imaging techniques (e.g. magnetic resonance imaging or computerized tomography). Nonetheless, small infiltrative neoplasms or areas of multifocal myocarditis or infarction will not be seen, and a wide variety of systemic illnesses affect the heart and circulation.

Myocarditis and myocardial necrosis are recognized sporadically in all species. Parvovirus, toxoplasmosis, and other infective agents may induce myocarditis. Idiopathic myocarditis has been recognized in boxers and bulldogs. Nonsuppurative myocarditis has long been recognized in cats and may be a component in the development of restrictive cardiomyopathy (see Chapter 18). Myodegeneration and necrosis secondary to selenium and/or vitamin E deficiency is well recognized as a generalized muscle disturbance in horses and farm animals. The definitive clinical diagnosis of myocarditis requires endomyocardial biopsy; however, diagnosis usually requires a level of clinical suspicion and exclusion of other possibilities.

Cardiac tumours may be primary or metastatic. Clinical manifestations usually include arrhythmia or conduction disturbance, obstruction to venous return, or pericardial haemorrhage with cardiac tamponade. Cattle and cats are prone to cardiac lymphosarcoma, while this occurs sporadically in dogs and horses. Haemangiosarcoma of the right atrium is common in dogs. Chemodectomas are frequently encountered in older brachycephalic breeds.

Heart function is also influenced by many metabolic and endocrine disorders. Hyperthyroidism (principally in cats) and hypothyroidism (notably in dogs) both affect cardiac contractility and heart rate. Hyperthyroidism is probably the most common endocrine-related cardiac disorder in the cat. This leads to marked cardiac hypertrophy. The resultant cardiomyopathy must be distinguished from primary myocardial diseases (e.g. hypertrophic cardiomyopathy). Failure to control the endocrinopathy may lead to inappropriate cardiac therapy. Advanced hyperthyroidism causes myocardial failure with biventricular congestive heart failure. Similar findings can occur in large animals with severe and chronic anaemia or with trace mineral disturbances.

Electrolyte disturbances affect particularly the cardiac rhythm (see Chapter 23). Hyperkalaemia and hypokalaemia, disorders often related to adrenal or renal diseases, have potent effects on rhythm and myocardial function. Pronounced hypocalcaemia or hypophosphataemia can impair myocardial contractility, and hypomagnesaemia (especially when combined with low potassium) can lead to refractory ventricular rhythm disturbances.

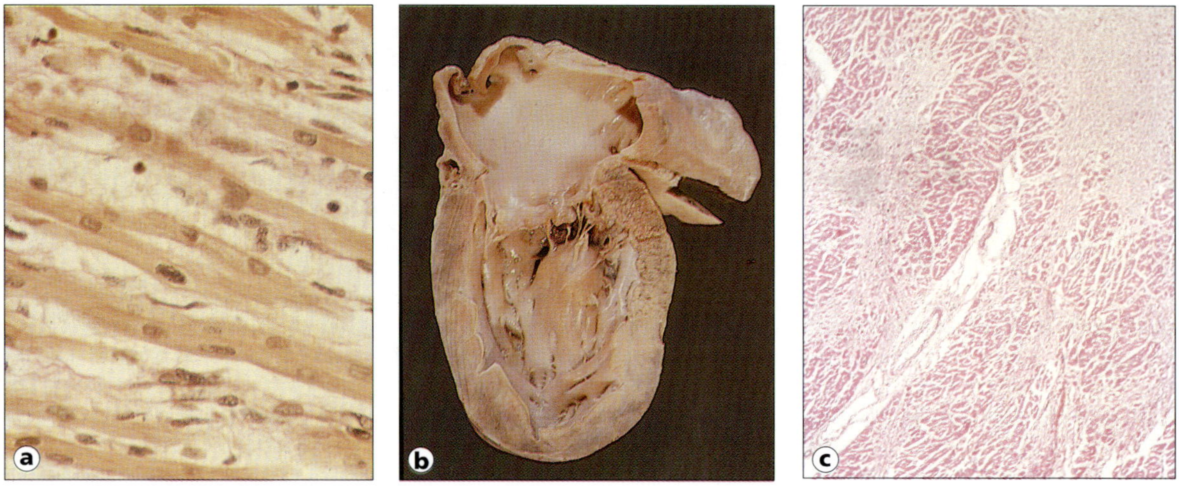

19.1 (**a**) Infection of the heart of young puppies with parvovirus can result in myocardial fibre injury. Infected cells develop large basophilic intranuclear inclusion bodies. More severe myofibre injury may be accompanied by cell loss, interstitial oedema and mild myocarditis. Affected puppies may die suddenly at this stage with ventricular fibrillation. (**b** and **c**) Puppies that survive the acute infection may develop myocardial scarring at the sites of earlier injury; these dogs may also die suddenly, or may develop chronic cardiac failure with patchy, randomly distributed myocardial fibrosis (from a 12-week-old cavalier King Charles spaniel).

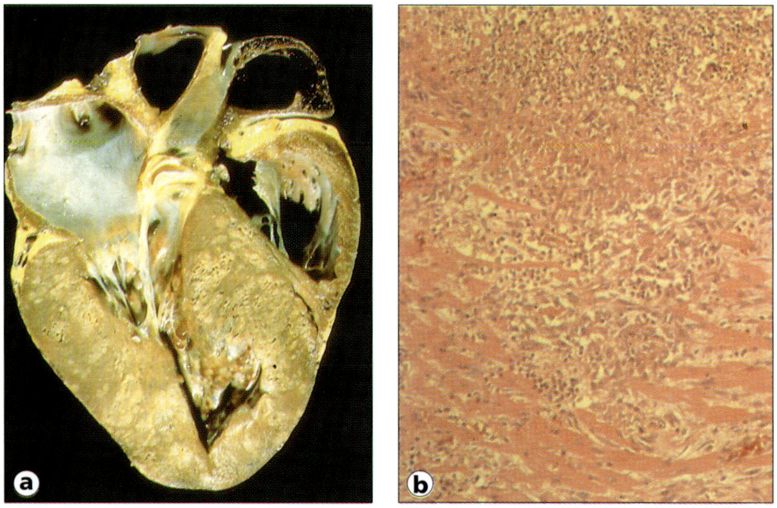

19.2 Granulomatous myocarditis in a 4-year-old German shepherd dog. (**a**) Multifocal discoloration of the myocardium due to cellular infiltration and necrosis secondary to infection by *Acremonium* sp (courtesy of Dr SE Johnson). (**b**) Microscopic section from the dog in **a** demonstrates disruption and necrosis of myocytes and marked granulomatous inflammation.

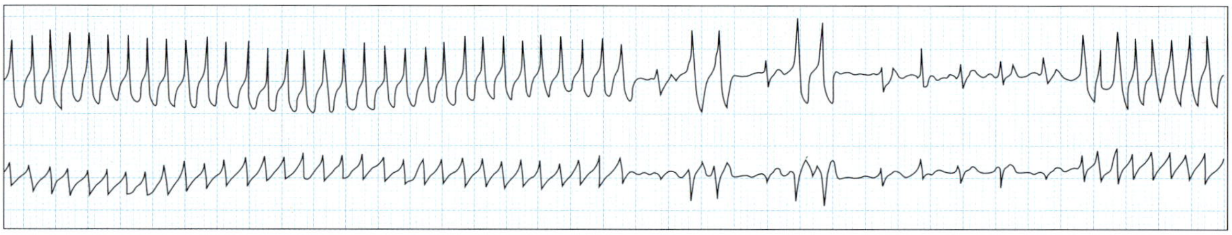

19.3 Sustained ventricular tachycardia in an English bulldog with arrhythmogenic cardiomyopathy recorded by Holter ECG during a period of collapse. The ventricular rate during the tachycardia is nearly 300bpm. Boxers, bulldogs, Doberman pinschers, German shepherds and mastiffs, among other breeds, may manifest a primary ventricular arrhythmia that is unrelated to myocardial failure or dilated cardiomyopathy.

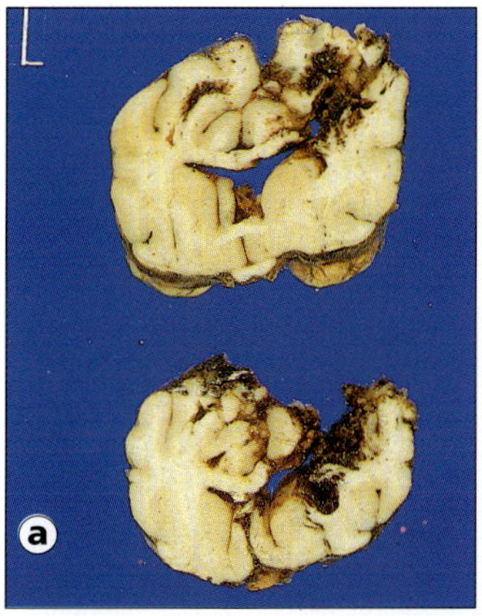
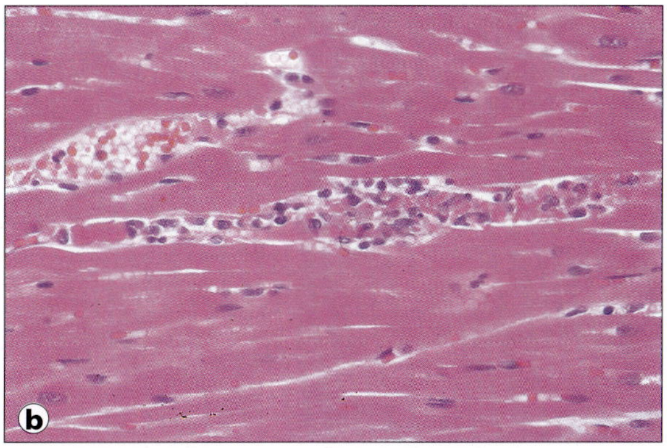
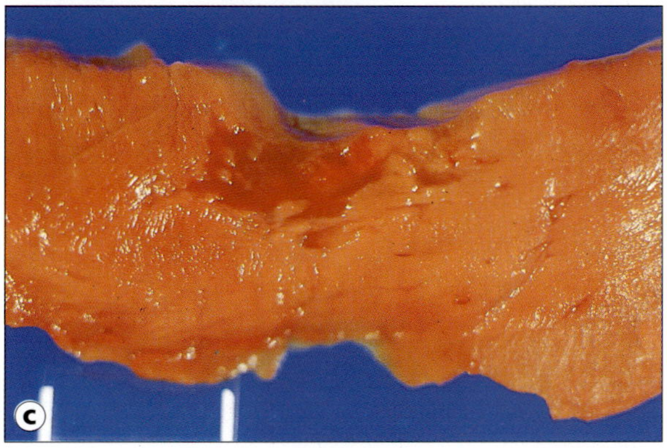
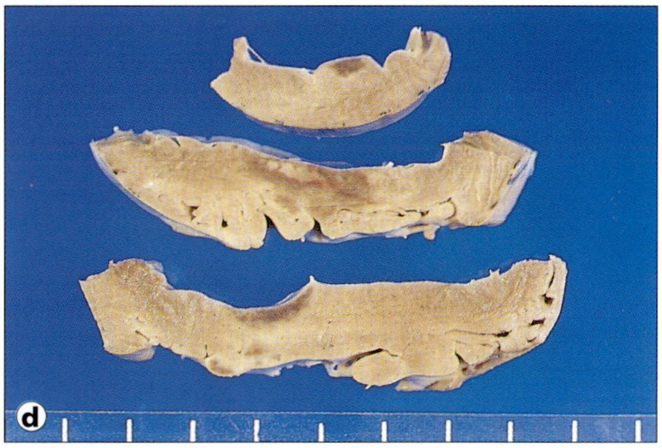
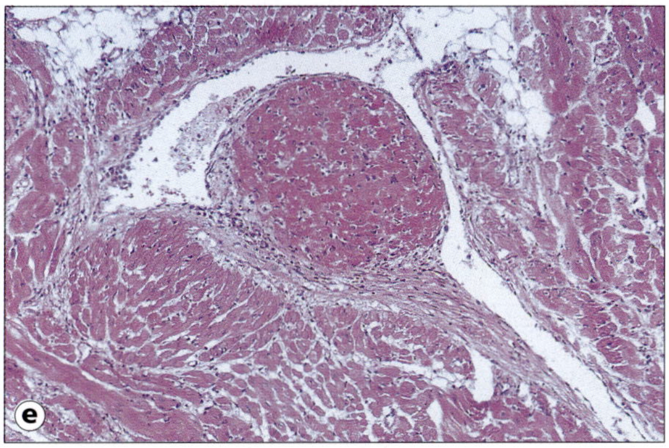

19.4 (**a** and **b**) Focal myocardial necrosis (FMN) associated with brain injury in a 3-year-old Doberman. (**a**) There is extensive laceration and haemorrhage in the cerebrum. (**b**) The photomicrograph shows FMN with minimal associated inflammatory reaction. This is a complication of increased catecholamine output. (**c**) Myocardial infarction in an 8-year-old standard poodle. In the interventricular septum there is a solitary, well circumscribed area of coagulative necrosis. (**d**) Multiple small and larger areas of myocardial infarction in the interventricular septum of a 5-year-old cross-bred dog. (**e**) Organizing mural thrombosis in the left atrium of a 4-year-old male Great Dane.

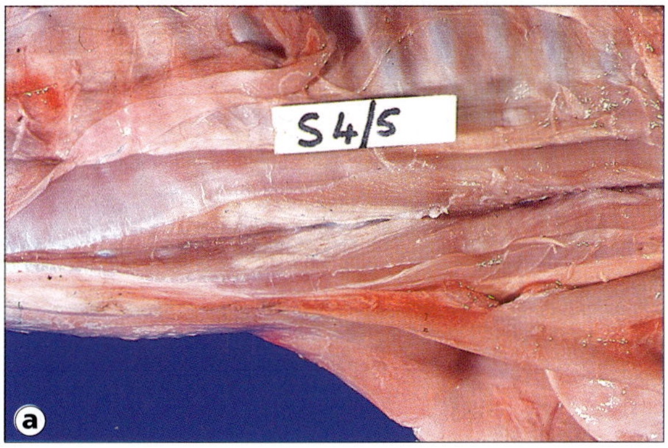
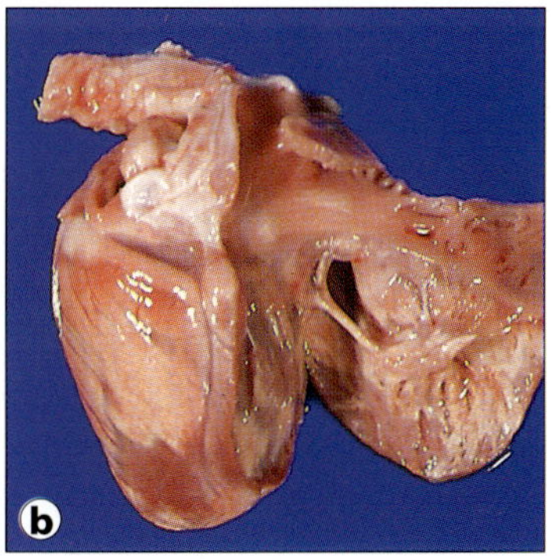

19.5 (**a**) Nutritional myopathy associated with antioxidant deficiency in a lamb. There is patchy necrosis and pallor of lumbar muscle. (**b**) In the heart there is more extensive coagulative necrosis and calcification of myocardium that produces a distinct white appearance.

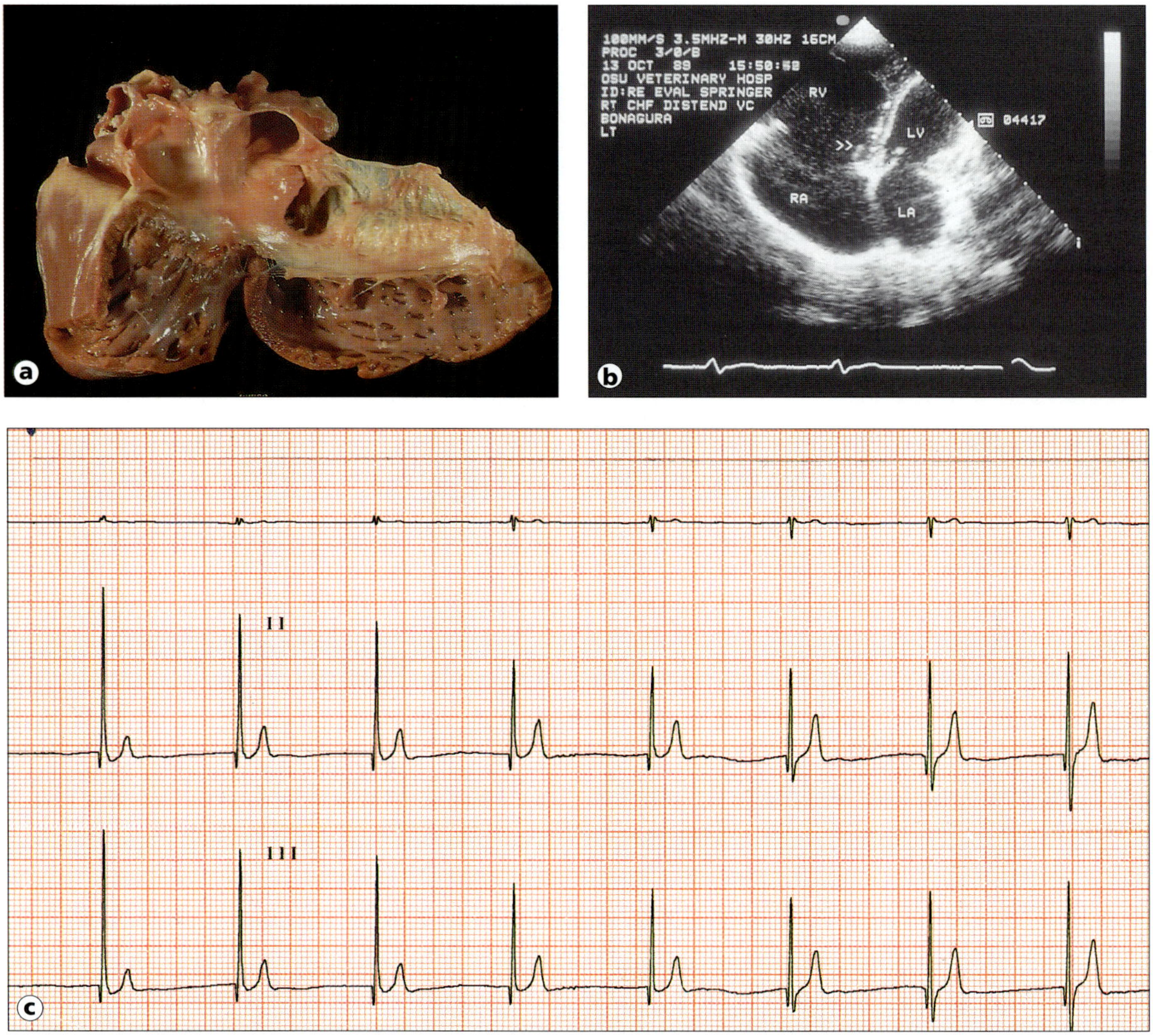

19.6 Silent atrium' syndrome in the dog. (**a**) Post mortem specimen from an English springer spaniel with silent atrium. The right atrium and right ventricle are opened. Note the marked loss of myocardial tissue in the right atrium giving a translucent appearance to the atrium. Eventually, sinus node function is lost or isolated from effective pathways and the heart must be driven by an escape rhythm. Cardiac dilatation occurs and right-sided cardiac failure is common in advanced cases. (**b**) Echocardiogram from another springer spaniel with silent atrium. Note the marked volume overload of the right atrium and right ventricle. These are consequences of the protracted bradyarrhythmia, loss of functional myocardium, secondary tricuspid regurgitation, and renal retention of sodium and water due to limited cardiac output. (**c**) ECG from a golden retriever with silent atrium and normal electrolyte levels. There is atrial standstill (no P wave) with a variable escape rhythm indicated by QRS waveform variations. (25 mm/sec; 10 mm/mV).

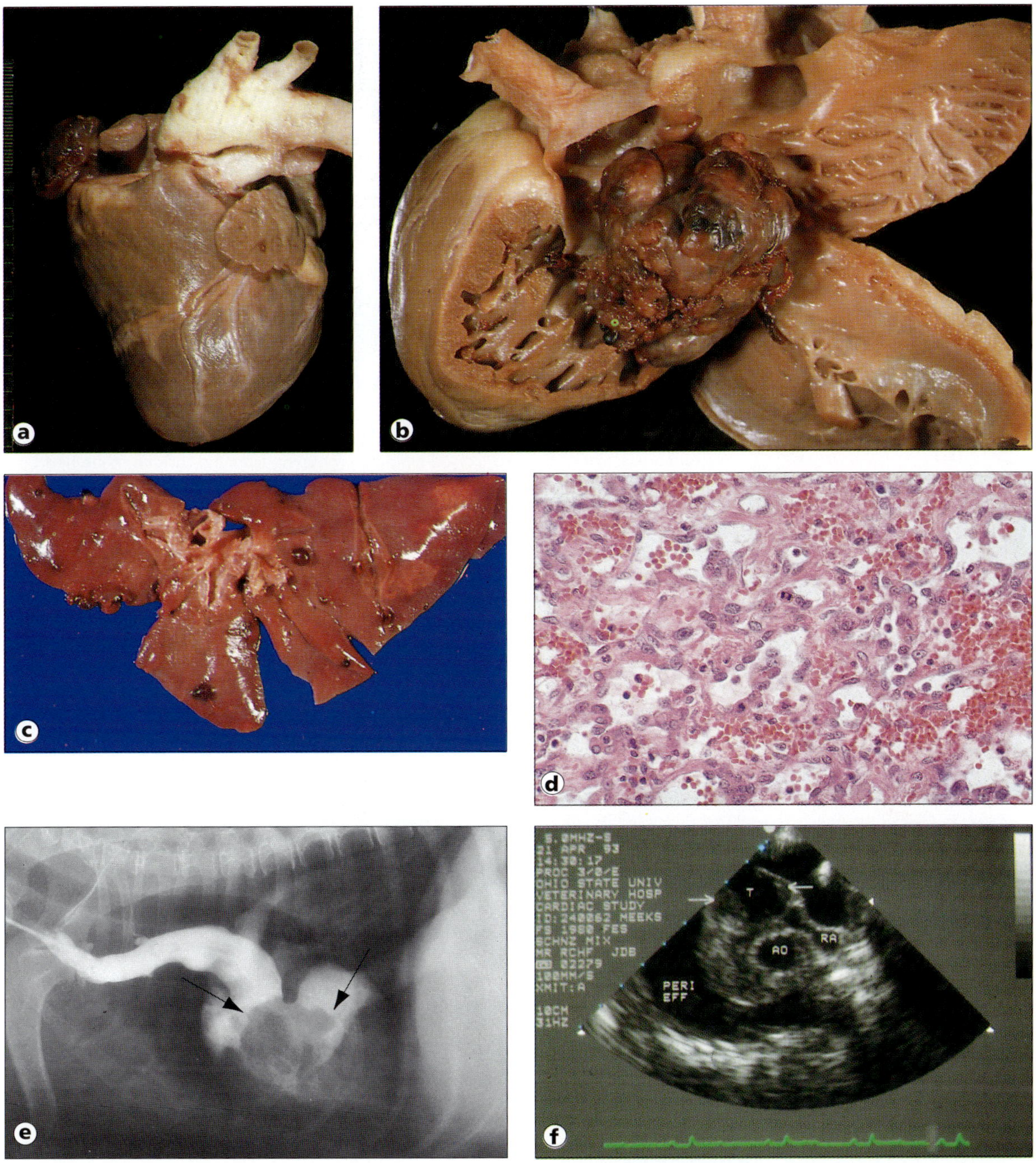

19.7 Haemangiosarcoma in a dog. (**a**) Typical extracardiac auricular location. (**b**) Large intraluminal tumour that obstructs venous return. This tumour arises either as a metastatic growth from splenic or hepatic primary tumours or as part of a 'multicentric' process. (**c**) Metastatic haemangiosarcoma in a liver. (**d**) Photomicrograph showing numerous vascular channels lined with neoplastic endothelial cells (**e**) The functional consequences of cardiac haemangiosarcoma can include obstruction to venous return, as shown here. This nonselective angiogram from the dog in (**b**) shows the filling defect (arrows) caused by a space-occupying lesion within the right ventricular inlet. Contrast medium that was injected into the cranial vena cava outlines the tumour. (**f**) Short-axis echocardiogram from an old dog with haemangiosarcoma of the right atrium. A pericardial effusion is evident around the heart (PERI EFF) while a large tumour is observed within the right atrium and extending into the wall of the right ventricle along the AV groove. The central tumour (arrows) is sonolucent (T) due to necrosis. The right atrial wall is collapsed owing to cardiac tamponade.

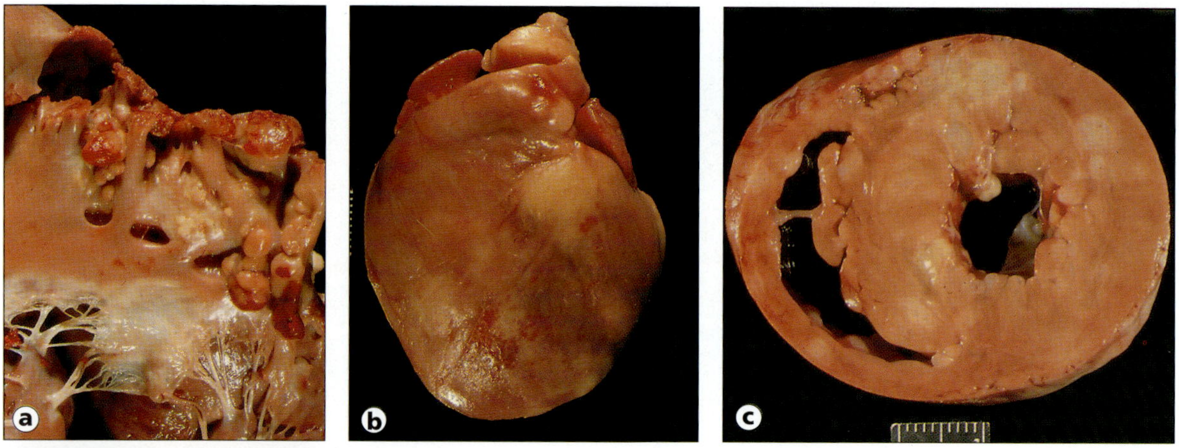

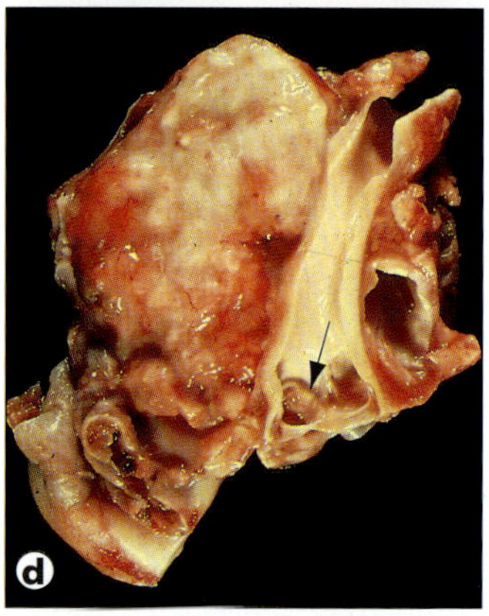

19.8 (**a**) Right atrial lymphosarcoma in a cow. Pericardial effusion or obstruction of venous return may develop in such cases. (**b**) Multifocal lymphosarcoma in a cat. Note the numerous, variably sized, raised tumours protruding from the surface of the heart. (**c**) Metastatic carcinoma in a dog is evident as multiple, well-demarcated areas of white discoloration in both ventricles. (**d**) Heart-base tumour, most likely to be a chemodectoma, in a dog. The tumour originates at the base of the aorta (arrow) which is cut in longitudinal section. These tumours are relatively common in older brachycephalic breeds.

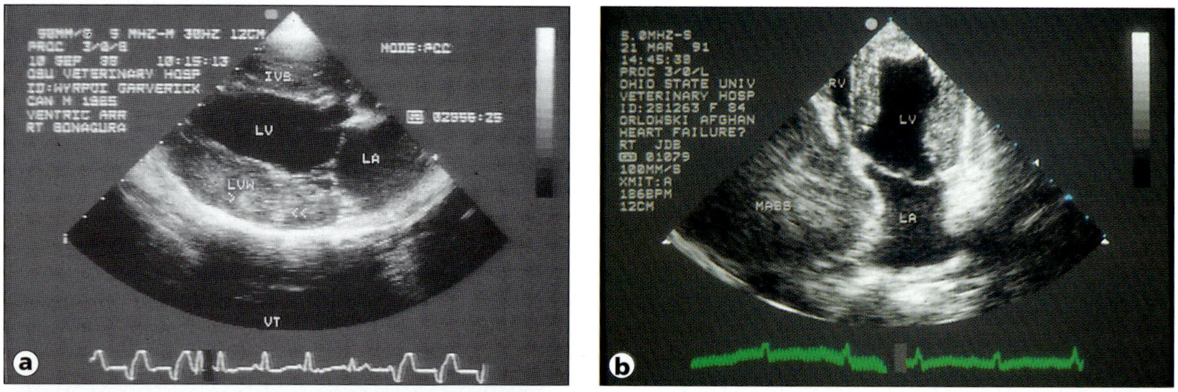

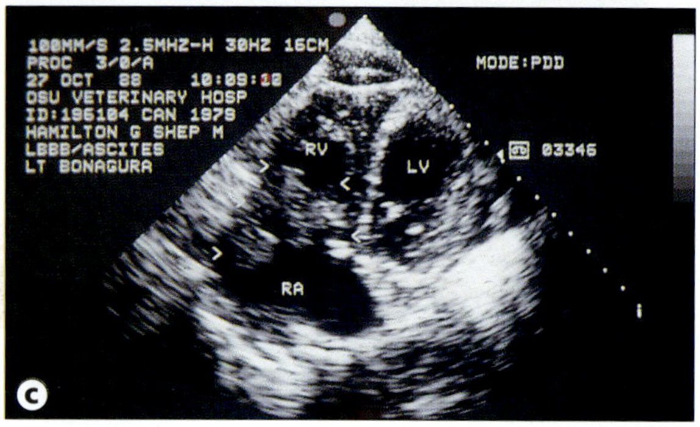

19.9 (**a**) Two-dimensional echocardiogram from a dog with suspected lymphosarcoma of the heart. In this view, the diffuse infiltration and areas of mixed echogenecity (arrowheads) are evident in the left ventricular free wall. Other views demonstrated tumours in the right ventricular wall. The dog was referred for evaluation of unexplained ventricular tachycardia.
(**b**) Echocardiogram from an Afghan hound with a large extracardiac mass which is compressing the left atrium. The tumour was an unusual, large, multilobulated mesothelioma.
(**c**) Echocardiogram from a German shepherd with a multifocal intracardiac tumour that is most evident in the inlet of the right ventricle. The mass obstructed the venous return and caused right atrial dilatation. There was also tricuspid valve regurgitation.

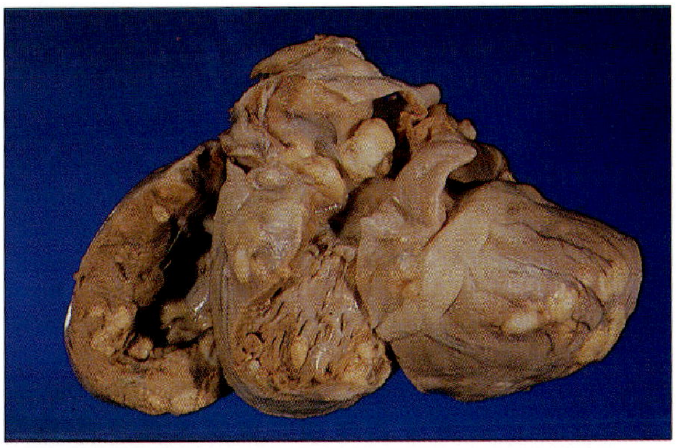

19.10 Metastatic rhabdomyosarcoma in a 6-year-old springer spaniel. The myocardium contains multiple secondary deposits of rhabdomyosarcoma that metastasized from the primary muscle tumour in a forelimb.

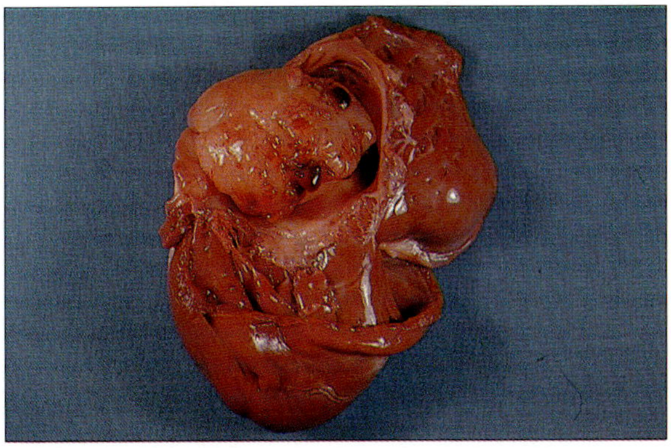

19.11 Cardiac myxoma in an 8-year-old male cocker spaniel. Within the right atrial lumen is a pedunculated pale myxoid mass that acts as a ball valve impeding atrial filling and causing right-sided congestive heart failure.

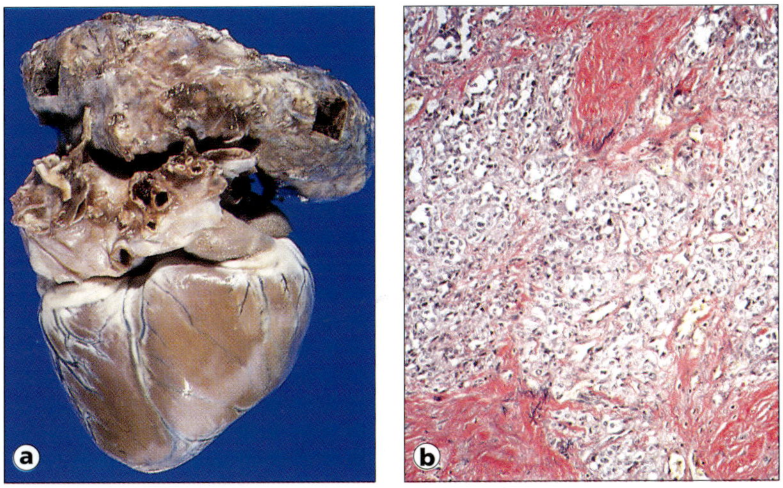

19.12 Heart-base tumours. (**a**) This large mass is situated dorsal to the heart base in a samoyed. These tumours may infiltrate locally and/or produce pericardial effusion.
(**b**) Photomicrograph showing organoid groups of chemodectoma cells separated by fine fibrous trabeculae (from a 6-year-old male English bulldog).

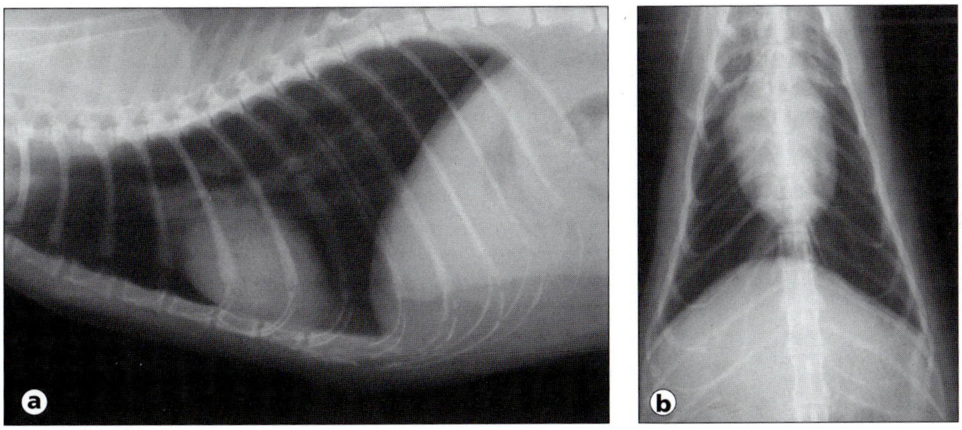

19.13 (**a** and **b**) Radiographs of a 12-year-old domestic short-haired cat with hyperthyroidism. Although there is no gross cardiomegaly, the cardiac outline appears slightly rounded.

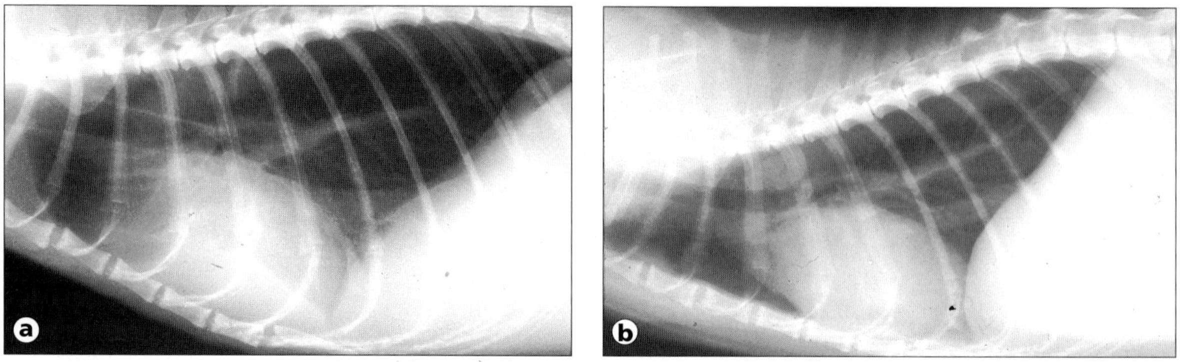

19.14 Radiographs of a cat with hyperthyroidism taken before (**a**) and after (**b**) therapy for congestive heart failure. A pleural effusion and cardiomegaly are obvious in (**a**). There is resolution of the fluid and reduced cardiac size after treatment with anti-thyroid medication and furosemide.

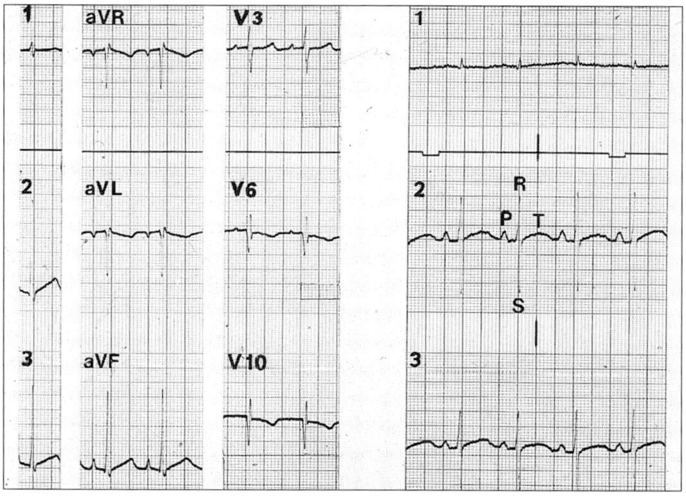

19.15 ECGs from two cats with hyperthyroid heart disease. The 9-lead ECG (left) demonstrates left ventricular hypertrophy characterized by large voltage R waves in leads II and aVF. In addition, prominent S waves in leads I and V3 suggest intercurrent right ventricular hypertrophy. The 3-lead ECG (right) shows markedly increased QRS voltages with terminal ventricular activity directed cranially and resulting in deep S waves in leads 2 and 3.

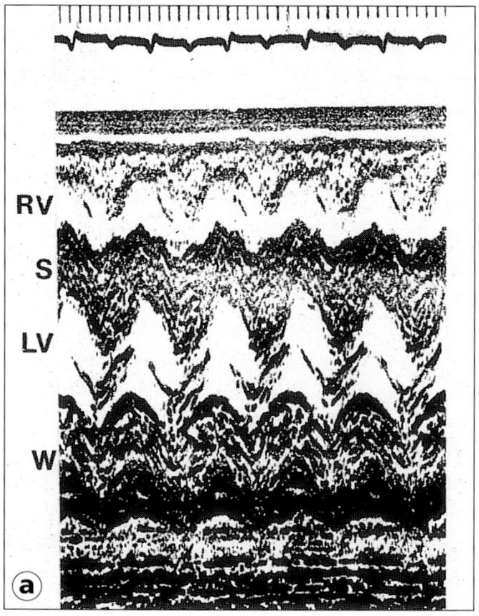

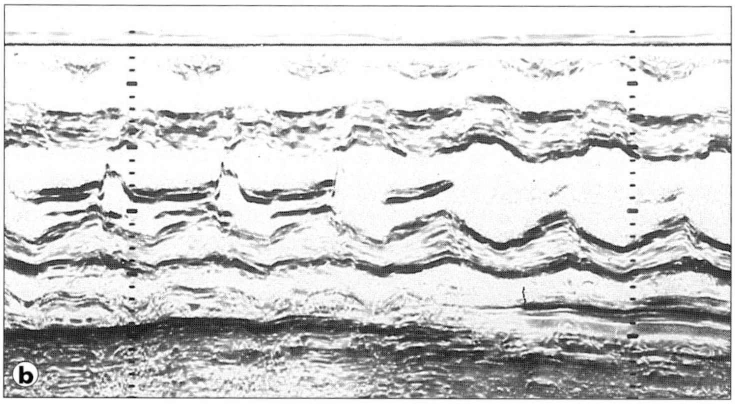

19.16 (**a**) M-mode echocardiogram from a hyperthyroidic cat with marked left ventricular hypertrophy. The left ventricle (LV) is hypertrophied and hyperdynamic. The M-mode (**b**) from the cat in **19.14** shows a pericardial effusion and a diminished left ventricular shortening fraction. The transducer was swept from the mitral level (left) to the chordal level.

20. Pericardial Diseases

The pericardium is not an essential structure, though it serves to protect the heart and influences ventricular diastolic function. The pericardial space (the cavity between the epicardium and the parietal pericardium) normally contains a few millilitres of lubricating fluid. Disorders of the pericardium can be congenital or acquired, and related clinical problems are generally associated with accumulation of fluid within the pericardial space (pericardial effusion), inflammation (pericarditis) or the effects of a space-occupying mass. Pericardial disorders generally lead to diastolic ventricular dysfunction. Thus, therapy for pericardial diseases typically involves removal of accumulated fluid or the surgical removal of a portion of the pericardium in order to prevent cardiac tamponade or progressive pericardial/epicardial constriction.

PERITONEOPERICARDIAL–DIAPHRAGMATIC HERNIA

Pericardial cysts, partial absence of the pericardium, and peritoneopericardial–diaphragmatic hernia (PPDH) are the most frequently encountered congenital lesions of the pericardium. Only the last of these is observed with any frequency. The PPDH is a congenital malformation of the embryonic septum transversum which results in a defect in the ventral portion of the diaphragm. Various abdominal tissues may enter the pericardial sac from this peritoneal communication, and these include mesentery, fat, stomach, intestines, liver or spleen. The condition is fairly common in cats in which the pericardium typically contains falciform fat and liver, but not intestines. Clinical signs are very variable according to the extent of herniation and the tissues involved. Animals can appear normal, with the hernia an incidental clinical finding, or there may be dyspnoea caused by hydrothorax or the effects of space-occupying herniated contents. Less often, there are signs of right-sided cardiac failure or of alimentary disturbances.

The diagnosis must be suspected if heart sounds are not heard in the normal location during routine cardiac examination. Radiography is quite helpful, and the diagnosis should be considered if a very large cardiac outline is present, especially when there is tissue inhomogeneity (fat or gas) over, or ventral to, the heart and continuity between the cardiac and diaphragmatic shadows. A xiphoid deformity is noted in some cases, and the dorsal border of the hernia (a persistent mesothelial remnant) may be evident on the lateral radiograph between the caudal border of the pericardium and the diaphragm. The presence of the hernia can sometimes be confirmed by barium contrast alimentary studies or by angiography of the heart, but the diagnosis is best secured by two-dimensional echocardiography. Surgical treatment is usually successful, though it may not be advisable or needed in some mature animals.

PERICARDIAL EFFUSIONS

Pericardial effusions develop in many species. Although the nature and cause of the pericardial effusions vary among the species, clinical findings are often similar, especially when pericardial pressures become critically high and exceed the filling pressures of the right side of the heart (cardiac tamponade). Acute cardiac tamponade usually causes hypotension and low-output signs such as weakness, collapse, syncope or death. In subacute or chronic cases of cardiac tamponade, fluid retention and right-sided cardiac failure develop and dominate the clinical presentation.

Pericardial effusions can be classified cytologically (**20.1**). In dogs, pericardial effusions are usually haemorrhagic, due to trauma, bleeding from neoplasms such as haemangiosarcomas or heart-base tumours, or are idiopathic. Golden retrievers appear to be predisposed to these haemorrhagic effusions. Suppurative pericarditis, which is relatively common in cattle, is much less frequent in other species. Serous effusions can be found in generalized oedematous disorders, including congestive cardiac failure and hypoalbuminaemia, and in some cases of neoplasia.

Clinical findings in pericardial effusion often include muffled or distant heart sounds, jugular venous distension, weak or variable arterial pulses, and signs of right-sided cardiac failure. Differentiation from dilated cardiomyopathy in dogs is helped by radiography, which shows a very sharp and rounded outline to the heart, together with signs of right-sided or biventricular cardiac failure. The ECG can also be useful, as it may demonstrate low voltages, and sometimes electrical alternans or S–T segment elevation. However, neither of these techniques is conclusive, and echocardiography provides the specific diagnosis for all species. Partial collapse of the right side of the heart may be observed by two-dimensional echocardiography in cases of tamponade.

Pericardiocentesis is essential for both diagnosis and treatment of pericardial effusion with tamponade. Even partial relief of the fluid distension will give rapid clinical improvement. Following pericardiocentesis, cytology should be carried out and culture of the fluid sample if infection is suspected. The risk of constrictive pericarditis in infective pericardial disease is great; accordingly, septic pericarditis in small animals is best treated with antibiotics and subtotal pericardiectomy with pleural drainage. Large animals can be treated with antibiotics and placement of one or more lavage tubes within the pericardial space. Idiopathic pericardial haemorrhage in dogs is treated initially by pericardiocentesis; however, recurrent pericardial haemorrhage calls for partial pericardiectomy to exclude a tumour, to prevent constriction, and to permit insidious haemorrhage into the thorax, where blood causes few further problems.

CONSTRICTIVE PERICARDIAL DISEASE

Constrictive pericardial disease is present when the parietal and visceral (epicardial) layers begin to adhere and lead to a constricting band that impairs diastolic filling of the heart. The condition is not common except in cattle where it is a consequence of infection, fibrinous or purulent inflammation, reabsorption of fluid, and fibrosis. Constriction can develop in dogs as a consequence of infective pericarditis or from recurrent pericardial haemorrhage. Most often this is a constrictive–effusive pericardial disorder. Constrictive pericardial diseases can produce clinical signs similar to those of pericardial effusion; however, the management is more difficult and the prognosis less favourable. Friction rubs (to-and-fro sounds synchronous with two or three phases of the cardiac cycle) may be heard. Echocardiography again assists the definitive diagnosis, but specific findings may also be made by cardiac catheterization. Suspected cases are best referred to a cardiologist or thoracic surgeon for evaluation prior to surgical intervention.

Clinical Associations with Pericardial Effusions

Transudation[a]
- Congestive heart failure (can be very severe in cats)
- Peritoneopericardial diaphragmatic hernia
- Pericardial cysts
- Hypoalbuminaemia
- Infections/toxaemia or other causes of increased vascular permeability
- Heart-base tumours that obstruct lymphatic drainage

Exudation
- Bacterial, septic, pericarditis in cattle related to wire perforation from the reticulum (traumatic reticulopericarditis or 'hardware disease')
- Septic pericarditis in horses due to extension of respiratory or pleural infections; far less often from gastric foreign body perforation or penetrating external wound (e.g. fence post)
- *Nocardia* infection or mixed aerobic/anaerobic pericarditis due to perforating plant, wood or metallic foreign bodies in dogs or cats
- Fungal involvement of the pericardium in dogs with coccidiomycosis
- Pericarditis from feline infectious peritonitis infection
- Pericarditis may develop in large animals with multisystemic infections and is usually characterized at necropsy by fibrinous exudation
- Idiopathic, sterile (granulomatous) pericarditis in the dog and horse

Intrapericardial haemorrhage[b]
- Idiopathic pericardial haemorrhage is the most frequent condition encountered in dogs
- Left atrial rupture in dogs with mitral regurgitation
- Blunt chest trauma or puncture of the heart (by knife, bullet, missile, thoracocentesis)
- Coagulopathy
- Intrapericardial rupture of the aorta in older stallions
- Neoplasia of the heart, heart base or pericardium frequently causes a haemorrhagic effusion; clinically important causes include:
  - **Haemangiosarcoma** of the right atrium (especially common in dogs over 8 years of age; including German shepherd dogs and golden retrievers; this tumour may be multicentric with splenic involvement)
  - **Chemodectoma** (aortic-body tumour) with invasion of the heart base (especially common in aged brachycephalic breed dogs)
  - **Thyroid carcinoma** (ectopic thyroid tissue at the heart base)
  - **Mesothelioma** of the pericardium
  - **Lymphosarcoma** of the right atrium and heart is the most important cardiac neoplasm in the cat and the cow; multicentric lymphoma can involve the heart of the dog
  - **Metastatic carcinoma or sarcoma** to the heart

[a]Such accumulations tend to be necropsy or ultrasound findings which do not impair heart function.
[b]With or without secondary pericardial reaction.

20.1 Clinical associations with pericardial effusions.

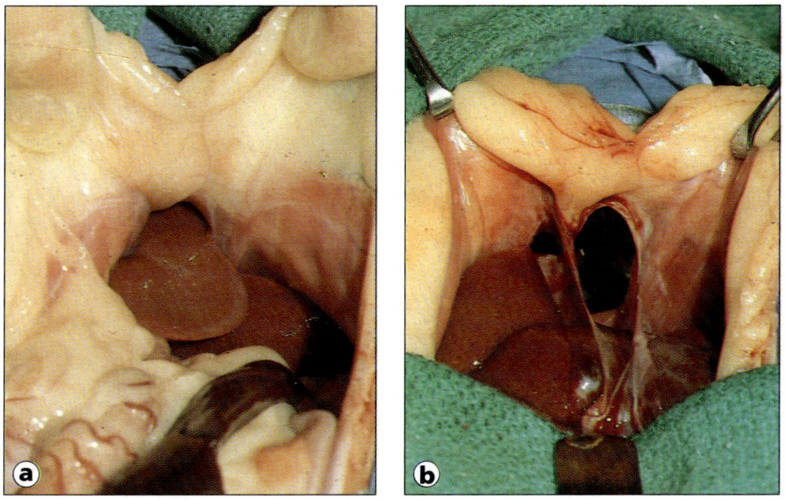

20.2 Congenital peritoneo-pericardial–diaphragmatic hernia in a cat. Before (**a**) and after (**b**) surgical reduction of the liver and falciform fat. The hernia was subsequently sutured to close the rent in the diaphragm.

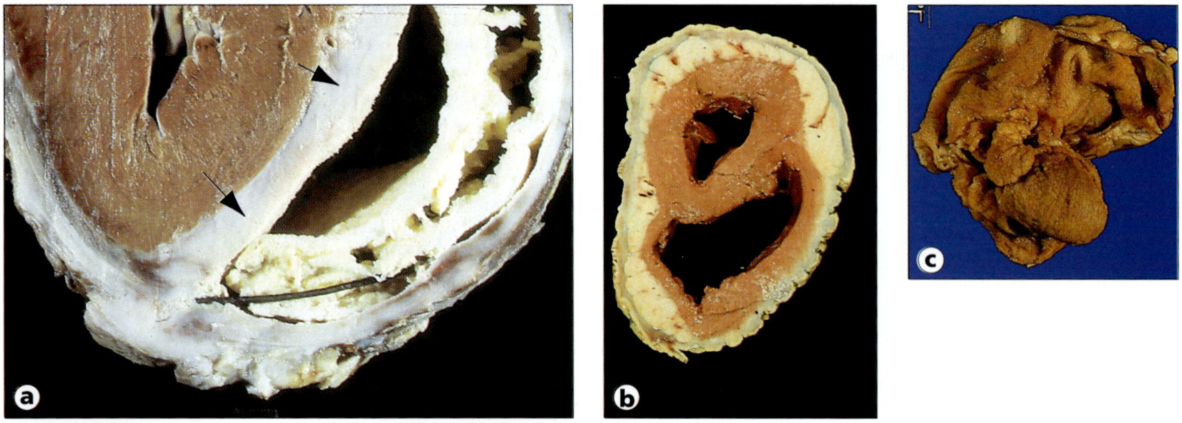

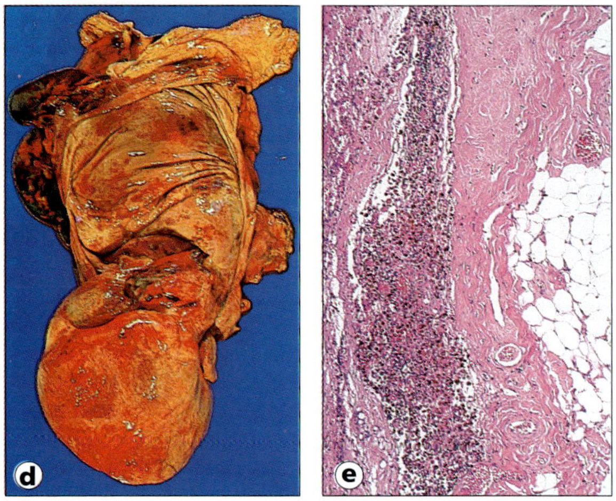

20.3 (**a**) Traumatic reticulopericarditis in a cow. The perforating wire and organized pericardial reaction (fibrin) are evident to the right of the left ventricle. The thickened fibrinous reaction has resulted in severe epicardial thickening (arrows). (**b**) Constrictive pericarditis in a cow due to chronic pericarditis. No fluid remains in the pericardial space, which has been obliterated by fibrous tissue. (**c**) Chronic active pericarditis in a 9-month-old cat with the 'dry' form of coronavirus infection (or feline infectious peritonitis). The pericardial sac is distended by fibrinous inflammatory exudate. The epicardial surface is roughened by inflamed graulation tissue. (**d**) Chronic haemorrhagic pericardial effusion in a 5-year-old male Saint Bernard dog. The opened, distended pericardial sac and the epicardial surface are patchily roughened and discoloured by haemosiderin that accumulates following recurrent idiopathic haemorrhage. (**e**) Section of a specimen taken at pericardectomy from a 9-year-old Labrador retriever dog with recurrent pericardial effusion. There is fibrous thickening, haemorrhage and haemosiderosis, and modest chronic inflammation.

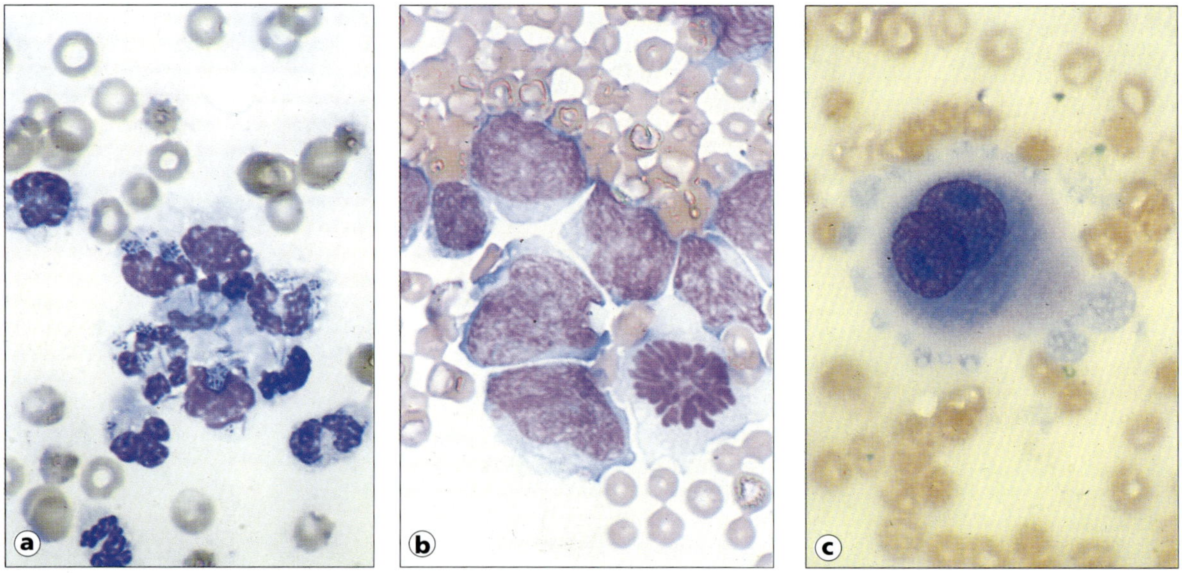

20.4 Cytology of pericardial aspirates. (**a**) Septic, suppurative pericarditis in a dog. (**b**) Lymphosarcoma and haemorrhage in a cow. (**c**) Idiopathic haemorrhagic pericardial effusion with a reactive mesothelial cell. This should not be misdiagnosed as a malignancy.

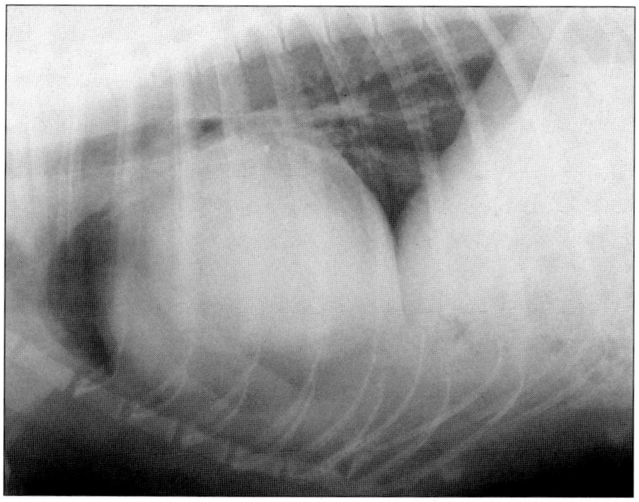

20.5 Lateral radiograph of a symptomless 4-year-old English setter in which a peritoneopericardial–diaphragmatic hernia was an incidental finding. There is continuity between the lower diaphragm and the heart, and the cardiac outline is very large and rounded, with variations in density of tissues over the heart. Omental fat sometimes helps to outline soft tissues (liver lobe) in the pericardial sac in this disease.

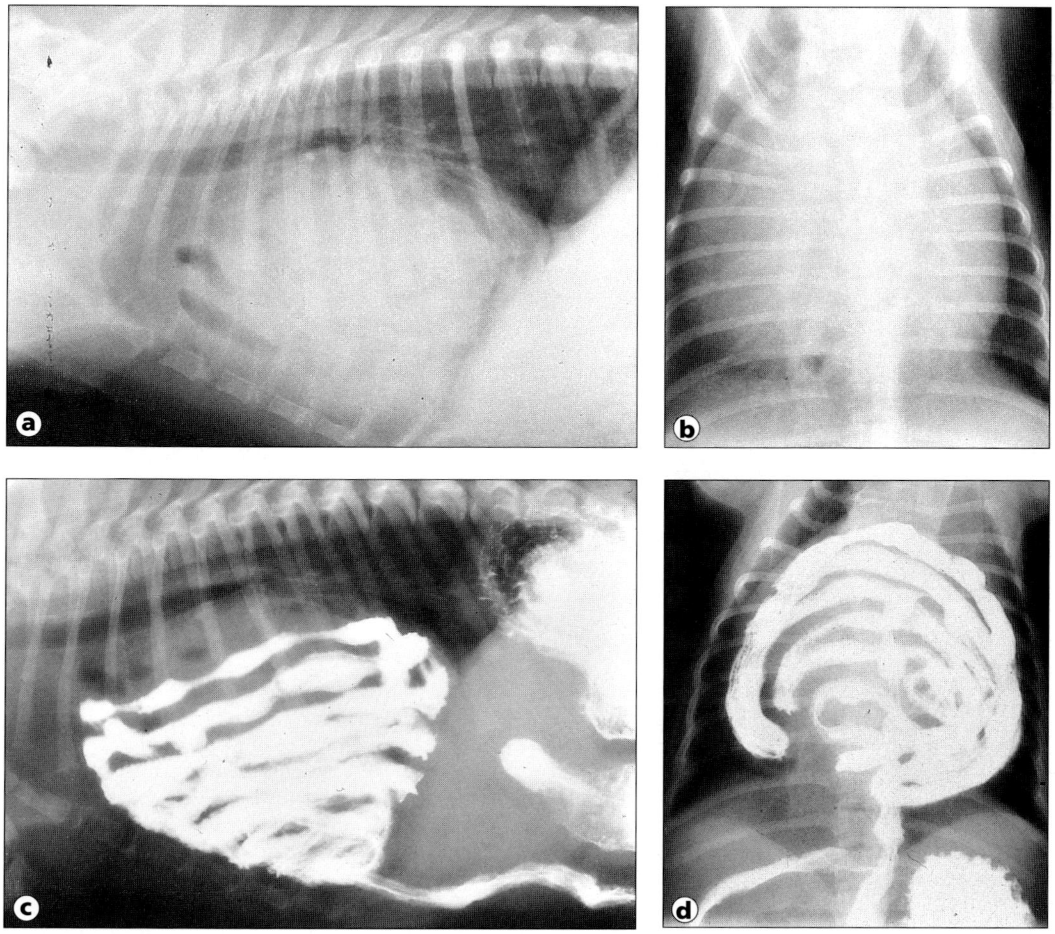

20.6 Peritoneopericardial–diaphragmatic hernia in a schnauzer puppy. (**a** and **b**) Survey radiographs indicate enlarged cardiac silhouette with gas-filled intestinal loops within the pericardial space. (**c** and **d**) A barium study indicates the communication of the small bowel with the pericardial space via a ventral hernia near the midline.

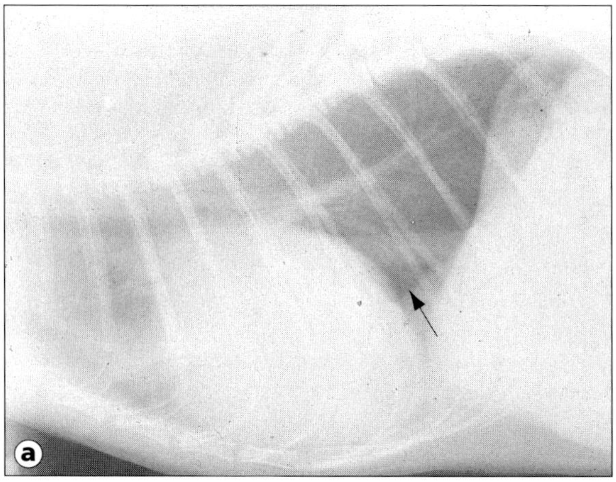

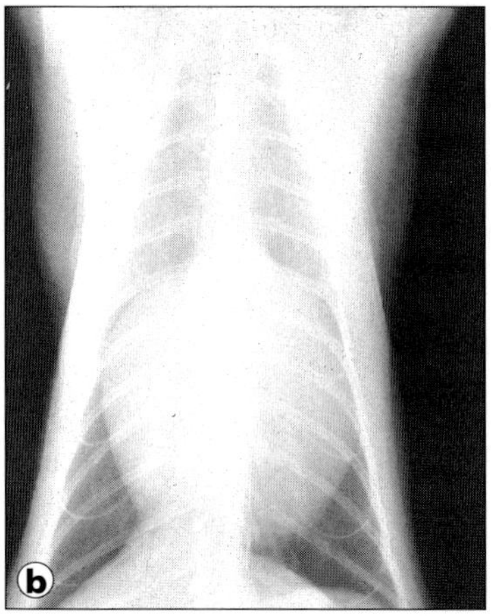

20.7 (**a** and **b**) Radiographs of peritoneopericardial–diaphragmatic hernia from a cat. Unlike the dog, the cat less often has bowel within the hernia sac. In this case the enlarged cardiac shadow could be confused with cardiomegaly. However, the persistent mesothelial remnant (arrow) is evident on the lateral film. This marks the dorsal border of the communication. The VD film shows potential continuity between the mediastinum and peritoneal space.

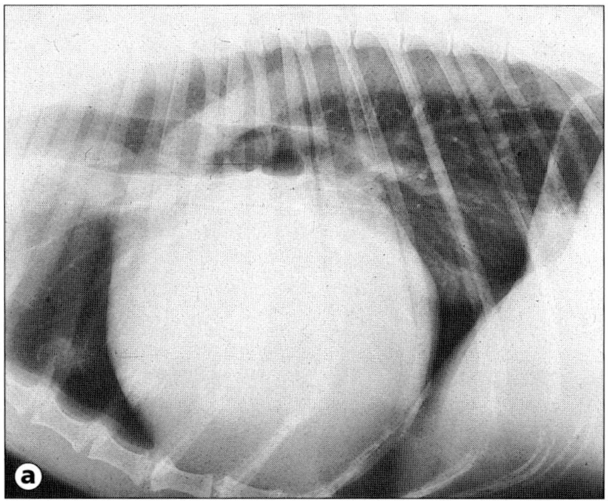

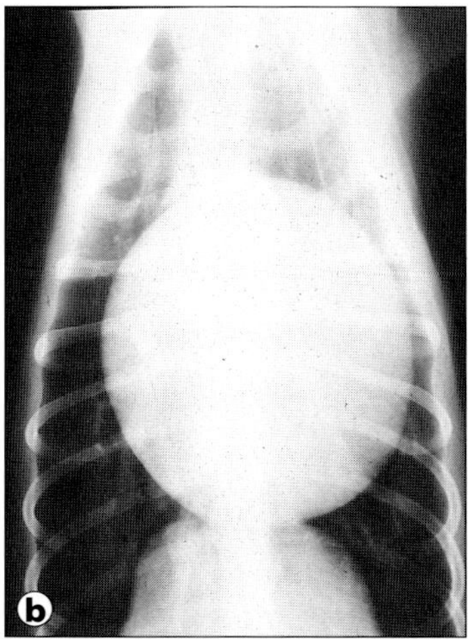

20.8 (**a** and **b**) Pericardial effusion in a dog secondary to coccidiomycosis with involvement of the pericardial space. Note the sharp edges of the rounded cardiac silhouette typical of decreased motion at the periphery of the distended sac. The left atrial shadow is now rounded and no angles are evident.

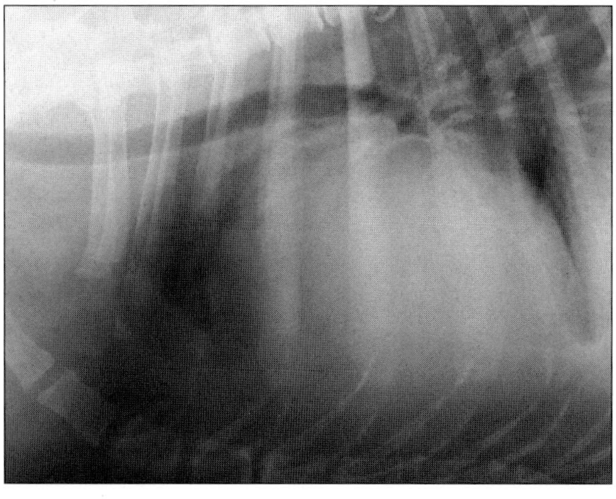

20.9 Radiograph of an 11-year-old male German shepherd dog with pleural effusion that partly obscures the cardiac outline. However, the cardiac outline appears to be generally enlarged and rather globular, and the caudal vena cava is very large – typical of the right-sided failure of pericardial effusion. A similar appearance could be seen with other diseases such as dilated cardiomyopathy.

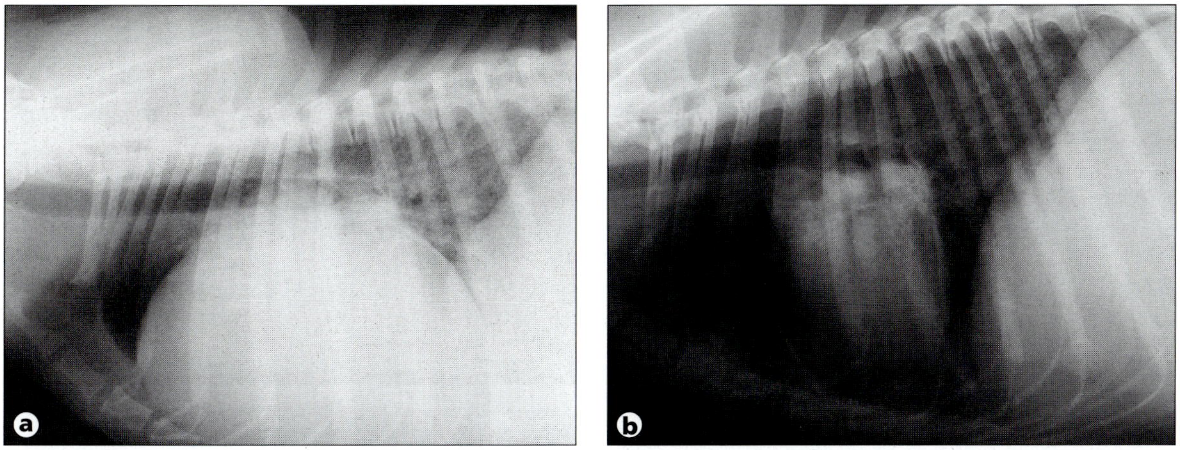

20.10 Radiographs of a 4-year-old standard poodle, (**a**) before and (**b**) after drainage of pericardial effusion. (**a**) A large and notably globular cardiac outline. There is also a diffuse and miliary interstitial pulmonary density. (**b**) A normal cardiac outline within the pericardial sac showing pneumopericardium after pericardiocentesis. The pulmonary pattern persists. An unclassified mycobacterium was isolated from the effusion in this case of pericarditis.

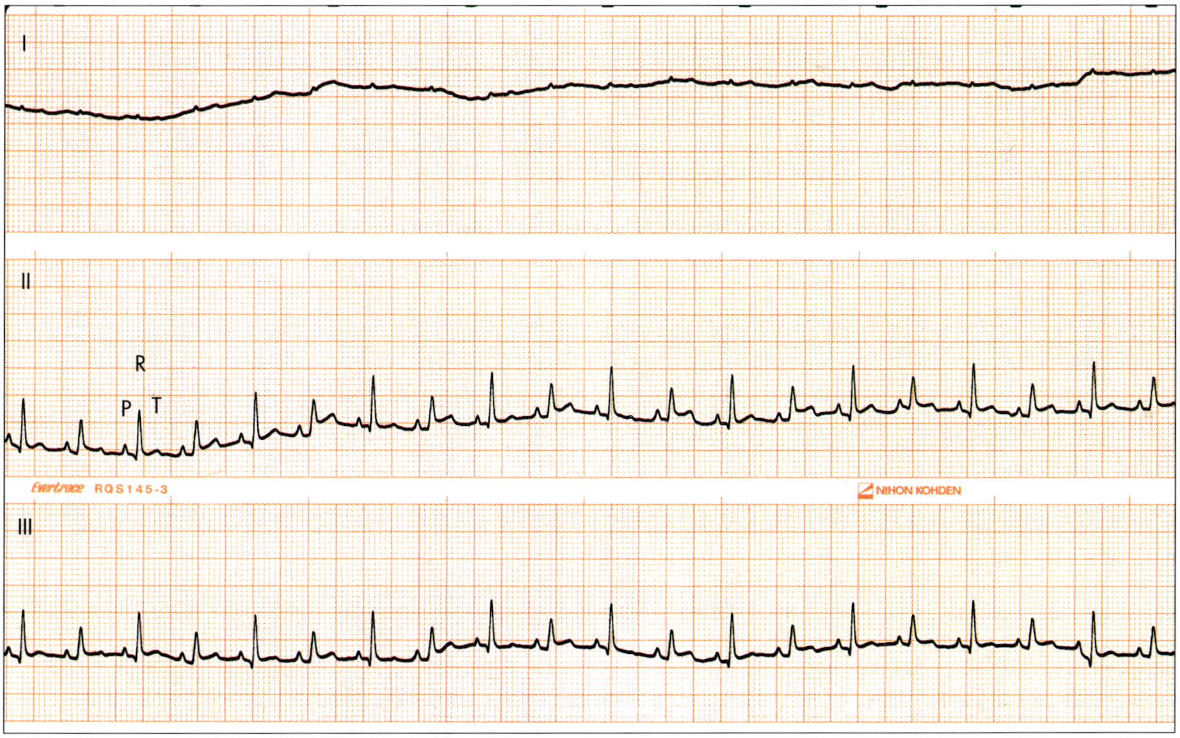

20.11 ECG (25 mm/sec; 10 mm/mV) from the German shepherd dog in **20.9**, showing regular sinus rhythm at a heart rate of about 140bpm. The ECG voltages are rather low and there are also electrical alternans and S–T elevation, all typical, but not inevitable, features of pericardial effusion. There was idiopathic haemorrhage in this case.

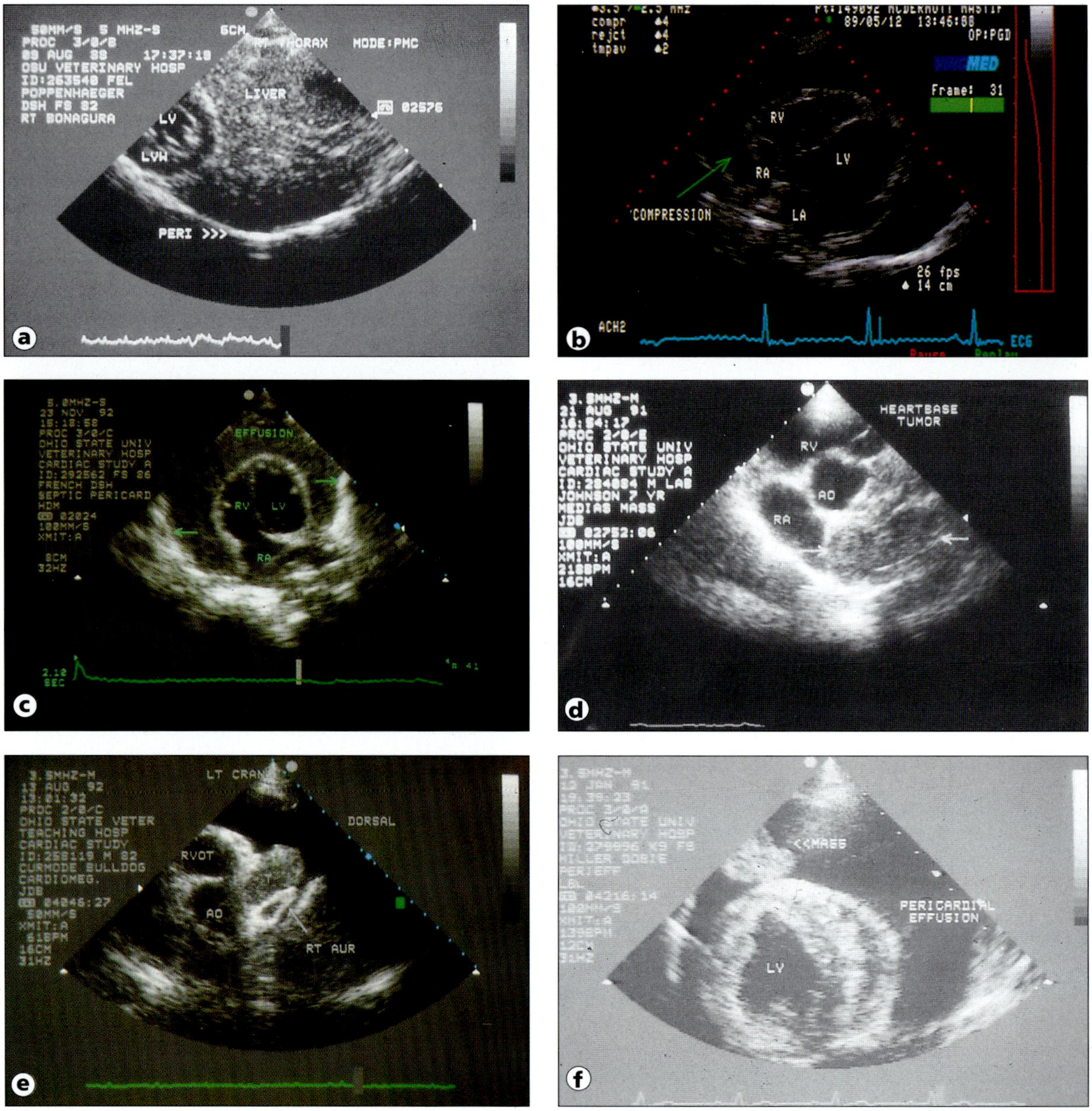

20.12 Echocardiography in pericardial disease. (**a**) A case of peritoneopericardial–diaphragmatic hernia in a cat shows liver within the delimiting membrane of the parietal pericardium (PERI>>>). The left ventricle and left ventricular wall are adjacent to the liver. (**b**) Right parasternal long-axis view of the heart of a mastiff with pericardial effusion, which is seen as an echo-free space around the heart. There is also right atrial compression (arrow). (**c**) Mixed echogenic appearance of septic pericarditis in a cat (left apical image plane). The parietal pericardium is shown (arrows). Acute haemorrhage may also result in an echogenic pericardial effusion. Most chronic, sterile effusions and haemorrhagic effusions are sonolucent. (**d**) Large heart-base tumour in a dog (arrows) evident around the base of the aorta and the atria. (**e**) A well-defined heart-base tumour in a bulldog with an extensive transudate in the pericardial sac. The tumour is evident between the right auricle and the aorta. The echo-free space around the mass and heart base is a pericardial effusion. (RVOT – right ventricular outflow tract.) (**f**) Pericardial effusion with right ventricular compression and a mass lesion in an unusual location near the apex of the heart and attached to the pericardium. This is typical of a blood clot. The 'mass' resolved spontaneously and was not evident on follow-up examinations. Differential diagnosis should include atypical tumour or metastatic neoplasm.

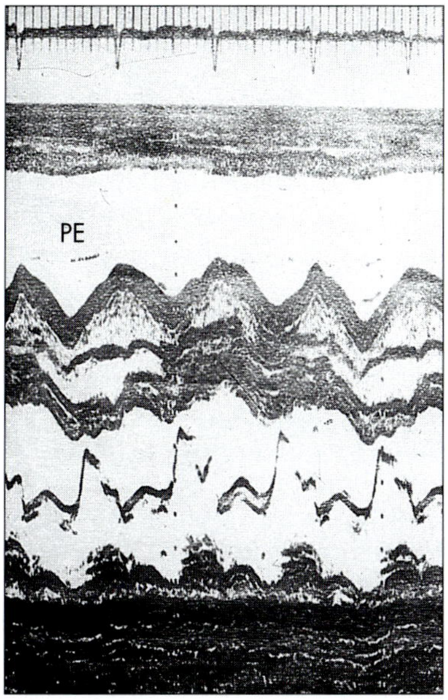

20.13 M-mode echocardiogram from a dog with pericardial effusion. The pericardial effusion (PE) is evident. There is respiratory variation in right ventricular filling that leads to varying size of the chamber. This can cause pulsus paradoxus.

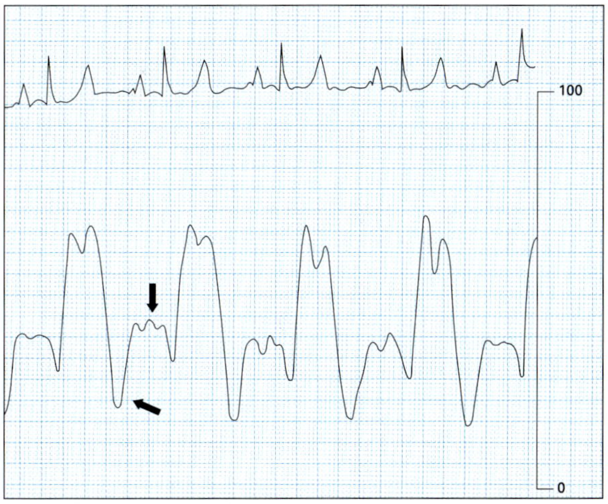

20.14 Dip and plateau (arrows) pattern in a pressure tracing from a horse with constrictive pericardial disease. The recording is from the right ventricle. Differential diagnosis should include infiltrative or restrictive cardiomyopathy.

21.

Vascular Diseases

Numerous disorders affect the arteries and veins of animals, and many of these are clinically relevant. This chapter covers some of the more important malformations and acquired conditions that affect arteries, veins and lymphatics.

PATENT DUCTUS ARTERIOSUS

Persistent patent ductus arteriosus (PDA) is encountered in most species, but it is clinically important only in the dog and, to a lesser degree, the cat. The prevalence of PDA is high and, with subaortic stenosis, is one of the most common cardiac congenital defects in the dog. Bitches are predisposed to PDA, with numerous breeds over-represented, including poodles, German shepherd, Maltese, chihuahua, Pomeranian, various spaniels, Shetland sheepdog, Yorkshire terrier and collies. The wall of the persistent PDA is abnormal, lacking the smooth muscle that causes a normal ductus to close within a few days following birth. Because there are marked differences between systemic and pulmonary pressures, continuous shunting occurs from the descending aorta to the pulmonary artery. This left-to-right shunt overloads the pulmonary circulation and the left side of the heart. Volume overload and progressive myocardial failure precipitate pulmonary oedema. Infrequently, the ductal diameter is so great that the high pulmonary flow causes pulmonary vascular disease, pulmonary hypertension, and shunting that is reversed from right-to-left; this leads to cyanosis in the caudal mucous membranes, polycythaemia and rear-limb weakness; these uncommon cases develop during the first 2–4 months of life, are irreversible and cannot be treated surgically.

Clinical signs of the typical left-to-right PDA depend on the magnitude of shunting (see Appendix A3, *Congenital Heart Disease in Animals*). Exercise intolerance and signs of left-sided cardiac failure are the most prominent features (see Chapter 1). The pulse is often bounding, owing to a large stroke volume and rapid collapse from release of pressure through the ductus. There may be a prolonged precordial thrill at the left dorsal heart base, and this is accompanied by a characteristic continuous 'machinery' murmur that waxes and wanes throughout systole and diastole. The ECG and thoracic radiographs show enlargement of the left atrium and ventricle. Atrial fibrillation may be observed in advanced cases. Radiographs usually show pulmonary overcirculation and widening of the descending aorta and pulmonary artery associated with high-volume, turbulent flow. Echocardiography demonstrates dilatation of the pulmonary artery and the left side of the heart, and can be used to assess left ventricular systolic function. The ductus may be visualized with two-dimensional echocardiography, but this is not very reliable. However, Doppler studies are sufficient to confirm the shunt and demonstrate the disturbed, retrograde flow in the pulmonary artery that is the hallmark of uncomplicated PDA. The prognosis for untreated PDA is poor and 50% or more of the cases are expected to die within a year of diagnosis. Fortunately, this condition is one of the few cardiac disorders that is readily amenable to surgical correction and prognosis following successful ligation is excellent. Surgery should not be delayed, as progressive myocardial failure is common. Sporadic cases of PDA are encountered in mature dogs and are best referred to a cardiologist.

VASCULAR RINGS

Abnormal development of the great vessels can entrap or compress the oesophagus within a *vascular ring*. The most common of these malformations is a right-sided aortic arch. Persistence of the embryonic right (as opposed to left) fourth aortic arch produces no circulatory disturbances. However, when the pulmonary artery and ligamentum arteriosum circle the descending aorta, a vascular ring constricts the oesophagus. Other vascular-ring anomalies include double aortic arches, normal great vessels with a right-sided ligamentum arteriosum, and a retro-oesophageal right subclavian artery (a minor problem). Clinical signs of vascular rings are usually related to alimentary dysfunction and include regurgitation of solid foods, aspiration pneumonia and failure to thrive. A barium contrast study will show gross dilatation of the oesophagus cranial to the heart base, and even plain films may demonstrate the accumulation of food material at this point. Treatment involves management of aspiration pneumonia and surgical relief of the obstruction, usually accomplished by ligating and dividing the ligamentum arteriosum. Prognosis is guarded and depends largely on attainment of normal oesophageal function.

OTHER CONGENITAL LESIONS

Other congenital vascular disorders include arteriovenous fistulae (see below), congenital portosystemic shunts (leading to hepatic encephalopathy) and persistent left cranial vena cava. The latter causes no functional disturbance, but is often encountered in dogs (especially German shepherds) with persistent right aortic arch, and must be retracted from the surgical field.

THROMBOSIS

Thrombosis refers to the presence of a formed coagulum in a blood vessel; the thrombus may obstruct blood flow. Thromboembolism refers to the sudden occlusion of an artery by a thrombus carried from one site to another via the circulation. Thrombus formation in a systemic vein or right side of the heart may obstruct systemic venous flow or be carried to the lungs and cause a pulmonary embolism. A thrombus or embolus that originates in the left side of the heart or in a systemic artery may obstruct systemic blood flow causing ischaemia and necrosis of tissues usually nourished by that occluded vessel. Venous thrombi are usually related to stasis of blood and activation of clotting factors. Deficiencies of plasma antithrombin-III predispose to thrombosis. Arterial thrombosis follows activation and aggregation of platelets and is frequently related to injury or disruption of vascular endothelium or endocardium. Thrombosis is less problematic in animals than in man, but it can be serious in all species. Aortic (iliac) thrombosis occurs in dogs, cats and horses. In cats, this disease is strongly associated with thrombus formation in the left atrium, which follows chamber dilatation, usually resulting from cardiomyopathy. Thrombosis in dogs is more often associated with hyperadrenocorticism,glomerular disease, haemolytic anaemia or dirofilariasis. Thrombosis in horses can result from damage to arteries, caused by migration of larvae of *Strongylus vulgaris*. Bacterial endocarditis causes thromboemboli in all species (see Chapter 14). Thrombosis can also develop around indwelling intravascular catheters, particularly in horses, and is exacerbated by phlebitis. Infection via the umbilical veins (omphalophlebitis or 'navel ill') is recognized in the newborn, especially in foals, as a hard, painful and possibly purulent umbilicus. Hepatic abscesses syndrome in cattle can be associated with caval thrombosis that may also lead to pulmonary thromboembolism. The pathophysiology and clinical signs depend on the acuteness of injury, location of obstruction, extent of thrombosis and the presence or absence of collateral circulation. Potential consequences related to site include:

- Myocardium – myocardial ischaemia causing infarction, arrhythmias, hypokinetic ventricular wall motion and myocardial failure. Clinical signs include discomfort and anxiety, ECG abnormalities (ST–T segment deviation, infarction patterns, ventricular arrhythmias), elevation of cardiac muscle enzymes (myocardial-MB-band of creatine kinase) and echocardiographic abnormalities such as regional hypokinetic wall motion.
- Limbs – muscle ischaemia, rhabdomyocytolysis, peripheral neuropathy. Signs include limb weakness, limb pallor, loss of pulse, ischaemic myopathy (pain, contracture, elevated serum muscle enzymes) and lower motor neurone neuropathy.
- Spinal cord – neuronal degeneration and ischaemic or haemorrhagic necrosis, causing segmental spinal cord disease (upper or lower motor neurone).
- Brain – haemorrhage, necrosis, and ischaemia-induced neuronal damage, causing ischaemic neuropathy or 'stroke' with attendant seizures or neurologic deficits.
- Kidney, adrenal gland, liver, spleen and skin – infarcts, haemorrhages and parenchymal necrosis, causing organ dysfunction or biochemical abnormalities.
- Systemic veins – obstruction to venous return and subsequent elevation of venous pressure (causing swollen cutaneous vessels that do not collapse and may be warm and painful – thrombophlebitis), oedema distal to the obstruction (a deep venous thrombosis may lead to bilateral limb oedema or thrombosis in the liver or spleen). Severe jugular thrombosis can extend into the heart and cause right-sided endocarditis or pulmonary thromboembolism.
- Lung – pulmonary thromboembolism (see Chapter 22).

The clinical diagnosis of thrombosis or embolism requires a high level of suspicion. A sudden onset of clinical signs is typical. Certain conditions (see above) predispose to thrombosis. Appropriate laboratory studies should be conducted for the suspected cause and regions of injury. Specialists should be consulted for radiographic, ultrasonic, angiographic, radionuclide (perfusion studies) and clinical laboratory tests. These studies may demonstrate changes attributable to decreased blood flow, organ ischaemia or tissue necrosis.

Treatment varies with the cause. Principles of therapy include removal or disintegration of the clot, control of the underlying disorder and supportive care to damaged tissues. A specialist (haematologist, internist or cardiologist) should be consulted prior to the use of thrombolytic therapy as treatment is aggressive with high morbidity and mortality. Tissue plasminogen activator and streptokinase are effective in dissolving some arterial thrombi and restoring tissue perfusion, particularly if used during the first 6 hours. Uncontrolled bleeding and metabolic disturbances can be complications. Surgical intervention is rarely employed. Anticoagulants (e.g. heparin) or drugs that interfere with platelet function (e.g. aspirin) do not dissolve thrombi, but are commonly administered to prevent further thrombosis.

OTHER ARTERIAL DISORDERS

In addition to thrombosis, various other arterial conditions are recognized. Some of these (arteritis, medial necrosis, dissection, arteriosclerosis, arterial mineralization, and vascular neoplasia) are illustrated in this chapter. *Arteritis*, inflammation involving arterioles or arteries, can be caused by various microorganisms and is often a component of multisystemic infections including feline infectious peritonitis (FIP) and Rocky Mountain spotted fever. Immune-mediated arteritis is believed to be important in systemic lupus erythematosus and idiopathic vasculitis, and with some drug reactions. A primary viral arteritis of horses may also be associated with abortion. Clinical signs of vasculitis are related to inflammatory mediators, increased vascular permeability and interruption of the vascular endothelial lining; they include fever, subcutaneous oedema, cutaneous haemorrhages, coagulation disorders (thrombocytopoenia, disseminated intravascular coagulopathy), thrombosis and ischaemic injury. Treatment of vasculitis depends on the underlying cause. Immunosuppressive doses of glucocorticoids are indicated in some cases. Thrombotic complications may require prophylactic heparin (10–100 i.u./kg q8h, subcutaneously).

Arteriosclerosis, a chronic degenerative lesion of arteries, is characterized by loss of elasticity, luminal narrowing, and proliferative and stenosing lesions of the intima and media. Atherosclerosis describes the disorder in which fat and cholesterol cause degenerative changes in the arterial wall. This is the typical underlying lesion of coronary artery disease in human patients, but it is relatively uncommon in animals. Microvascular coronary arteriosclerosis (often involving amyloid) is prominent in older dogs with endocardiosis, and it results in small areas of left ventricular myocardial fibrosis. This is presumably due to ischaemic degeneration of myocytes secondary to reduced perfusion of the inner myocardium. Similar stenosing myocardial lesions are also observed in the left ventricle of dogs with congenital subaortic stenosis, pulmonic stenosis or diabetes mellitus, and in cats with hypertrophic cardiomyopathy.

HYPERTENSION

An elevation in systemic arterial blood pressure is termed *systemic hypertension*, which can be systolic or diastolic, or both. Identification of systemic hypertension is impeded by technical aspects of blood pressure determination in animals and the wide variation of normal values (see Chapter 3). Hypertension occurs secondary to renal disease (especially in cats), Cushing's disease, phaeochromocytoma, hyperthyroidism, drugs (e.g. alpha-adrenergic agonists), CNS disease and laminitis. The pathogenesis of hypertension in animals is unresolved and, as in human patients, is probably multifactorial. Clinical signs of hypertension most often affect the following target organs: eyes, heart, kidneys and brain. Retinal oedema, haemorrhage and detachments causing blindness are among the most devastating complications. Left ventricular hypertrophy may be observed, though congestive heart failure is uncommon. Progressive renal injury may occur. Diagnosis of hypertension requires either arterial puncture or an indirect determination that is repeatable with a reliable technique. Oscillometric methods and Doppler flow methods have been used successfully in dogs and in cats. Systolic pressures exceeding 160 mmHg and diastolic pressures exceeding 95 mmHg are generally considered abnormal in the resting dog and cat with a normal heart rate.

Unless urgent treatment is needed to manage retinal detachments (vasodilators plus diuretics), therapy for systemic hypertension in dogs and cats usually involves a step-wise method of treatment which is currently empirical and based more on experience than on controlled studies. Commonly used treatments (see Appendix A2) include:

- Management of the underlying problem (e.g. treat hyperthyroidism).
- Dietary sodium restriction, usually with modest diuretic therapy (furosemide 1–2 mg/kg or 2–4 mg/kg of combined hydrochlorothiazide–spironolactone).
- Angiotensin-converting enzyme inhibitor (enalapril).
- Beta-adrenergic blocker (propranolol).

- Direct-acting arteriolar dilator (hydralazine 1–2 mg/kg q12h).
- Calcium-channel blocker (e.g. diltiazem); in cats, amlodipine (0.625 mg daily) is the agent of choice.
- Alpha-adrenergic blocker (prazosin 1–2 mg q8–12h).

ARTERIOVENOUS FISTULAE

An *arteriovenous fistula* is a congenital or acquired communication between artery and vein. Congenital lesions tend to be multiple and involve limbs, while a post-traumatic fistula is usually a single direct connection associated with trauma and inappropriate healing of the injured blood vessels. Declawing operations have been associated with AV fistula formation in cats. Thyroid carcinoma in the dog may lead to a cervical AV communication. Hepatic AV fistula represents a special type of congenital vascular malformation. This condition is usually associated with portal hypertension and ascites. The clinical findings in arteriovenous fistula include local vascular changes (due to venous hypertension) and cardiac manifestations (due to increased cardiac output required to perfuse the shunt). A continuous murmur (bruit) is often detectable over the affected area as blood shunts continuously through the fistula. A positive Branham sign may be present in large shunts (slowing of the heart rate following digital occlusion of the artery). Diagnosis is made by clinical signs, ultrasonography (including Doppler studies) and angiography. Ligation of the shunt can be accomplished surgically. However, surgery for congenital fistulae can be problematic.

LYMPHATIC DISORDERS

Various *lymphatic disorders* are recognized in animals. These include congenital lymphatic dysplasia and acquired lymphatic disturbances, causing protein-losing enteropathies and chylothorax, lymphatic obstruction from neoplasia, and lymphangitis. Occlusion of lymphatic vessels invariably alters microcirculation and results in oedematous swelling or effusions.

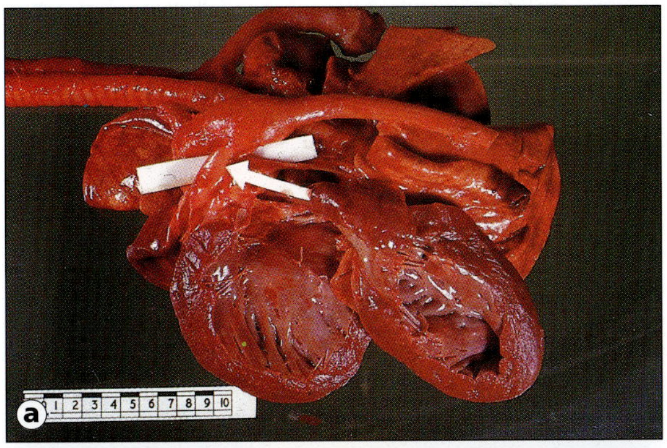

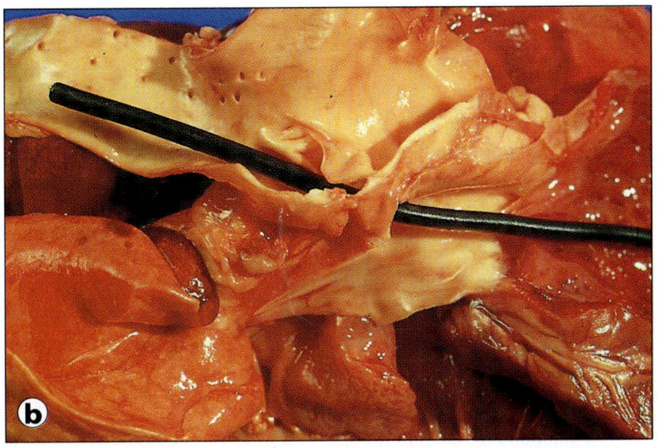

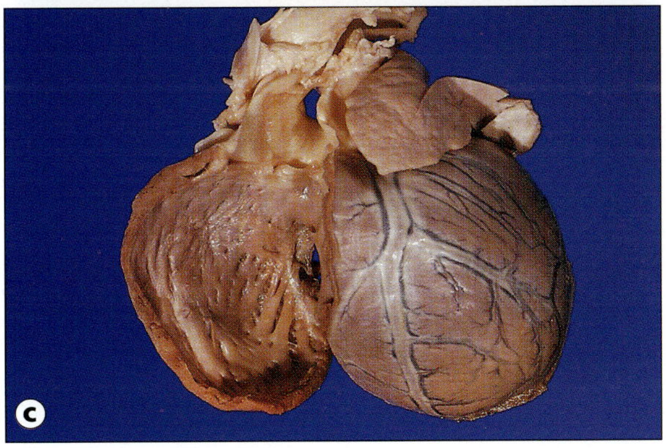

21.1 (**a**) Patent ductus arteriosus in a 6-year-old male greyhound. (**b**) Patent ductus arteriosus in a 16-week-old female cross-bred dog. The probe indicates a widely patent communication between the aorta and the pulmonary artery. The patent ductus arteriosus led to hyperperfusion of the pulmonary arterial bed by blood from the left ventricle. (**c**) Patent ductus arteriosus in a 4-month-old male springer spaniel. The opened pulmonary artery reveals the large circular ductus arteriosus that allows blood from the left ventricle to perfuse the lung through the pulmonary artery (left-to-right shunting).

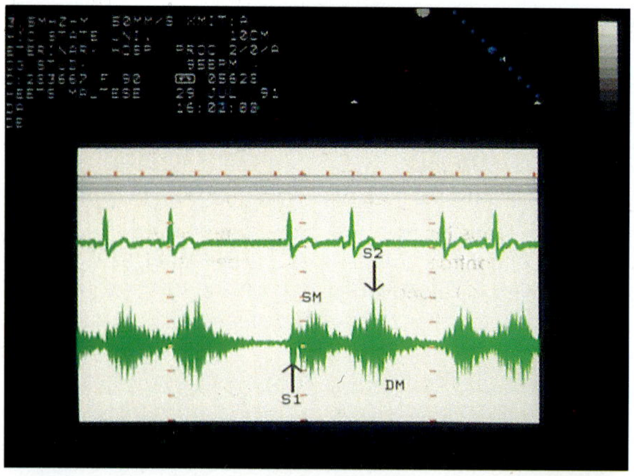

21.2 Phonocardiogram from a dog with patent ductus arteriosus. The timing of the first (S_1) and second (S_2) heart sounds is shown. The murmur is both systolic (SM) and diastolic (DM).

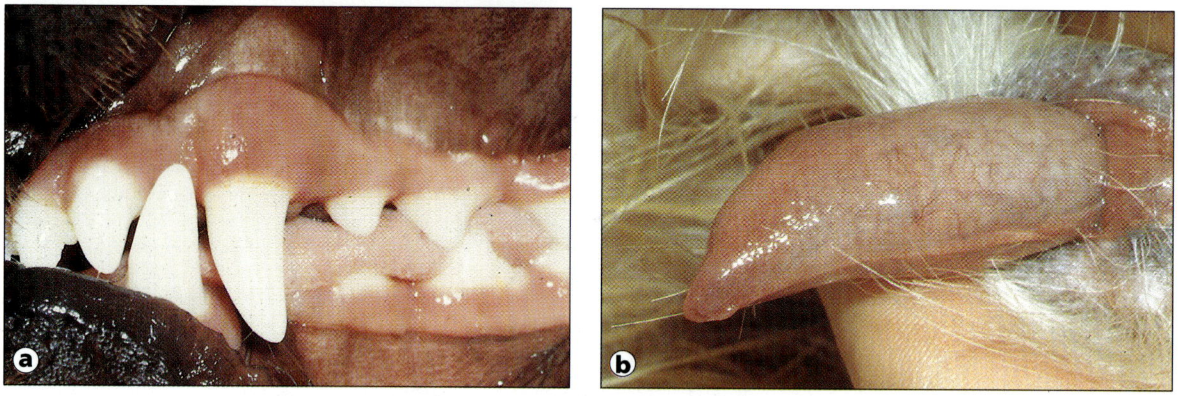

21.3 Differential cyanosis in a dog with reversed PDA due to pulmonary hypertension. (**a**) The cranial systemic circulation is derived from the left ventricle prior to the entrance of the shunting blood, and oral mucous membranes are pink. (**b**) Right-to-left shunting from the pulmonary artery to the descending aorta leads to cyanosis of the caudal mucous membranes.

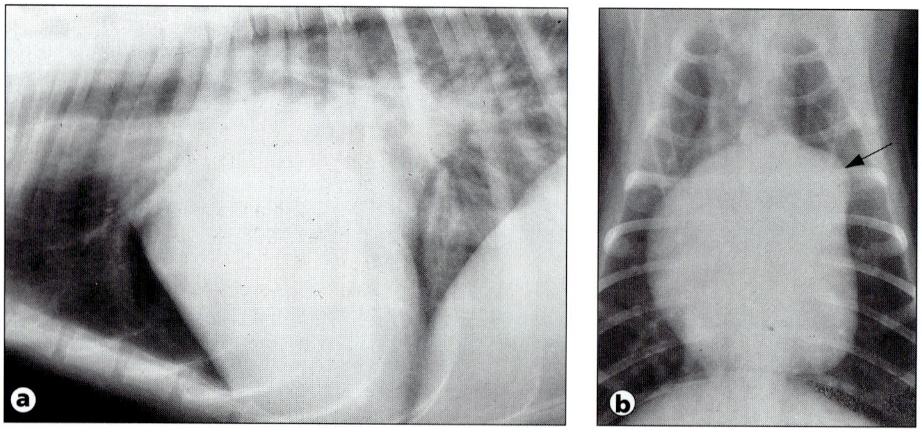

21.4 (**a**) Radiograph of a dog with PDA showing severe cardiomegaly, especially left ventricular (cardiac elongation) and left atrial dilatation. Pulmonary circulation is increased, typical of left-to-right shunts. (**b**) Radiograph of a different dog with reversed PDA. The right ventricle is hypertrophied and the main pulmonary artery dilated (arrow) owing to pulmonary hypertension. The lung in this case is not overcirculated.

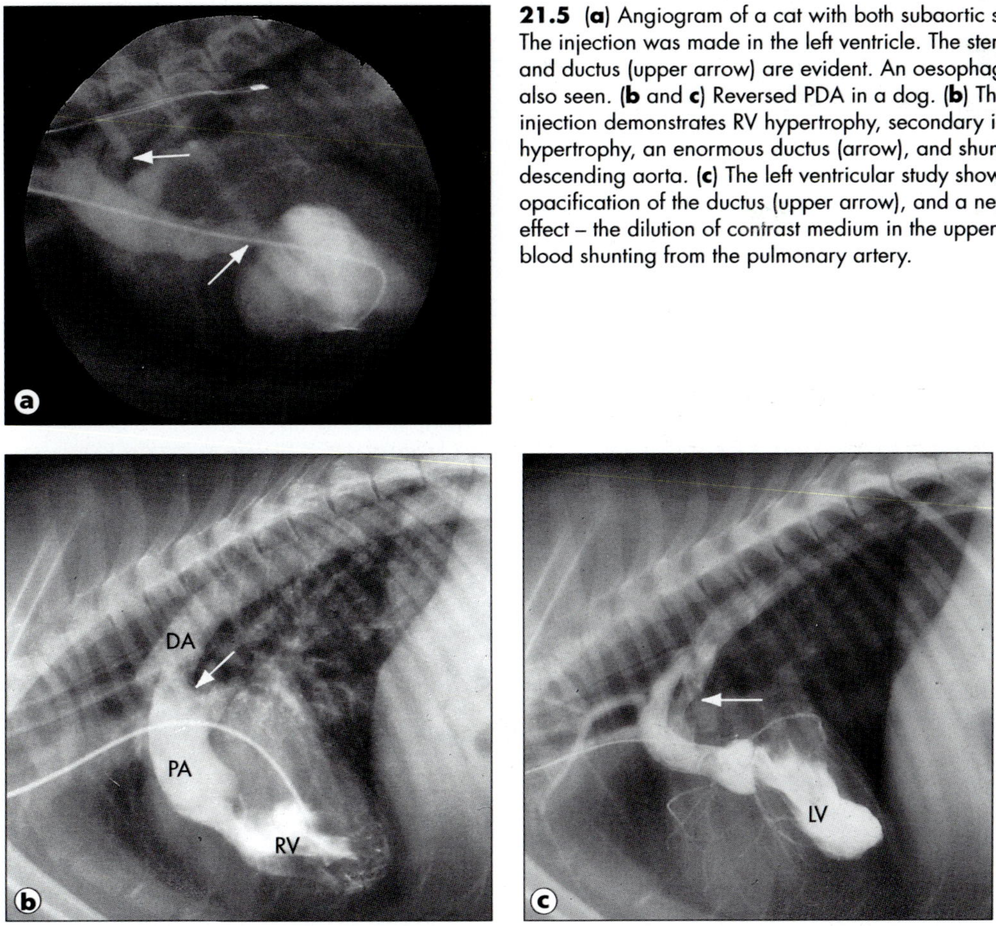

21.5 (**a**) Angiogram of a cat with both subaortic stenosis and PDA. The injection was made in the left ventricle. The stenosis (lower arrow) and ductus (upper arrow) are evident. An oesophageal stethoscope is also seen. (**b** and **c**) Reversed PDA in a dog. (**b**) The right ventricular injection demonstrates RV hypertrophy, secondary infundibular hypertrophy, an enormous ductus (arrow), and shunting into the descending aorta. (**c**) The left ventricular study shows a small ventricle, opacification of the ductus (upper arrow), and a negative contrast effect – the dilution of contrast medium in the upper ventricle from blood shunting from the pulmonary artery.

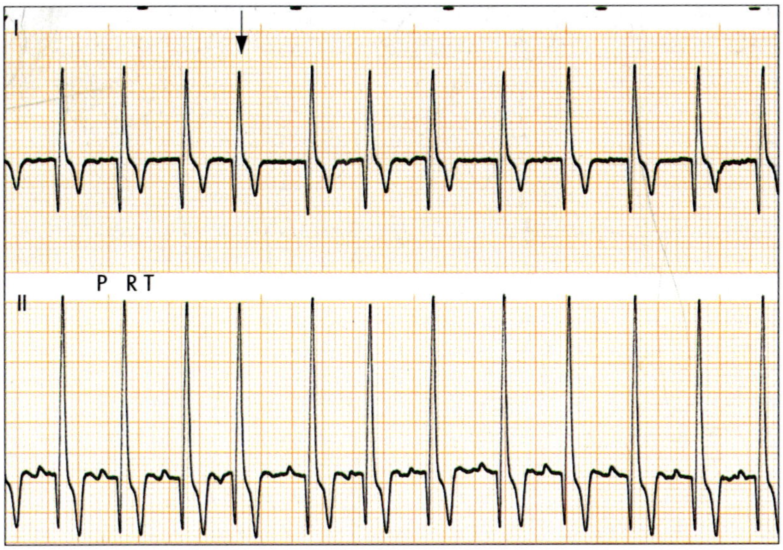

21.6 ECG (leads I and II) from a 7-month-old springer spaniel with a patent ductus arteriosus. There is sinus rhythm at a heart rate of about 150bpm, with atrial premature complexes (one is arrowed). There are also deep Q waves and tall R waves in lead II (2.8 mV) and a prolonged QRS complex (0.08 sec) and S–T coving, all typical features of the left ventricular dilatation found with severe shunting. The APCs are probably associated with left atrial dilatation.

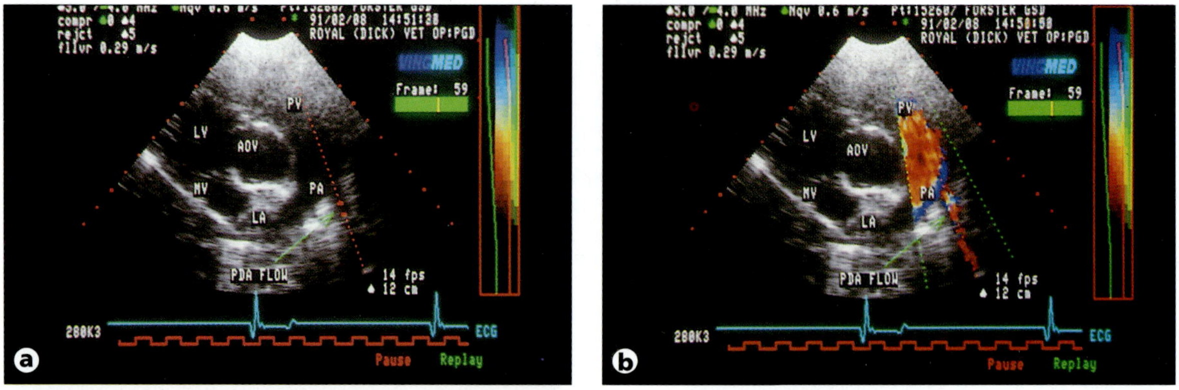

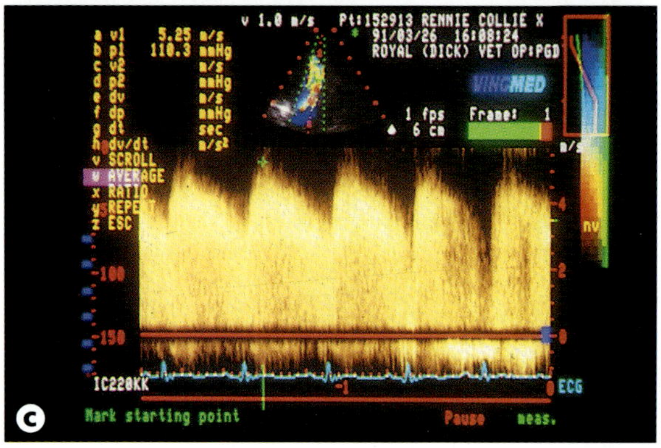

21.7 (**a**) Two-dimensional, short-axis view of the heart base from a young German shepherd dog, showing a patent ductus arteriosus. (**b**) Colour-flow Doppler recording of flow through the patent ductus shown in (**a**). The flow through the ductus is towards the transducer (coded red) and retrograde in the pulmonary artery. (**c**) HPRF pulsed-wave spectral Doppler recording of the flow in a patent ductus arteriosus in a collie-cross. Note the varying velocity of flow, maximal in systole, and declining in diastole, with a maximum velocity of about 5.25 m/sec, which represents a pressure gradient between aorta and pulmonary artery of about 110 mmHg (by the Bernoulli equation), indicating that this is a restrictive ductus, without pulmonary hypertension.

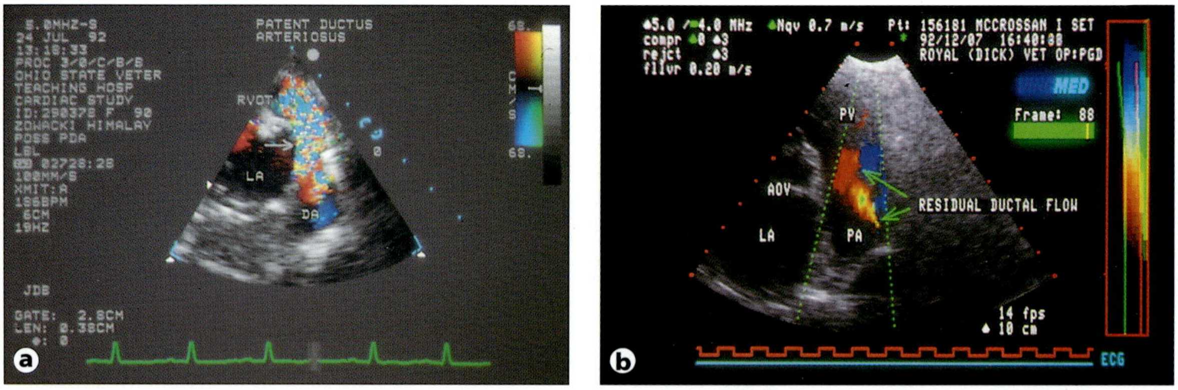

21.8 (**a**) Colour-flow echocardiogram from a cat with PDA. The image of the pulmonary artery, obtained from the left base, demonstrates a turbulent mosaic of flow returning from the ductus. (DA – descending aorta.) (Courtesy of Dr Linda B. Lehmkuhl.) (**b**) A jet of residual flow through a ductus arteriosus after ligation in a young Irish setter. Residual flow can be demonstrated by colour-flow Doppler after successful surgery in some cases, even in the absence of an audible murmur, as in children. However, the volume of flow is usually insignificant.

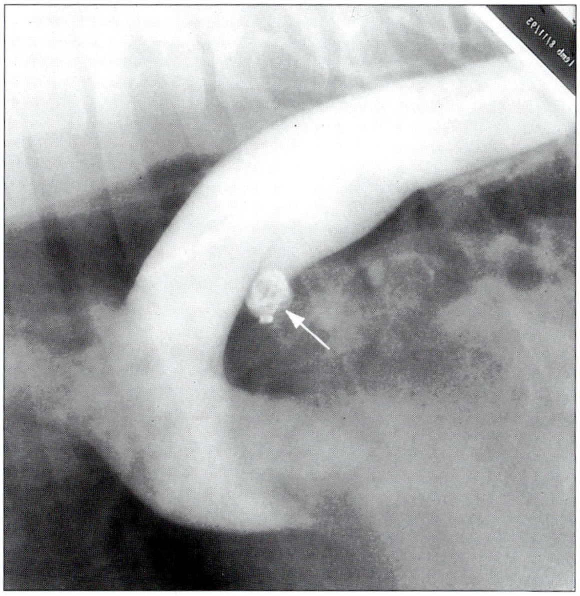

21.9 A Gianturco coil occlusion (arrow) of a patent ductus in a dog. (Courtesy of Dr Matt W. Miller.)

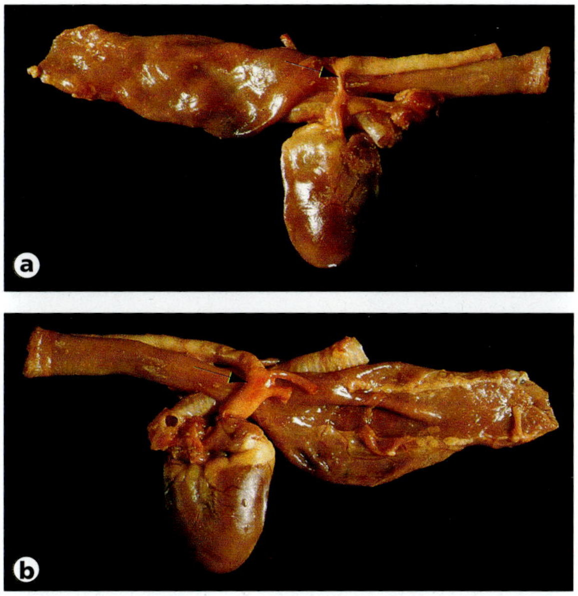

21.10 (**a** and **b**) Persistent right fourth aortic arch viewed from the left (**a**) and the right (**b**). The vascular ring in this cat was formed by the heart base, ductus arteriosus (arrow in **a**), right aortic arch (arrow in **b**) and trachea. The cat died of septic complications from dilatation, necrosis and rupture of the oesophagus which is evident cranial to the heart.

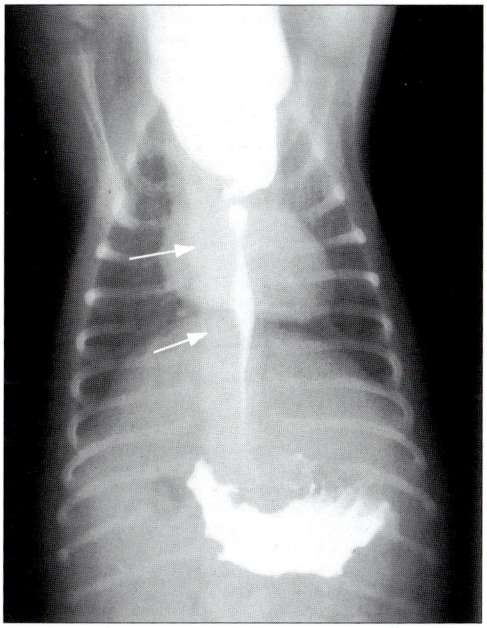

21.11 Radiograph taken after the administration of a barium meal to an 8-week-old cross-bred pup with persistent regurgitation of solid foods. The oesophagus is clearly obstructed at the base of the heart, and a dextroposed aorta can be seen (arrows) with a vascular ring stricture.

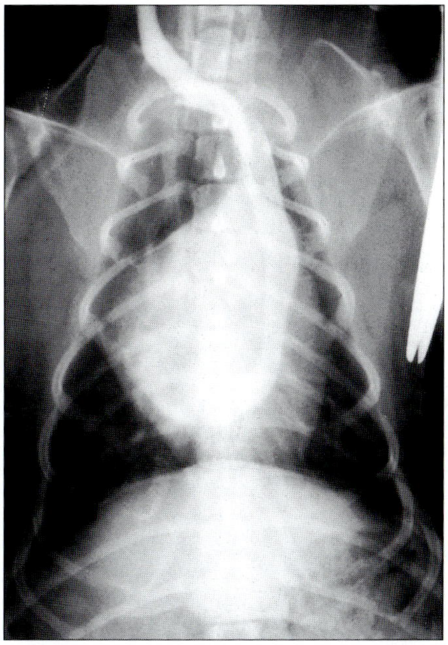

21.12 Angiogram following the injection of contrast medium into the right cranial vena cava of a cavalier King Charles spaniel with concomitant patent ductus arteriosus. The contrast medium flows through a left-sided cranial vena cava that tracks around the left atrium to enter the right atrium caudally.

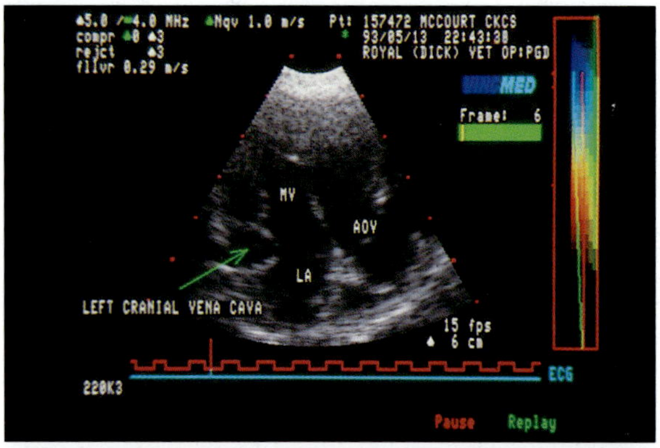

21.13 Two-dimensional image of the persistent left cranial vena cava as it tracks behind the left atrium to enter the right atrium, in the dog in **21.12**.

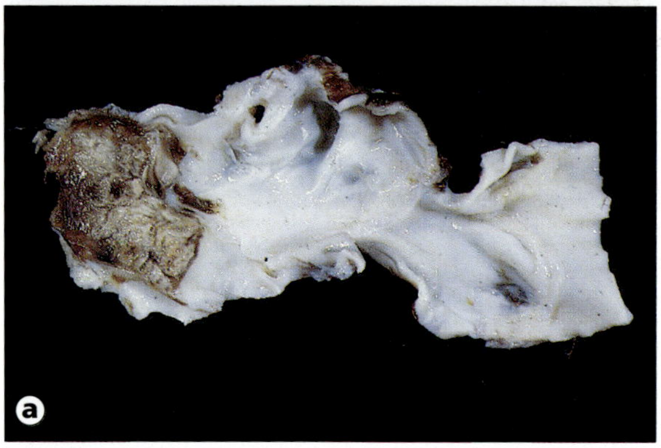

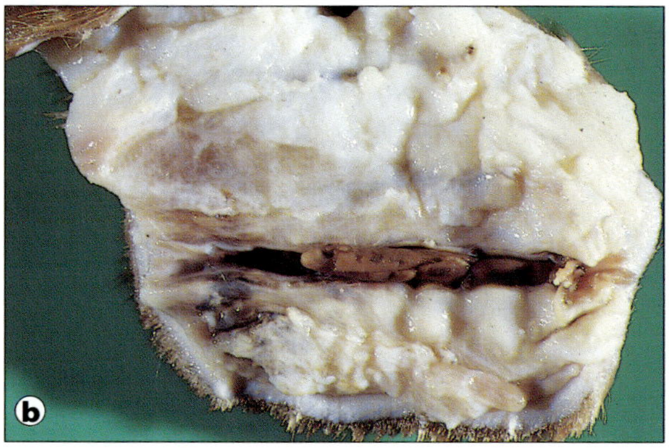

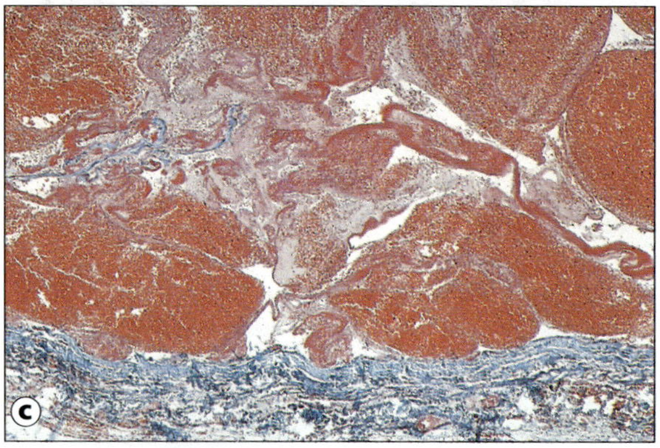

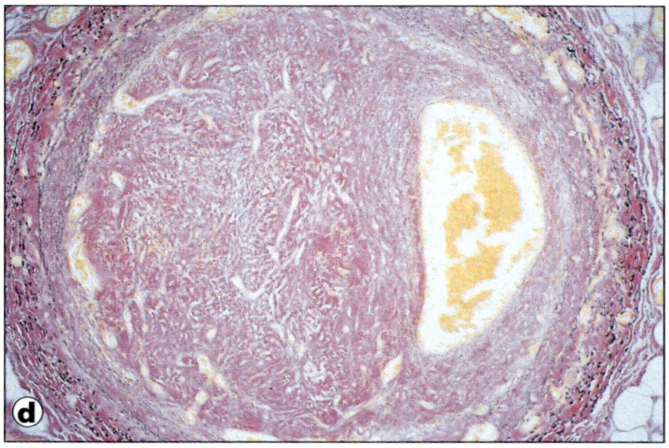

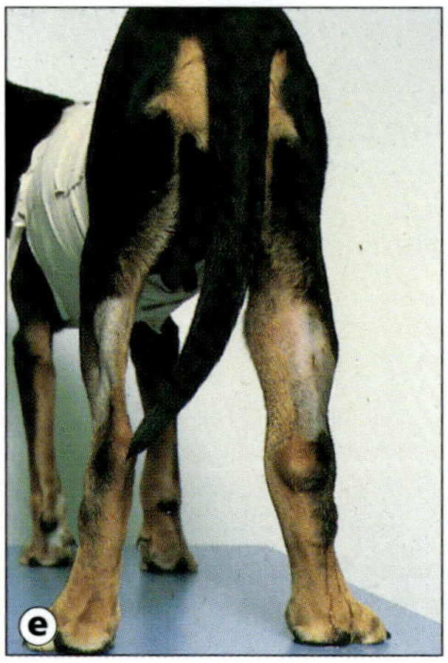

21.14 (**a**) Jugular vein from a cow showing normal pale intima and valves, and a large adherent thrombus. Such lesions can occur as complications of venepuncture and iatrogenic infection. (**b**) A length of cephalic vein from a dog, showing extensive occlusion by thrombus. Such lesions can occur as complications of cannulation or injection of irritant fluids. (**c**) Section of lamellated thrombus in the cranial vena cava of a dog. Thrombosis resulted from initial damage produced by an indwelling catheter. (**d**) Section of a cephalic vein from a dog that had an earlier thrombosis. This is now organized and recanalized (EVG stain). (**e**) Severe limb oedema in a dog with a thrombosed femoral vein caused by an indwelling intravenous catheter.

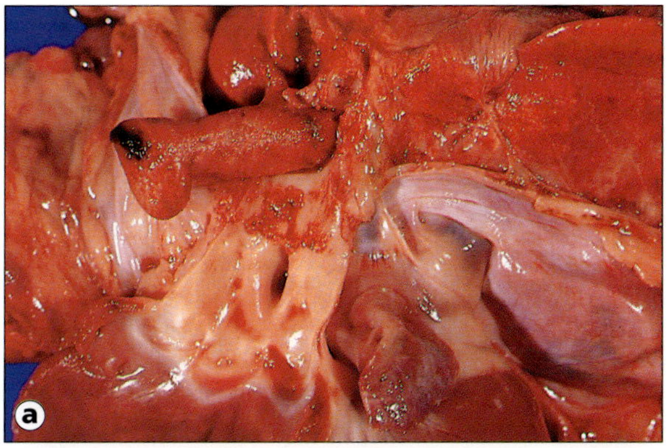

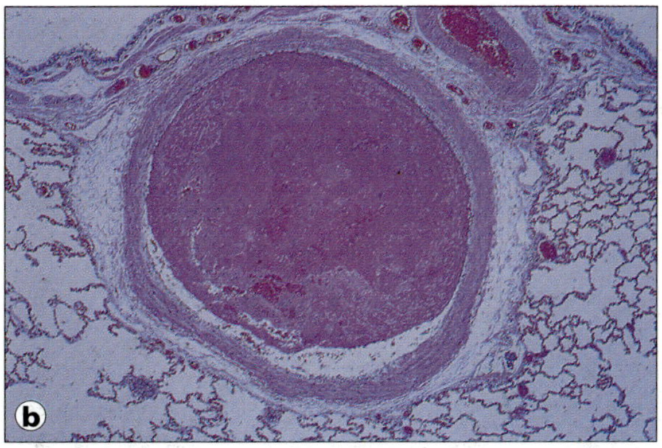

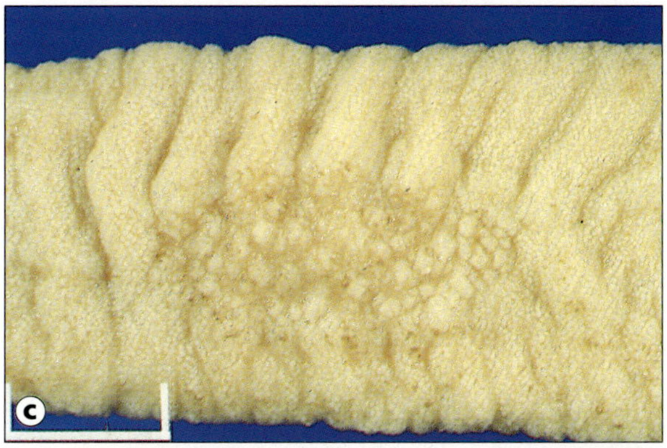

21.15 (**a**) Pulmonary arterial thrombosis in a 2-year-old springer spaniel with renal amyloidosis. There is complete occlusion of the outflow tract from the right ventricle. (**b**) Section of lung from a 3-year-old springer spaniel showing a thrombosed pulmonary artery. Such lesions can be associated with a number of disorders, including amyloidosis, protein-losing enteropathy of the thrombus or even hyperadrenocorticism. There is propagation of the thrombus and eventually occlusion of the main pulmonary arteries. (**c**) Small-intestinal mucosa from a 3-year-old springer spaniel with lymphangiectasia, severe protein-losing enteropathy and pulmonary arterial thrombosis.

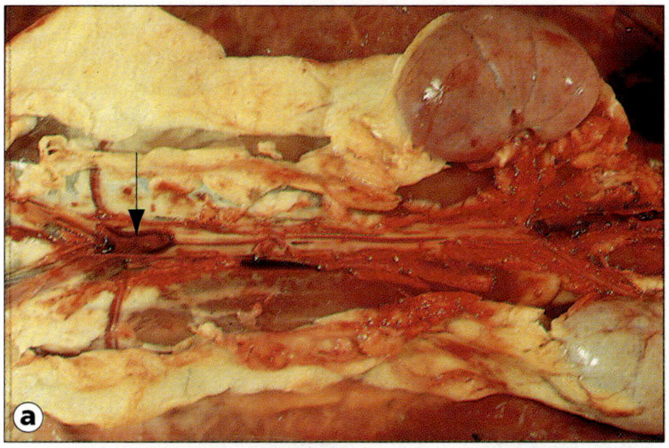

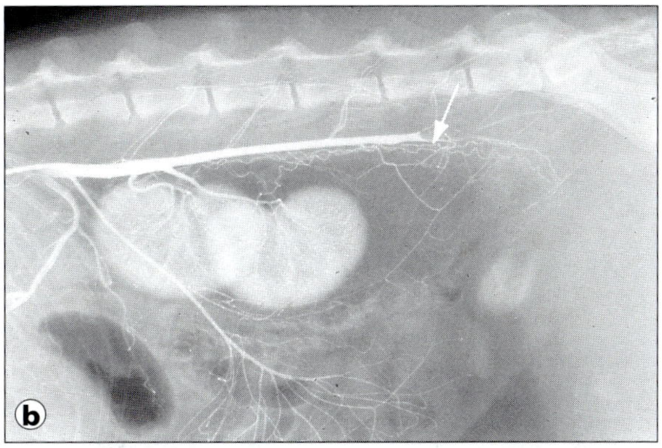

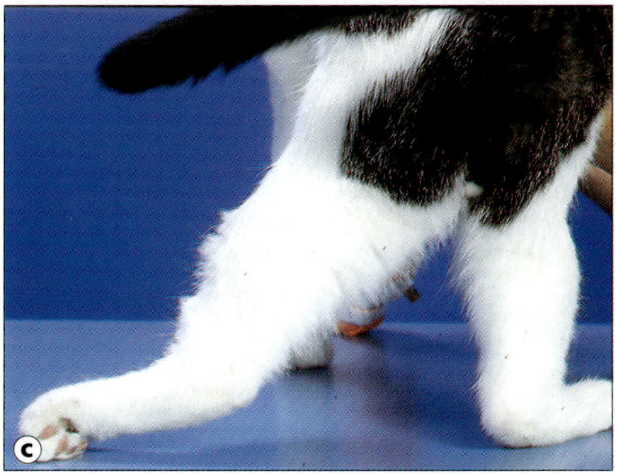

21.16 (**a**) Aortic thromboembolism in a 5-year-old Siamese cat with cardiomyopathy. The distal aorta is occluded by a massive thrombus derived from the left atrium. (**b**) Aortic thrombus (arrow) in a cat. The angiogram illuminates the abdominal aorta, renal circulation, and obstruction (arrow). There is scant collateral circulation caudally, with vasoconstriction likely to be a result of vasoactive chemicals released by the clot. (**c**) A cat recovering from aortic thromboembolism. The left rear limb has severe motor deficits. There is extensor weakness of the right rear limb.

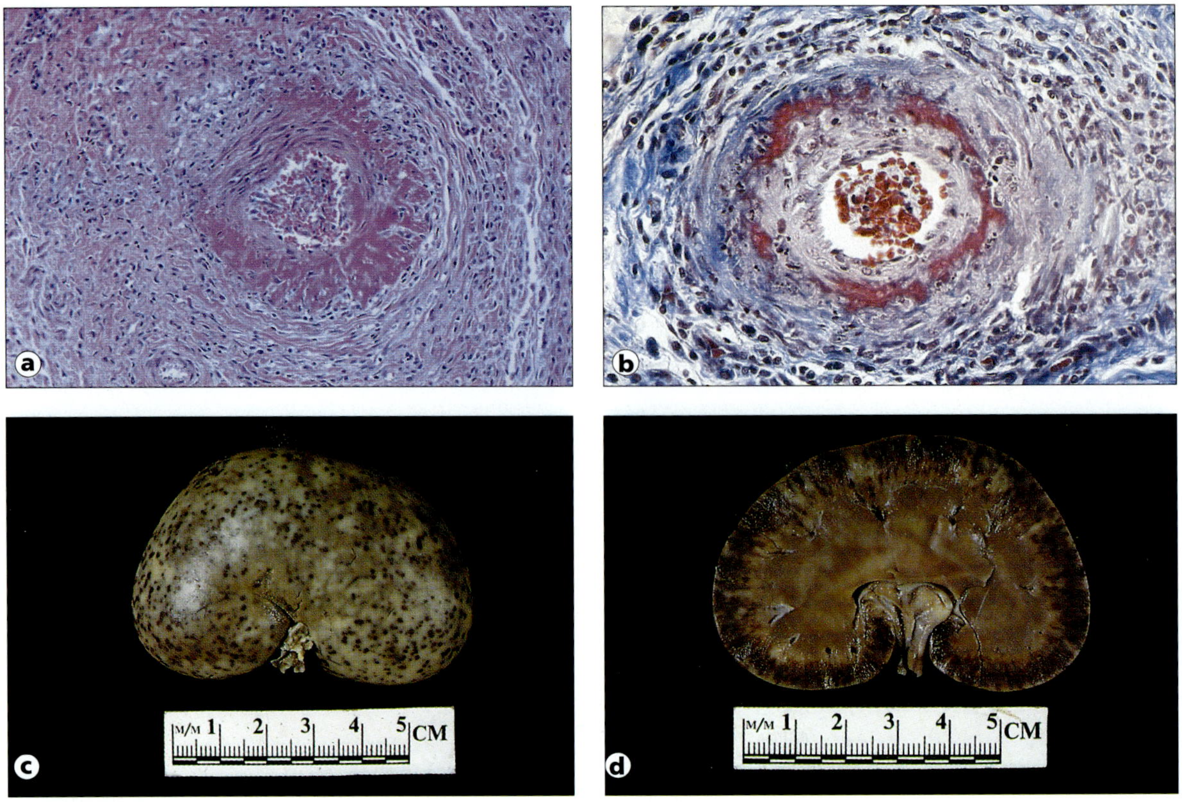

21.17 (**a**) Polyarteritis in a 10-month-old golden retriever. Photomicrograph showing florid necrotizing arteritis in the thyroid. There is extensive necrosis of the medial smooth muscle. (**b**) Polyaerteritis. Photomicrograph of a mediastinal artery, showing fibrin insudation into the injured tunica intima. (**c** and **d**) Kidney from a 7-year-old dog with polyarteritis, showing multifocal subcapsular petechial haemorrhages. (**d**) Cut surface of the kidney showing the extensive cortical haemorrhage.

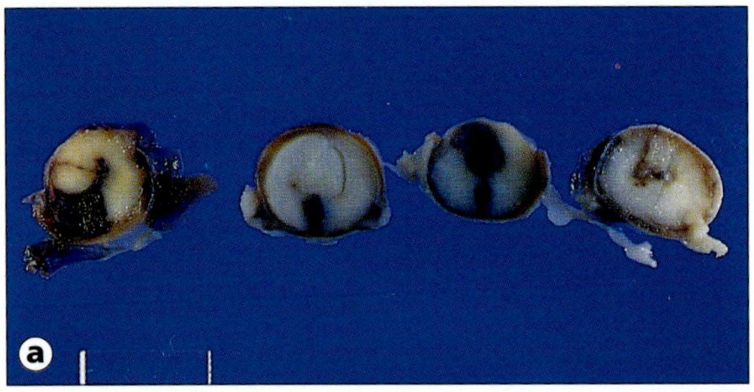

21.18 (**a** and **b**) Spinal arteritis and haematomyelia in a 10-month-old golden retriever. (**a**) Coronal sections of the spinal cord, showing subdural and intraspinal haemorrhage. The thrombosis results from severe necrotizing arteritis that appears, paradoxically, to be largely confined to the meningeal vessels. (**b**) Photomicrograph of the spinal cord. The central subdural artery has extensive severe necrotizing arteritis, with haemorrhage into the adjacent subarachnoid space. (**c**) Spinal arteritis in a 17-month-old Afghan hound. There is almost total necrosis of the tunica media with perivascular inflammation and haemorrhage.

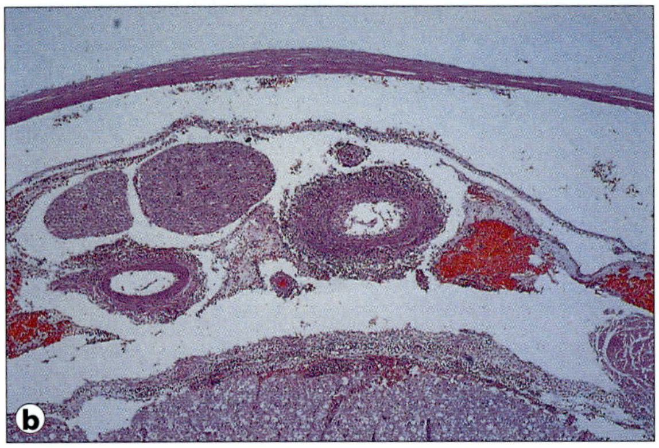

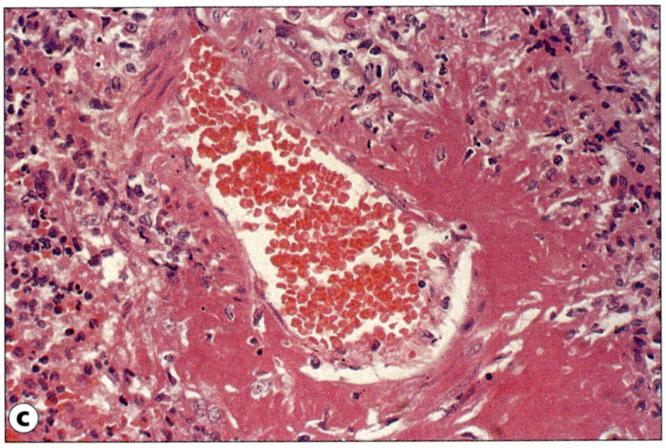

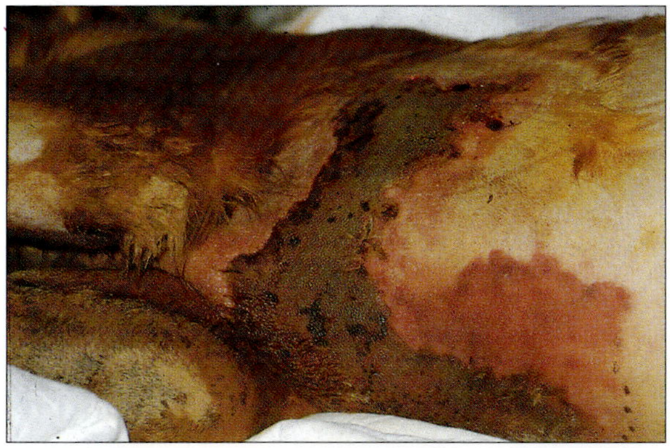

21.19 Large ecchymoses in a dog with histologically confirmed vasculitis.

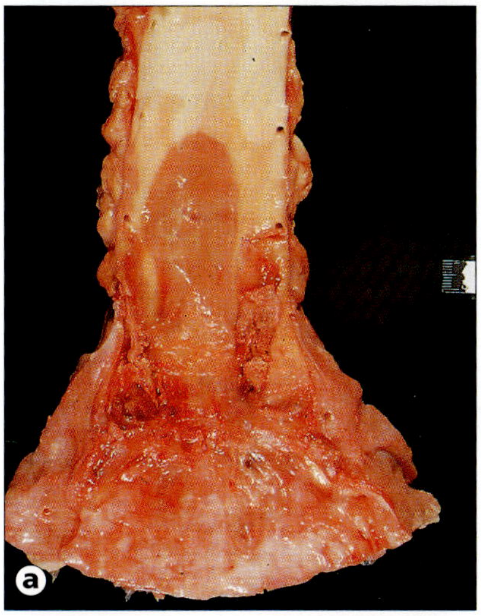

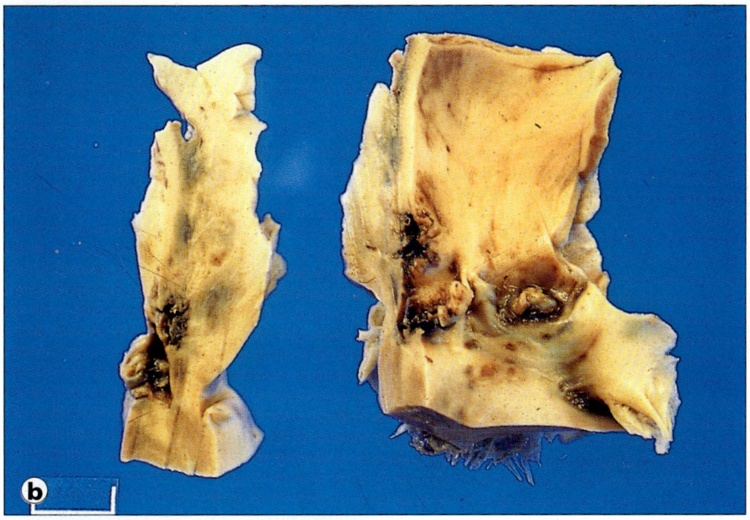

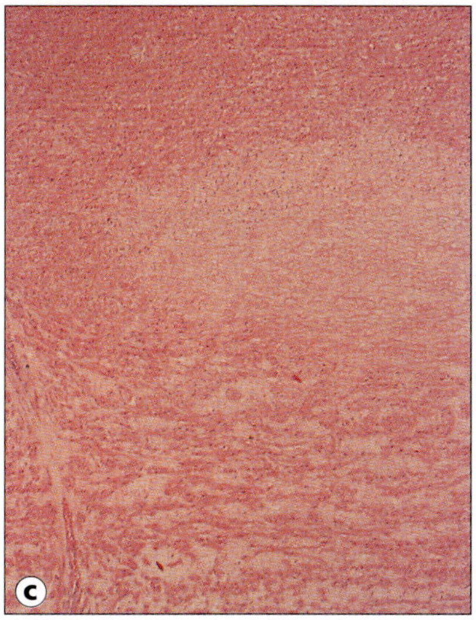

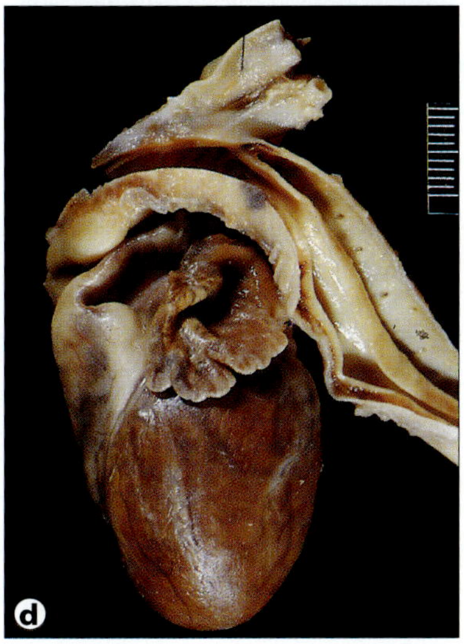

21.20 (**a**) Aortic necrosis in a horse. The cause was unknown, though streptococcus was isolated from the intimal inflammation. (**b**) Necrosis and rupture of the aorta adjacent to bacterial endocarditis of the aortic valve in a male German shepherd dog. (**c**) Photomicrograph of a section of aorta showing a central region of ischaemic necrosis. If there is anaemia or reduced perfusion this central region may undergo hypoxic necrosis. (**d**) Dissection of the aorta in a cat. The blood has been removed from the false lumen which had dissected through an intimal tear (not shown) and separated the media and adventitia. The inner tube is the true aortic channel. (Courtesy of Dr Linda B. Lehmkuhl.)

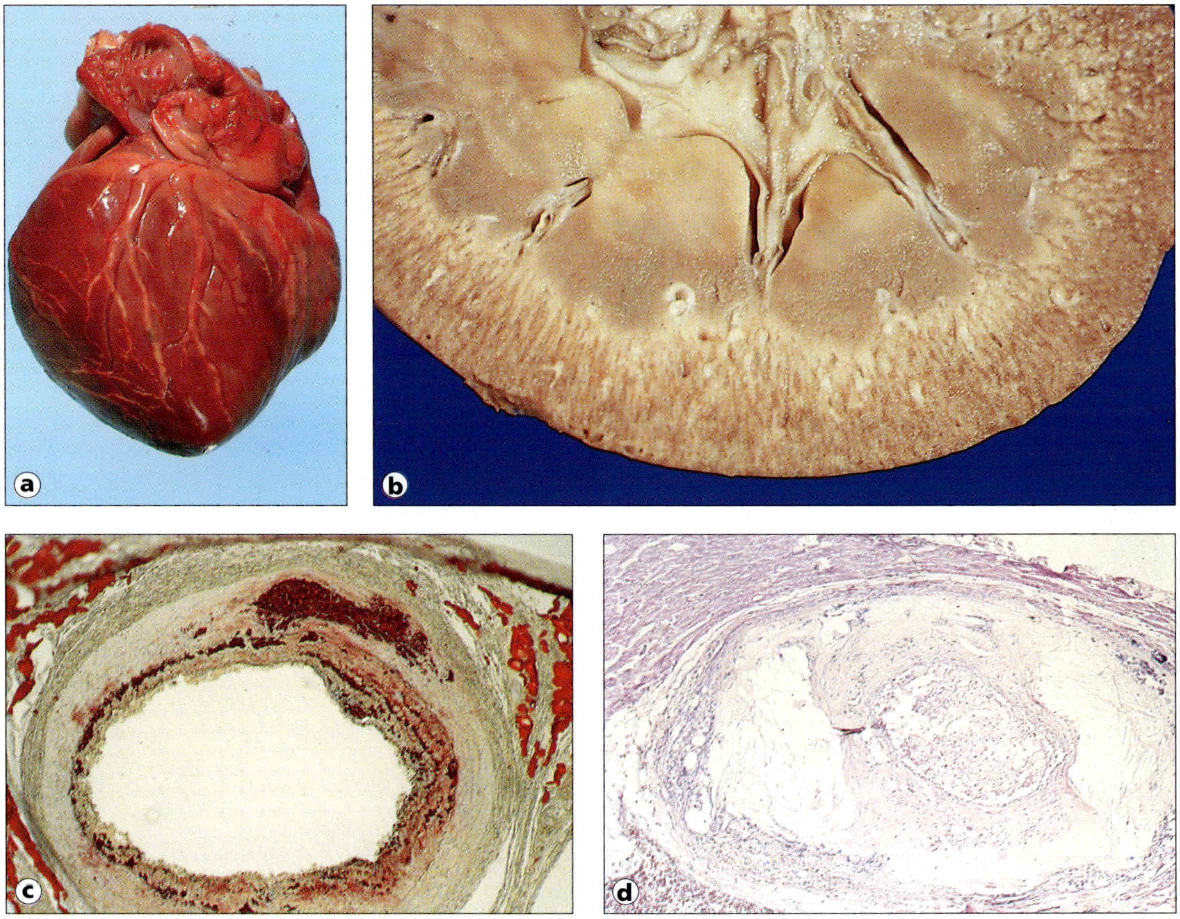

21.21 (**a**) Coronary atherosclerosis in a German shepherd dog. Extramural coronary arteries are thick and yellow/white because of lipid accumulation within their walls. (**b** and **c**) Atherosclerosis in a 6-year-old German shepherd dog. (**b**) The cut surface of the kidney reveals extensive thickening and pallor of the atherosclerotic intrarenal arteries. (**c**) Photomicrograph of a frozen section of coronary artery showing extensive lipid in the intima and tunica media. (**d**) Photomicrograph of a coronary artery showing the tunica media replaced by lipid. The lumen also contains lipid-laden macrophages.

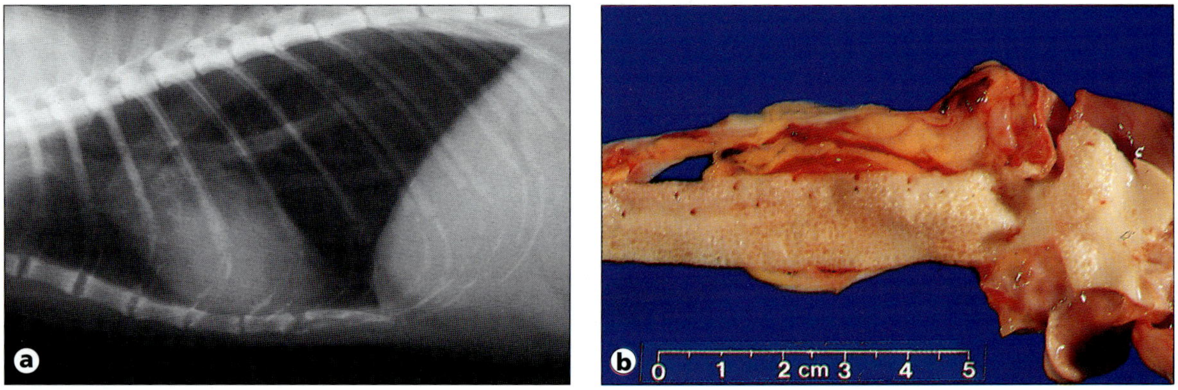

21.22 (**a**) Radiograph of a 12-year-old domestic short-haired cat after excessive dietary supplementation with calcium and vitamin D for many months. This therapy was instituted to counteract hypocalcaemia due to inadvertent removal of parathyroid tissue with a thyroid tumuor. There is mineralization of the aorta, the brachiocephalic arteries and the pulmonary artery. (Courtesy of Mr D. Foster.) (**b**) Extensive roughening and calcification of the aortic intima in a 10-year-old male cat with chronic renal failure.

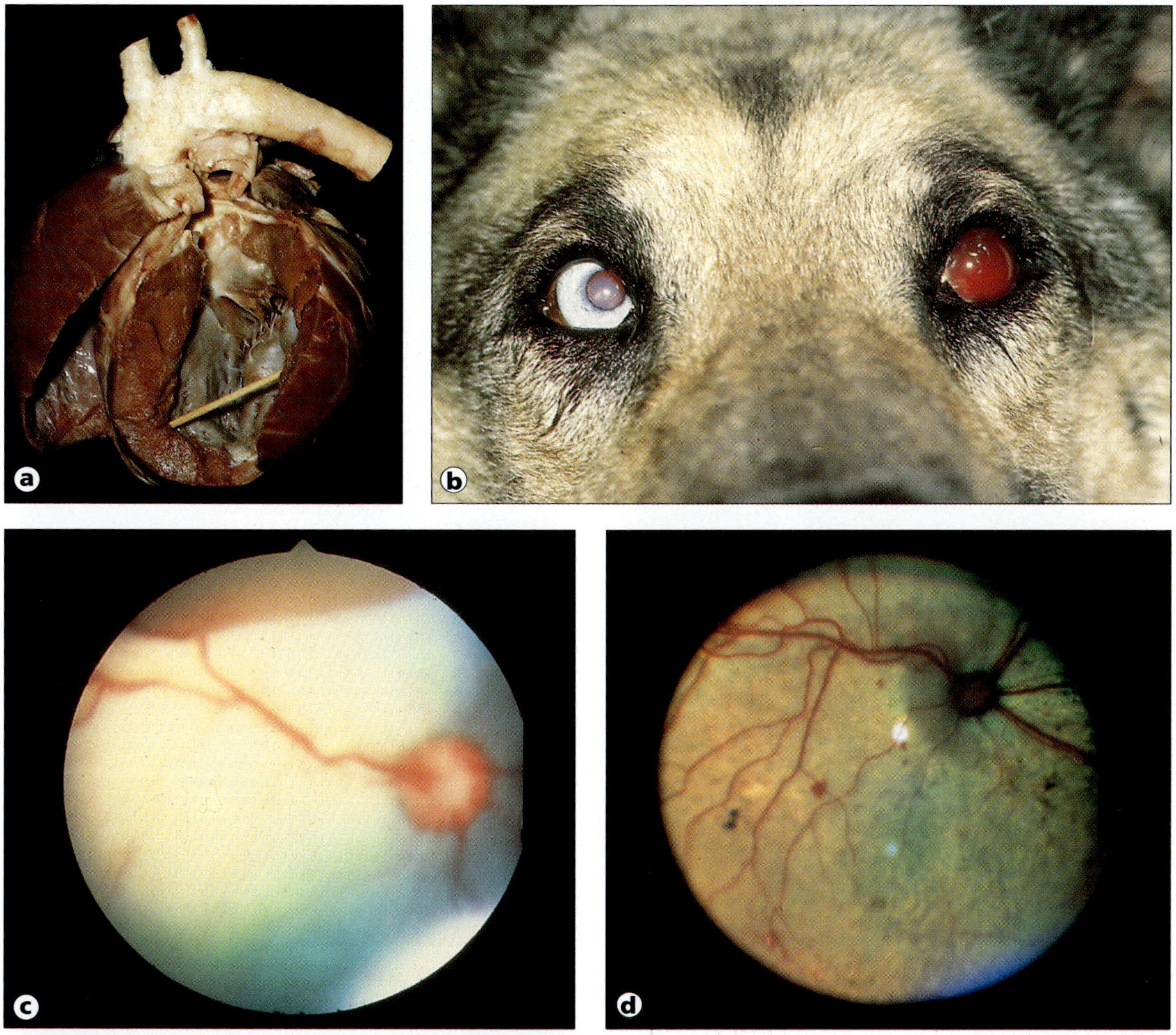

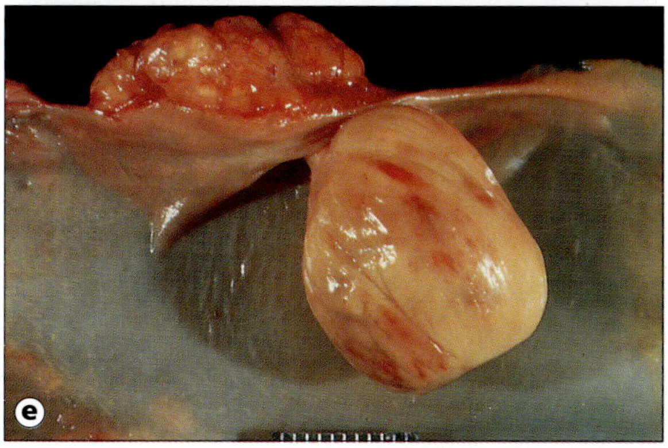

21.23 (**a**) Left ventricular hypertrophy in a dog with chronic and severe systemic hypertension related to renal disease. (**b**) Hyphaema in a dog with severe systemic hypertension. (**c** and **d**) Retinal detachment (**c**) and retinal haemorrhages (**d**) in cats with systemic hypertension. This species is most often affected with clinical consequences of systemic hypertension. (**d** – courtesy of Dr Dan Wolf.) (**e**) A phaeochromocytoma in a dog. The tumour may lead to localized obstruction of blood flow or elaborate catecholamines to produce a paraneoplastic syndrome.

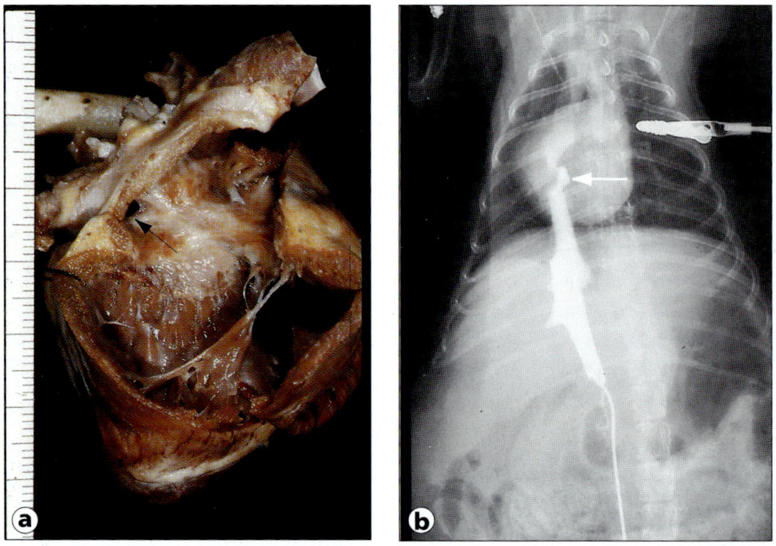

21.24 (**a** and **b**) Vena caval obstruction in an older schnauzer with ascites caused by fibrosis at the entry of the vessel into the caudal right atrium (arrow). (**b**) An angiogram demonstrates the narrowing and obstruction to blood flow (arrow). Differential diagnosis in a young dog should include cor triatriatum dexter, a malformation that leads to obstructive partitioning of the right atrium.

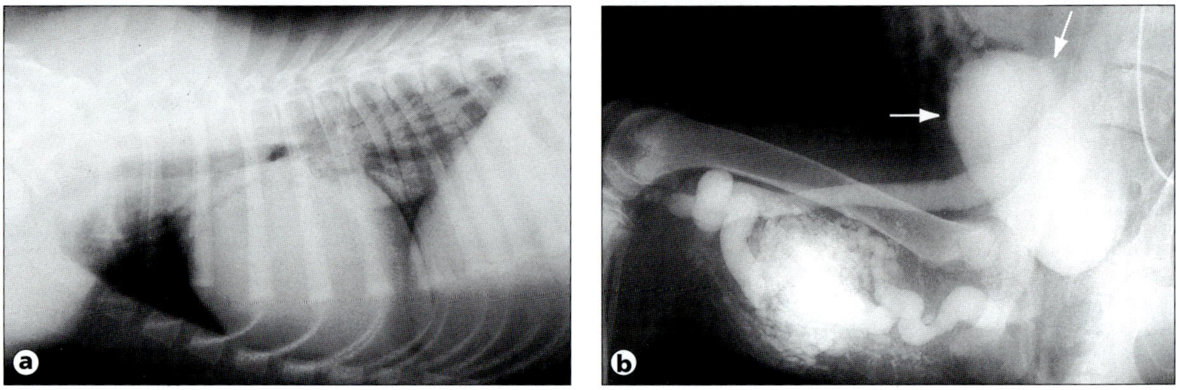

21.25 (**a**) Lateral thoracic radiograph from a 5-month-old greyhound with a hindlimb arteriovenous fistula of unknown aetiology. There is moderate cardiomegaly affecting particularly the right ventricle and enlargement of the caudal vena cava and pulmonary vessels. This volume overload is due to increased venous return from the peripheral shunt. (**b**) Following an injection of contrast medium into the femoral artery, tortuous tracts to the caudal vena cava can be seen. The bladder is filling with contrast medium (arrows) following excretion of dye from previous injections.

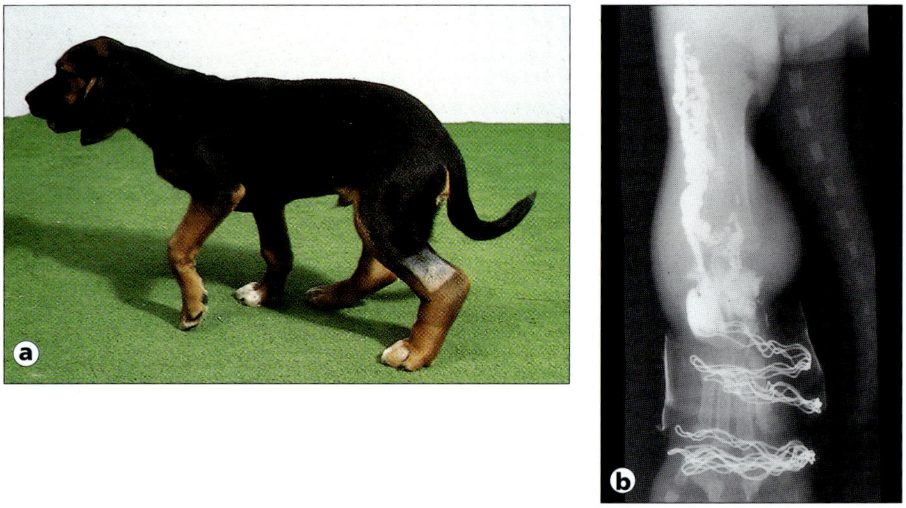

21.26 Congenital lymphoedema in a dog. (**a**) The oedema in this case affected the rear limbs. (**b**) Lymphangiography shows dilated, blindly ending lymphatics. (Note: opaque surgical sponges are apparent over the distal limb; lymphangiogram by Dr C. Wendy Myer). This dog gradually improved over a number of months and has survived to over 9 years of age, though being prone to hind limb infections.

22.

Cor Pulmonale

Cor pulmonale refers to right-sided heart enlargement that develops secondary to respiratory disease or pulmonary vascular disease. The condition is closely linked with pulmonary hypertension which is the underlying haemodynamic stimulus for the right ventricular hypertrophy and dilatation. Essential to an understanding of pulmonary hypertension is appreciation of the relationship:

$$\begin{bmatrix} \textit{Pulmonary} \\ \textit{artery} \\ \textit{function} \end{bmatrix} = \begin{bmatrix} \textit{Cardiac} \\ \textit{output} \\ \textit{flow} \end{bmatrix} x \begin{bmatrix} \textit{Pulmonary} \\ \textit{vascular} \\ \textit{pressure} \end{bmatrix}$$

Pulmonary vascular resistance depends on the following factors: left-sided heart function, pulmonary vascular anatomy and lesions, and pulmonary arterial reactivity. A significant reduction in total pulmonary cross-sectional arterial vascular area (usually > 50%) is needed to produce pulmonary hypertension. The pulmonary arterial tree also responds to local hypoxia by restriction. Thus, any primary pulmonary disease that reduces ventilation and lung function can lead to pulmonary arterial vasoconstriction. There are clear species differences in the responsiveness of the pulmonary vasculature to hypoxia-induced vasoconstriction. Ruminants are particularly sensitive to this reflex, followed by cats, horses and dogs. The pressure achieved in the pulmonary arteries to overcome high resistance must be generated by the right ventricle, which responds poorly to increased work. Mild-to-moderate cor pulmonale is associated with right-sided enlargement, subtle reductions in cardiac output, and exercise intolerance that might simply be attributed to the pulmonary disorder. Moderate-to-severe cor pulmonale usually causes marked right ventricular enlargement, with severe exercise intolerance and signs of right-sided congestive heart failure (see Chapter 1).

There are many causes of pulmonary hypertension and cor pulmonale, but among the most important clinically are:

- Dirofilariasis in dogs and cats.
- Pulmonary embolism – especially in dogs and cattle.
- Severe pulmonary disease (e.g. interstitial pneumonia or fibrosis, severe bronchial disease, chronic obstructive pulmonary diseases) in all species.
- Reactive pulmonary vasoconstriction due to low inspiratory oxygen tension – especially in ruminants grazing at high altitude.
- Idiopathic (primary pulmonary hypertension) – recognized in dogs.

It should also be emphasized that severe or chronic left-sided heart failure and congenital left-to-right shunts that cause pulmonary vascular injury (e.g. reversed PDA) can cause severe pulmonary hypertension; however, in these disorders the term 'cor pulmonale' is not generally used.

Clinical findings of cor pulmonale are usually dominated by the associated pulmonary disease or cardiac findings. Potential clinical signs include:

- Exercise intolerance.
- Abnormal heart sounds (loud or split second heart sound, tricuspid regurgitation, arrhythmias).
- Tachypnoea and dyspnoea, coughing, abnormal lung sounds, cyanosis and haemoptysis.
- Hypoxaemia (low arterial PaO_2).
- Radiographic or echocardiographic evidence of right-sided heart enlargement and dilatation of the pulmonary arteries.
- Increased pulmonary parenchymal densities (depending on the underlying cause).
- Right ventricular or atrial hypertrophy or dilatation or cardiac arrhythmias demonstrated by ECG (e.g. atrial or ventricular premature complexes, atrial fibrillation, junctional tachycardias).
- Shock (massive pulmonary embolus – see below)

Pulmonary hypertension can be diagnosed definitively only by cardiac catheterization or through Doppler echocardiographic methods that quantify the velocity of any associated tricuspid or pulmonary valve regurgitation. Systolic pulmonary artery pressures > 30 mmHg are generally considered significant. Noninvasive diagnosis can be made readily in most cases by a careful clinical and cardiac examination (see Chapters 3–7) coupled with a complete evaluation of the respiratory system.

The parasite *Dirofilaria immitis* is responsible for heartworm disease. In many parts of the world, this condition is very important in the dog and is also of clinical relevance in the cat. The parasite undergoes an indirect life cycle, involving many species of mosquito. The total life cycle takes about 200 days to complete, with the first 15–20 days spent within a mosquito. Once an infected mosquito takes a blood meal and introduces larvae (L_3) onto the skin of the canine or feline host, the parasites burrow into the subcutaneous tissues and moult twice over the next 2 months. It is this stage that is susceptible to preventive therapy with ivermectin, milbemycin or diethylcarbamazine. If uninterrupted by chemoprophylaxis, the fifth-stage larvae migrate into veins and are swept into the pulmonary arteries where they grow to mature adults, moving towards the heart as their length increases. A patent infection produces microscopic offspring (microfilaria) which circulate widely and are eventually taken into the intermediate host during a blood meal (completing the life cycle). The maturing worms and adults provoke a pulmonary vascular response, including arteritis, endarterial fibrosis and thrombosis. Should sufficient pulmonary injury occur, high vascular resistance develops, leading to pulmonary hypertension and cor pulmonale. Systolic pulmonary artery pressures that consistently exceed 60–70 mmHg are likely to provoke congestive heart failure. Many dogs never develop overt heart failure, but are incapacitated by a limited cardiac output or by pulmonary parenchymal complications. Lung lesions can include infarction, intrapulmonary bleeding from ruptured vessels, and pneumonitis in response to microfilarial antigens. Typical clinical features are illustrated in this chapter and are similar to those with cor pulmonale. Therapy involves anthelmintic treatment using a standardized protocol with an arsenical compound (thiacetarsemide sodium ormelarsomine dihydrochloride [RM-340]. Microfilaria can be killed with suitable dosages of oral ivermectin (50 mcg/kg – not to collie dogs) or milbemycin oxime (0.5 mg/kg). Pulmonary parenchymal complications are managed with anti-inflammatory dosages of prednisolone. Therapy for cats with dirofilariasis is undertaken infrequently, because of complications of arsenical therapy, though the clinical signs of this disease (vomiting and coughing in cats) can respond partly to prednisolone.

Pulmonary thrombosis or embolism represents another cause of significant cor pulmonale. Recurrent small emboli lead to clinical signs previously described for cor pulmonale. A massive pulmonary thrombosis or embolus can obstruct the left or right pulmonary artery leading to severe resistance to right ventricular ejection, low cardiac output, hypotension, myocardial ischaemia and cardiac arrest. Embolization of lobar vessels can initiate the release of vasoactive chemicals and cause noncardiogenic pulmonary oedema, pulmonary inflammation, and vascular narrowing with increased pulmonary vascular resistance. The most common causes of pulmonary embolism in animals include:

- Heartworm death following adulticidal therapy or spontaneous worm death in cats.
- Air embolus from injudicious air-contrast radiography or IV administration.
- Hypercoagulable states such as renal amyloidosis, glomerulonephritis, protein-losing enteropathy and Cushing's disease in dogs (reduction of antithrombin III activity).
- Autoimmune haemolytic anaemia in dogs.
- Liver abscess, caval thrombosis and pulmonary thromboembolism in cattle.
- Right-sided bacterial endocarditis in large animals.

Therapy for pulmonary embolism or pulmonary hypertension always involves treatment of the underlying condition. Oxygen therapy and improvement of pulmonary ventilation may decrease pulmonary arterial pressure if there is associated reactive pulmonary arterial vasoconstriction. Corticosteroids sometimes produce clinical benefit, probably by reducing pulmonary parenchymal reaction and ventilation:perfusion inequalities. Vasodilator drugs in general are dangerous for pulmonary hypertension as severe systemic hypotension may develop; accordingly, such therapy should not be undertaken without consulting a specialist with the ability to measure blood pressure. Heparin (50–100 i.u./kg, IV or SQ q8h) may be used in dogs and cats to prevent further thrombosis. If available, catheter retrieval, under fluoroscopic guidance, is probably the best treatment for a large, organized thrombus in the small animal. Shock therapy (fluids and dopamine infusion) may be needed to maintain blood pressure; however, excessive fluid therapy can increase pulmonary oedema.

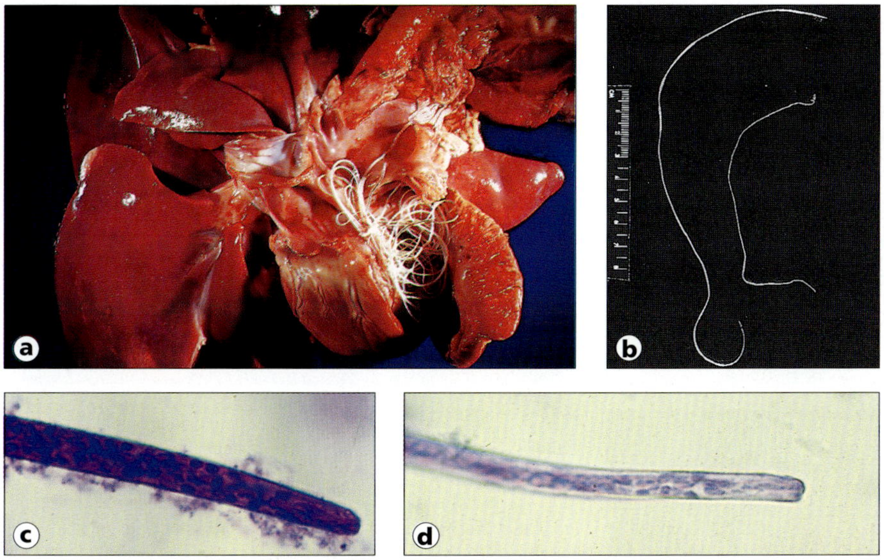

22.1 (**a**) Canine heartworm infestation. The heart is opened to reveal a mass of adult worms in the lumen of the right ventricle. (**b**) Adult *Dirofilaria immitis* (heartworm) parasites. The male is smaller and has a curled end. (**c** and **d**) Microfilaria of *D. immitis* and the nonpathogenic subcutaneous worm *Dipetalonema reconditum*. The microfilaria of *D. immitis* are wider and have a tapered head (**c**) whereas *D. reconditum* is more narrow with a blunted head (**d**).

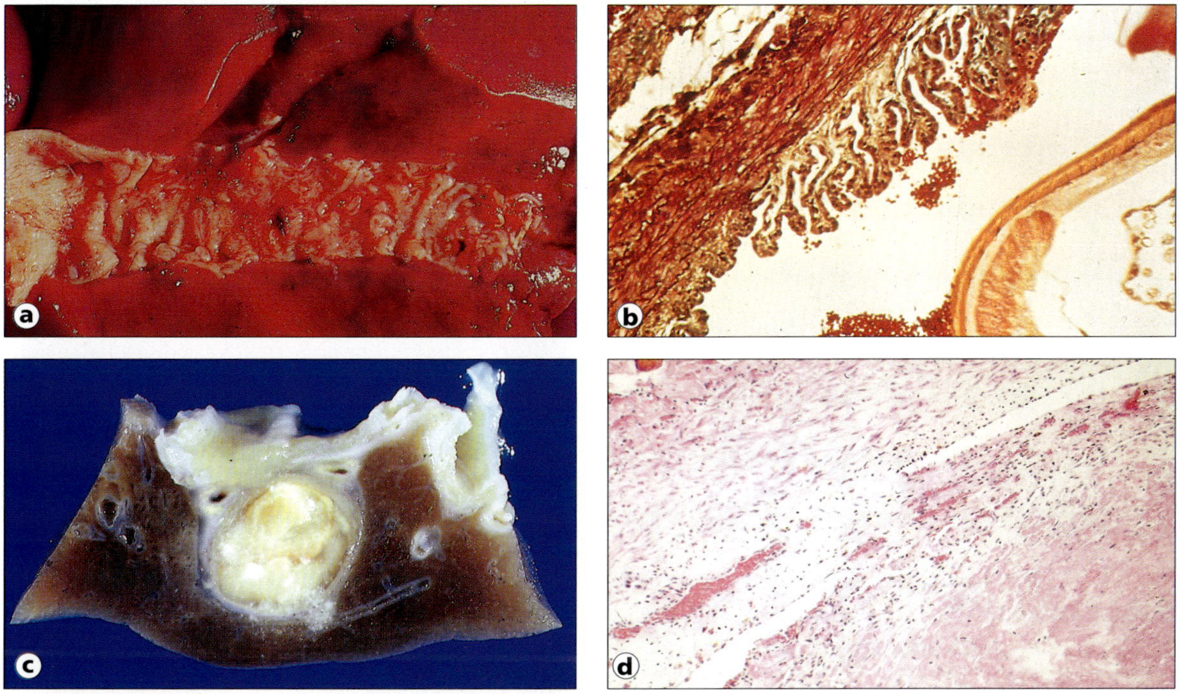

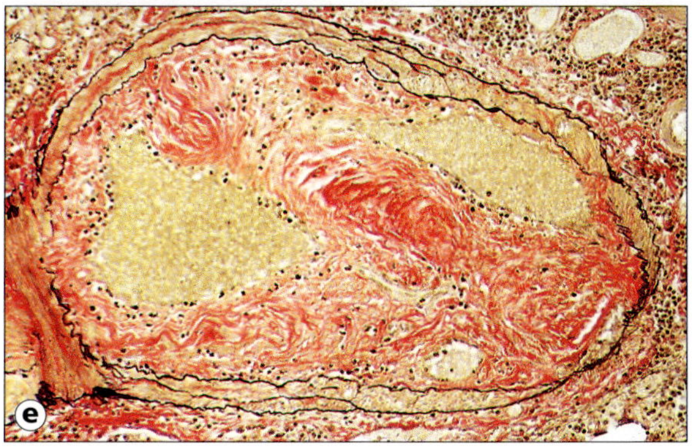

22.2 (**a**) The intima of the main pulmonary arterial trunk has villous projections formed by reaction to adult heartworms. (**b**) Endarteritis of the pulmonary artery caused by an adult heartworm. Note the villous pattern of endothelial reaction. (**c**) Pulmonary heartworm infestation showing a thrombosed pulmonary artery. (**d**) Photomicrograph showing pulmonary artery with recanalization following earlier thrombosis associated with heartworm infestation. (**e**) Photomicrograph showing a recent thrombus adhering to intima of a pulmonary artery from the same dog as in **c**.

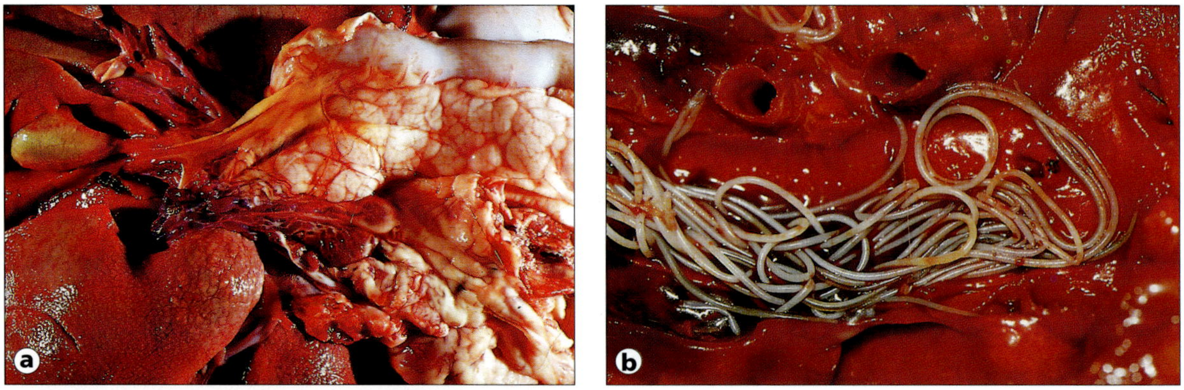

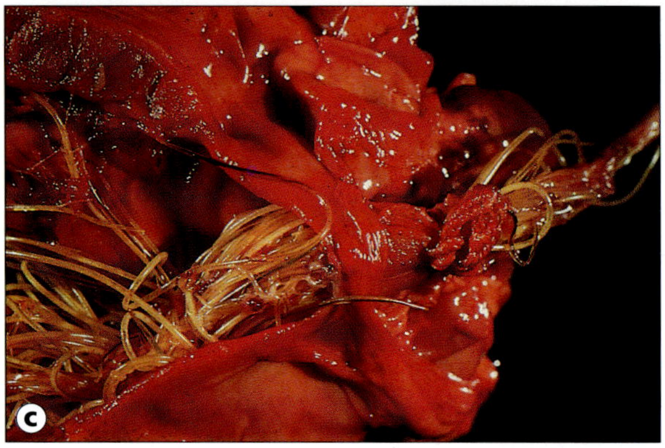

22.3 Canine heartworm infestation. (**a**) Right-sided cardiac failure showing venous congestion and liver swelling. (**b**) Mass of dead heartworms after adulticidal therapy to kill the worms. The massive pulmonary embolism leads to shock and sudden death. (**c**) Caval syndrome in a dog with heartworm disease showing a mass of adult worms.

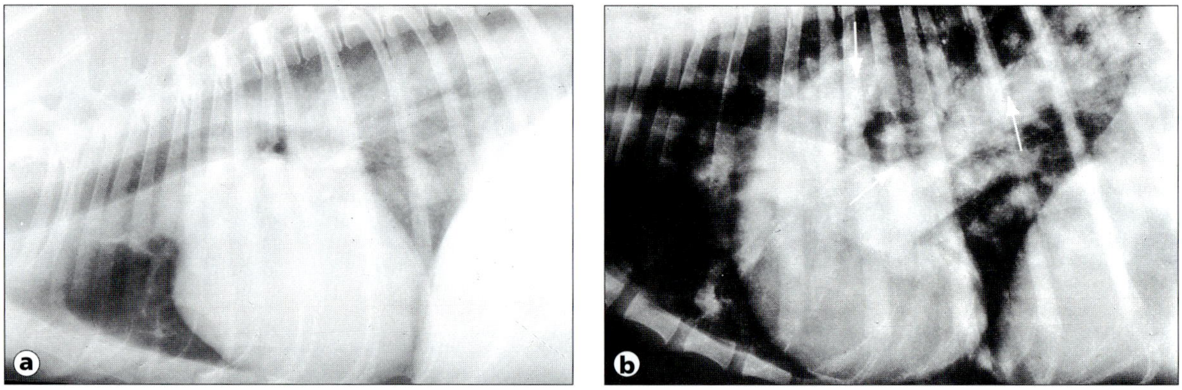

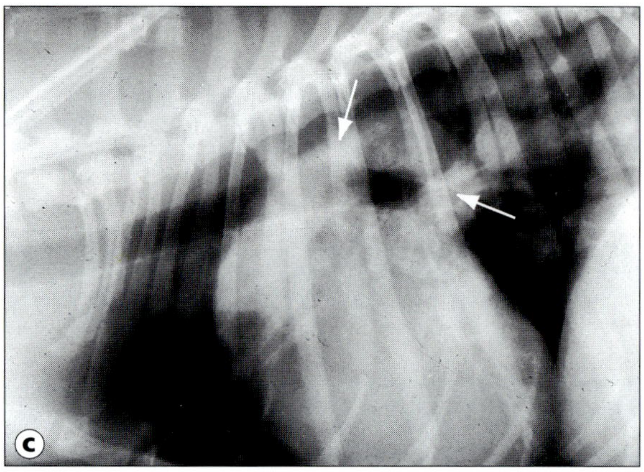

22.4 (**a–c**) Radiographs from three dogs with heartworm disease. Right-sided enlargement with displacement and elevation of the left apex is obvious in **a** and **c**. A pulmonary interstitial density typical of microfilaria or heartworm-related pneumonitis is evident in **a**. Severe dilatation of pulmonary arteries to the caudal lobes is observed in **b** and **c** (arrows).

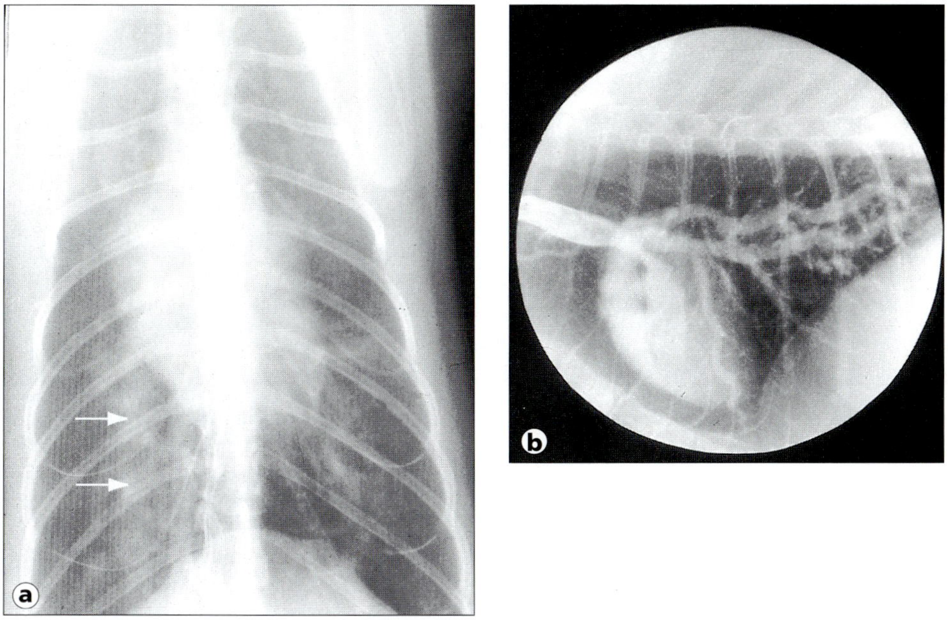

22.5
(**a**) Radiograph from a cat with heartworm disease. Note the large right caudal lobar artery (arrows). (**b**) Nonselective angiogram from another cat with heartworm disease. Note the tortuous caudal lobe pulmonary vessels.

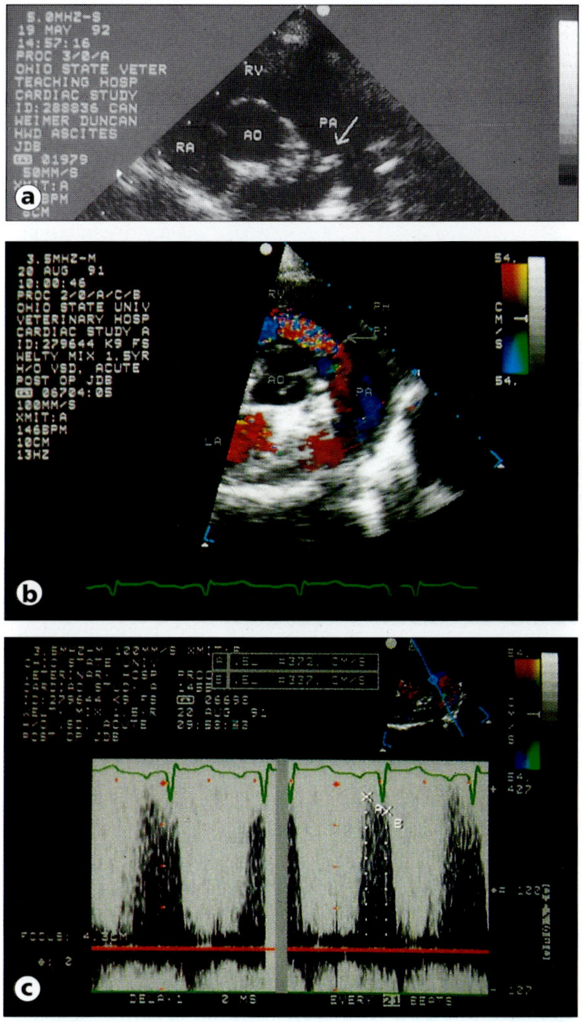

22.6 (**a**) Echocardiogram of the pulmonary arteries of a dog showing dilatation due to pulmonary hypertension. The arrow points to targets that are probably adult heartworms. (**b**) High-velocity pulmonary insufficiency in a dog with heartworm disease and pulmonary hypertension. The turbulent mosaic is typical of high-velocity regurgitation. The main pulmonary artery (PA) is dilated. (**c**) The continuous-wave Doppler study from the dog in (**b**) indicates a high-velocity jet of >3.7 m/sec. In contrast, physiologic pulmonary insufficiency is normally of low velocity (see Chapter 6).

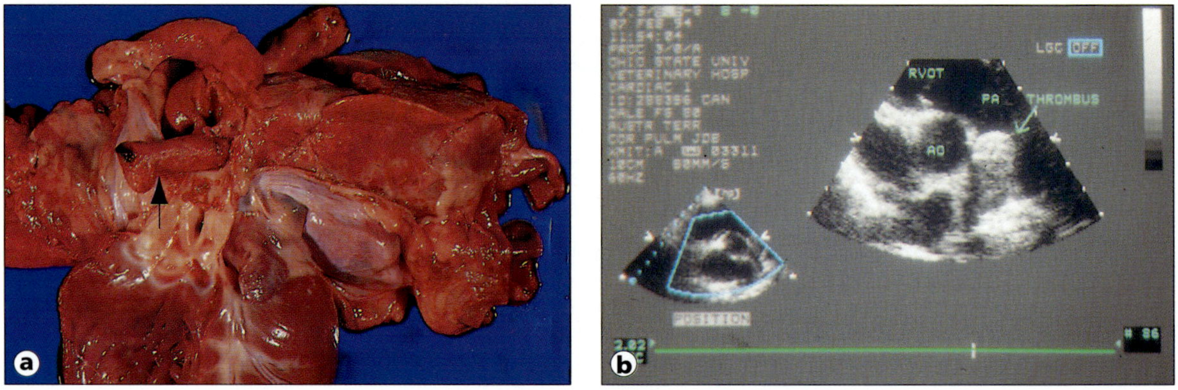

22.7 (**a**) The main pulmonary artery of a 2-year-old springer spaniel with renal amyloidosis is occluded by a lrage thrombus (arrow). (**b**) Pulmonary embolism (arrow) detected by two-dimensional echocardiography in a dog with chronic renal disease.

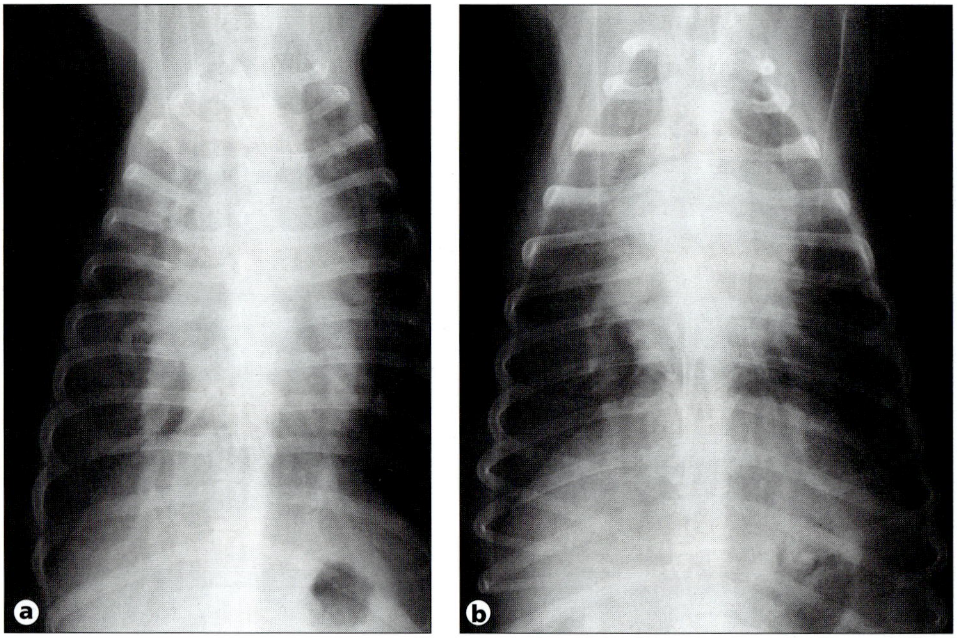

22.8 (**a** and **b**) Dorsoventral radiographs of a 9-year-old springer spaniel with diffuse pulmonary interstitial disease, showing evidence of cor pulmonale, before and after therapy. (**a**) There is gross dilatation of caudal lobe pulmonary arteries and (**b**) an obvious dilatation of the main pulmonary artery, with increased tortuosity of the caudal lobe arteries. There is also a suggestion of right ventricular enlargement.

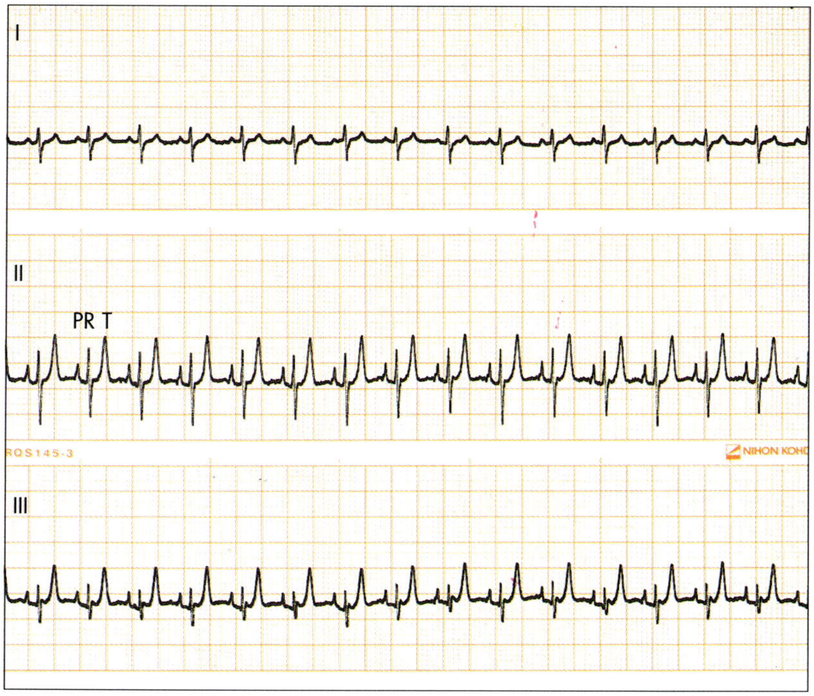

22.9 ECG from a cross-bred collie with interstitial pneumonia and cor pulmonale. Although the mean electrical axis is indeterminate, the deep S wave in the limb leads is consistent with right ventricular overload. The P wave is also peaked, although not out of the normal range.

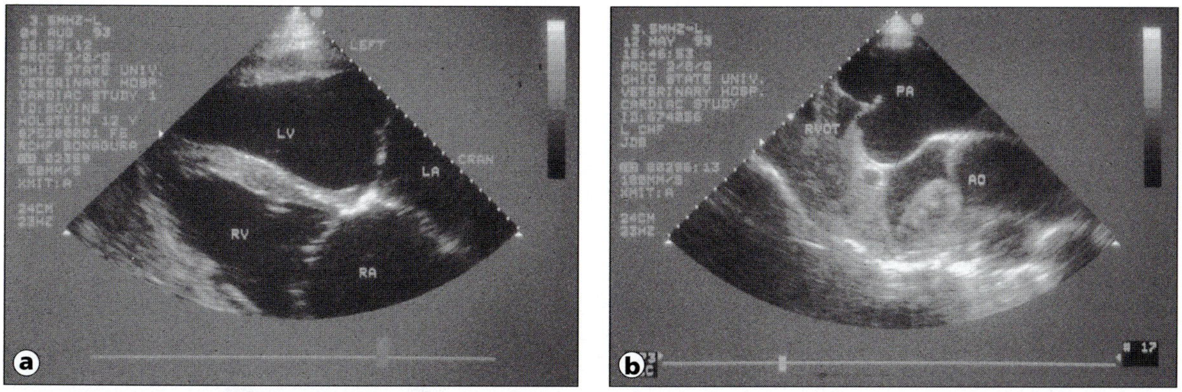

22.10 Right atrial, right ventricular (**a**) and pulmonary artery (**b**) dilatation in a cow with severe cor pulmonale due to pulmonary disease. Ruminants are very sensitive to local pulmonary hypoxia, resulting in vigorous constriction of pulmonary arteries. This leads to pulmonary hypertension and cor pulmonale. (**b**) An angled view to show the pulmonary valve and a dilated pulmonary artery.

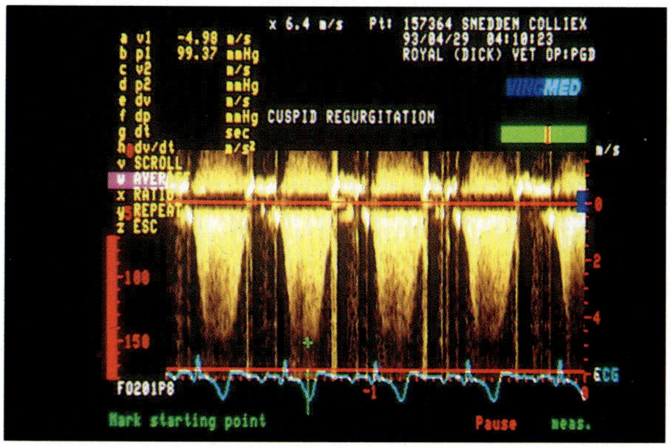

22.11 Continuous-wave spectral Doppler recording from the tricuspid valve of the collie in **22.9**, showing regurgitation at a velocity of 4.98 m/sec. This represents a pressure gradient across the valve of about 100 mmHg (by the Bernoulli equation), demonstrating elevated right ventricular systolic pressure. In the absence of pulmonary outflow obstruction, this strongly suggests cor pulmonale with pulmonary hypertension.

23. Cardiac Dysrhythmias

NORMAL CARDIAC RHYTHMS

Normal cardiac rhythms include *normal sinus rhythm* (regular rhythm of sinus node origin) and *sinus arrhythmia* which is cyclical and often synchronous with respirations – **23.1**). Sinus arrhythmia in normal dogs and in horses is often associated with a wandering sinoatrial pacemaker which is characterized by a recurrent variation in the P-wave morphology. Sinus bradycardia and sinus tachycardia may represent either physiologic rhythms – as with sleeping or exercise – or pathologic disorders of impulse formation (**23.2**). In horses, first- and second-degree atrioventricular (AV) block can be considered normal, particularly when the P–R interval varies progressively. Sinus arrhythmia and second degree AV block in these instances are vagally mediated; accordingly, exercise or excitement leads to a regular sinus rhythm.

ECG waveforms during normal cardiac rhythms are influenced by a number of autonomic, metabolic, thoracic and cardiac variables, including cardiomegaly, myocardial disease, pleural or pericardial effusions, obesity and hypothyroidism. Potassium disturbances, pericarditis, ischaemia, hypoxia and cardiac glycosides can deviate the S–T segment or alter the morphology of the T wave. Sympathetic activity can lead to physiologic alterations in the ST segment and T wave, especially in horses. Hypocalcaemia or hypokalaemia may prolong the Q–T interval.

BRADYDYSRHYTHMIAS

Disorders of sinus node impulse formation or of AV nodal impulse transmission are usually characterized by the presence of bradycardia which is transient or persistent and often by the appearance of escape complexes. Escape complexes of junctional origin generally lead to a normal but delayed lead II QRS complex which is often preceded or followed by a negative P wave (from retrograde conduction to the atria).Ventricular escape complexes are also delayed but are characterized by abnormal morphology and prolonged QRS–T complexes. Suppression of escape beats should never be attempted, as they may be critical for the animal's survival.

A number of atrial bradydysrhythmias are encountered in clinical practice (**23.1**). *Sinus arrest* is caused by a failure to initiate impulses. This leads to pauses which vary in length but are considerably longer than the normal P–P interval. Escape complexes may be evident. Recurrent sinus bradycardia, block or arrest may be associated with weakness or syncope in the so-called *sick sinus syndrome*, a term used to represent a diffuse electrical disorder which is seen particularly in certain small canine breeds. Affected animals (often miniature schnauzers) may also demonstrate periods of supraventricular tachycardia or AV block. *Atrial standstill* refers to a condition where the atrial muscle lacks excitability, P waves are absent, and QRS complexes are variable, depending on the site of impulse formation and path of impulse conduction. Atrial standstill develops readily with moderate to severe hyperkalaemia. The sinus node may continue to discharge across internodal pathways, causing a 'sinoventricular' rhythm (sinus in origin but without P waves). Should this fail, subsidiary junctional or ventricular escape pacemakers are usually recruited. Other ECG features of hyperkalaemia include progressive widening of the QRS complex, increased amplitude of the T waves, shortening of the ST–T interval, a sine-wave morphology QRS–T complex and eventually ventricular fibrillation.There will be other clinical signs related to the underlying cause (**23.2**). Persistent atrial standstill is uncommon but related to muscular dystrophy (notably in springer spaniels), severe dilated cardiomyopathy in cats and diffuse atrial myocarditis. Therapy for these conditions is summarized in **23.3**.

Atrioventricular blocks fall into three categories: first degree, in which the P–R interval is prolonged beyond the normal range and AV conduction is present but delayed; second degree, in which intermittent failure of AV conduction results in some P waves that lack QRS complexes; and third degree (complete) AV block, in which there is complete failure of atrioventricular impulse propagation and therefore no association between P waves and QRS complexes. In the latter case, QRS complexes are escape beats originating from tissues below the block and are usually of abnormal morphology. Such rhythms discharge slowly and usually regularly. Advanced second or third degree AV block often leads to low cardiac output with syncope (**23.2**, **23.3**).

PREMATURE COMPLEXES AND TACHYDYSRHYTHMIAS

Impulses that arise from sites outside the sinus node are termed ectopic and may develop through various mechanisms of re-entry or automaticity. Diseased atrial or ventricular myocardial tissues are prone to ectopic impulses, particularly with cardiomyopathy, ischaemia, fibrosis or cardiac dilatation. Premature impulses and tachyarrhythmias can be related to the effects of drugs, dysautonomia, hypoxia, endocrinopathies or metabolic disturbances (**23.2**). Any animal with tachydysrhythmia should be evaluated thoroughly for hypotension, drug toxicosis or evidence of cardiac, endocrine, systemic or metabolic diseases.

Premature complexes or *extrasystoles* can arise from the atria, AV junction or ventricles. Isolated *supraventricular* (usually atrial) ectopic complexes appear as premature QRS complexes of reasonably normal appearance, for which the P wave is also premature and usually of abnormal waveform. However, this P wave is often partly hidden in the preceding S–T segment or T wave, and a careful search may be required to demonstrate it. *Ventricular premature complexes* appear early in the cardiac cycle, show a QRS complex of bizarre waveform (which is usually prolonged), and have no associated, antecedent P wave. The distributional pattern of isolated premature complexes may be haphazard or regular, causing couplets (two ectopics), triplets or alternating normal and premature complexes (bigeminal rhythm).

Abnormal repetitive or sustained *supraventricular tachycardias* include atrial tachycardia, atrial flutter, atrial fibrillation (AF), junctional (nodal) tachycardia and AV nodal re-entrant tachycardia. These rhythm disturbances often indicate structural heart disease, and must be distinguished from sinus tachycardia. The AV node plays a pivotal role in each of these dysrhythmias as ventricular rate and response are governed by conduction of impulses across this structure. Accordingly, vagal manoeuvers (e.g. ocular pressure) or drugs that impede AV nodal conduction usually slow (and infrequently convert) supraventricular tachyarrhythmias.

Atrial tachycardia and *atrial flutter* have the same clinical significance as the AF discussed below. Atrial tachycardia represents rapid discharge due to an ectopic pacemaker or a circuit (re-entry) mechanism located within the atria. The atrial rate in both dysrhythmias is usually faster than during sinus tachycardia and is grossly inappropriate for the level of activity and physiologic state. These tachycardias can be paroxysmal or sustained, and the ventricular rate response regular or irregular.

Atrial fibrillation is clinically the most important of the sustained supraventricular tachyarrhythmias. It is often associated with atrial enlargement and congestive failure. However, AF can also be found in clinically normal animals, especially in horses and giant canine breeds. The rhythm is manifested as irregular QRS complexes of essentially normal configuration, indicating conduction of many of the fibrillation waves through the AV node. There are no identifiable P waves but, in their place, random undulations of the baseline ('f' waves) may be observed. The heart rate is often fast, particularly when there is structural heart disease, high sympathetic tone or heart failure, and slight beat-to-beat variations in QRS voltage may be observed.

The clinical management of supraventricular tachyarrhythmias depends on the exact rhythm diagnosis and the clinical circumstances, and details are summarized in **23.3**. Treatment of sinus tachycardia essentially involves management of the underlying condition (e.g. treat fever, correct hypovolaemia, control pain, manage heart failure). The management of sustained atrial tachycardia and atrial flutter is similar to that described below for AF. Frequent atrial premature complexes or paroxysmal atrial tachycardia may respond to treatment of the underlying condition and the addition of either a beta blocker or a calcium-channel blocker or digoxin if there is heart failure. If supraventricular tachycardia is related to AV nodal re-entry and an accessory (bypass) AV pathway it is treated initially with a calcium-channel blocker; thereafter a cardiologist should be consulted.

Atrial fibrillation may spontaneously convert to normal sinus rhythm, especially in cattle with potassium imbalances and in some horses with exercise-induced (paroxysmal) AF. In horses which have AF without heart failure, it is often converted with quinidine or digoxin with quinidine, and dogs with AF without heart failure or obvious structural heart disease may sometimes be converted to sinus rhythm using quinidine, diltiazem, or verapamil. The therapeutic aim in structural heart disease or congestive heart failure is control of the ventricular response to AF and prevention of excessive tachycardia during exercise or stress. Initially digoxin is administered, to be followed by either a calcium-channel blocker (diltiazem) or a beta-blocker (e.g. propranolol or atenolol). Often, chronic combination therapy – digoxin plus a beta or calcium-channel blocker – is employed with the admonition that the negative inotropic effects of the receptor blockers require careful titration of the eventual daily dosage.

Ventricular tachycardia (VT) is a repetitive discharge of premature ventricular complexes. When very rapid, VT can result in hypotension, myocardial ischaemia, further ventricular electrical instability and ventricular fibrillation. Sometimes VT develops at a relatively slow rate (e.g., 60–120 bpm in the dog; 60–90 bpm in the horse; 150–200 bpm in the cat) – a condition referred to as idioventricular tachycardia or accelerated ventricular rhythm. There may be frequent fusion QRS complexes caused by simultaneous depolarization of the ventricular muscle by the ectopic and sinus impulses. Relatively slow tachycardias are well tolerated if the volume status, blood pressure and serum potassium and magnesium are corrected. Faster VT represents a more serious problem; electrical and haemodynamic embarrassment may become manifest as hypotension, depression, weakness, collapse, syncope or death.

The clinical management of frequent ventricular extrasystoles or of ventricular tachycardia is not always straightforward, as treatment can be ineffectual or actually worsen the arrhythmia ('proarrhythmia'). However, when VT is sustained, very rapid, multiform in morphology or causes hypotension, therapy is recommended (**23.3**). Sustained VT in the dog usually responds to intravenous lidocaine (lignocaine) or procainamide, and may respond variably to one of a number of other agents (**23.3**). The horse with VT may be better treated with infusions of electrolytes containing potassium chloride and a magnesium salt, although low IV doses of lidocaine or quinidine gluconate may be effective. Cats with sustained VT should be treated with oxygen, and serum potassium should be corrected. Should these measures fail, low doses of lidocaine, procainamide or propranolol can be tried. Long-term antiarrhythmic therapy for ventricular arrhythmias requires careful consideration, ideally in consultation with a cardiologist. Animals prone to chronic symptomatic ventricular arrhythmias (e.g. boxer dogs and English bulldogs with arrhythmogenic cardiomyopathy) may need life-long therapy with an antiarrhythmic drug plus a beta blocker.

The lethal ventricular rhythm, *ventricular fibrillation*, can develop from VT, or it can occur spontaneously. This dysrhythmia appears as random undulations of the ECG baseline, with no consistent, recognizable waveforms. Therapy for ventricular fibrillation involves cardiopulmonary resuscitation with external or internal electrical defibrillation.

INTRAVENTRICULAR CONDUCTION DISTURBANCES

Disturbances of conduction through the ventricular Purkinje system are termed *intraventricular conduction disturbances*. These disorders are most easily recognized in dogs and cats because horses and ruminants have a more elaborate Purkinje network, and discrete blocks are not readily recognized. The principal conduction disturbances observed in clinical cases are right-bundle branch block, left-bundle branch block, left anterior fascicular block and left posterior fascicular block. Principal ECG features are prolongation of ventricular depolarization and dominance of terminal ventricular depolarization towards the blocked bundle. Right-bundle branch block is characterized by right-axis deviation in the frontal plane, prominent S waves in leads I, II, III and aVF and in the lower left precordial leads. Left-bundle branch block shows a similar or greater prolongation of the QRS complex (beyond 0.07 seconds) with a normally orientated QRS complex, tiny or absent Q waves in lead II, and often a notching of the R wave. Left anterior fascicular block is characterized by a left cranial frontal axis with prominent S waves in Leads II, III and aVF and a prominent qR complex in leads I and aVL. The diagnosis of left posterior fascicular block in animals cannot be made with certainty. There is no specific therapy for these conduction disturbances; however, recognition of the clinical associations of them is important (**23.2**).

Ventricular *pre-excitation* (including the Wolff–Parkinson–White and related syndromes) is found relatively rarely in animals. These conditions are caused by an accessory AV conduction pathway that bypasses the AV node and conducts more rapidly than the normal AV nodal tissues. The ECG is characterized by a shortened P–R interval during sinus rhythm. The accessory pathway predisposes the animal to circuit (re-entry) supraventricular tachycardias in which the impulse descends the AV node towards the ventricle while simultaneously re-emerging in the atrium via the accessory pathway. This appears to be more common in canine breeds predisposed to tricuspid valve dysplasia, especially Labrador retrievers.

Sinus Mechanisms	**Ventricular Rhythm Disturbances**
Normal sinus rhythm	Ventricular escape complexes
Sinus arrhythmia	Ventricular escape rhythm (idioventricular rhythm)
Sinoatrial block/arrest	Ventricular premature complexes
Sinus bradycardia	Accelerated ventricular rhythm (idioventricular tachycardia)
Sinus tachycardia	Ventricular tachycardia
Atrial Rhythm Disturbances	Ventricular flutter
Atrial escape complexes	Ventricular fibrillation
Atrial premature complexes	**Conduction Disturbances**
Atrial tachycardia – nonsustained and sustained	Sinoatrial block
Atrial flutter	Atrial standstill (hyperkalaemia)
Atrial fibrillation	Atrioventricular blocks
Re-entrant supraventricular tachycardia	first degree
Junctional Rhythm Disturbances	second degree
Junctional escape complexes	third degree (complete)
Junctional escape rhythm (idionodal rhythm)	
Junctional premature complexes	
Junctional ('nodal') tachycardia	
Re-entrant supraventricular tachycardia	

23.1 Cardiac rhythms.

Sinus Rhythms

- Normal sinus rhythm: A regular rhythm of sinus node origin – normal in all species
- Sinus arrhythmia: A normal rhythm, but uncommon in the cat
- Sinus bradycardia: Increased vagal tone; elevated cerebrospinal fluid pressure; brain stem lesions; head trauma; gastrointestinal disease; hypothermia; hypothyroidism; hyperkalaemia; sinus node disease; dilated cardiomyopathy (cats); administration of beta blockers, digitalis or inhalation anaesthetics
- Sinus tachycardia: Increased sympathetic tone; fear; excitement; pain; hypovolaemia; hypotension; anaemia; heart failure; hyperthyroidism; administration of vagolytic drugs, such as atropine, or sympathomimetics
- Sinus arrest: Sick sinus syndrome, high vagal tone; digitalis, surgical manipulation; can alternate with supraventricular tachycardia in sick sinus syndrome; over-administration of anaesthetic or antiarrhythmic drugs

Supraventricular Arrhythmias

- Supraventricular (atrial and junctional) premature complexes: Atrioventricular valve regurgitation; cardiomyopathy; hyperthyroidism; congenital heart diseases; chronic pulmonary disease; hypoxia; anaemia; digitalis intoxication; increased sympathetic tone; administration of anaesthetic agents; 'toxaemia'; hypokalaemia; atrial tumours
- Supraventricular tachycardia: As for supraventricular premature complexes; also atrial septal defect; tricuspid valve dysplasia; accessory atrioventricular pathway (re-entrant tachycardia); electrocution; cardiac catheterization
- Atrial tachycardia, flutter and fibrillation: Atrial dilation; cardiomyopathy; AV valvular insufficiency; untreated congenital heart disease; cardiac catheterization; trauma; drug administration; functional heart disorder in some large animals; electrolyte (K^+) disorders in large animals; vagomimetic tone or drugs (neostigmine) following respiratory infections (horses)
- Junctional escape rhythm: A protective rhythm associated with sinus bradycardia, sinus arrest, and atrioventricular block

Ventricular Arrhythmias

- Ventricular premature complexes/tachycardia: Cardiomyopathy; heart failure; endomyocarditis; chronic valvular heart disease; pericarditis; neoplasia; congenital heart disease; hypoxia; anaemia; acidosis; hypokalaemia; hypomagnesaemia; autonomic imbalance; thoracic and abdominal trauma; gastric dilatation-volvulus; sepsis and infections; pulmonary disease; digitalis intoxication; hyperthyroidism; administration of anaesthetics or sympathomimetics
- Ventricular escape rhythm: As per junctional escape

Conduction Blocks

- Atrial standstill: Hyperkalaemia; hypoadrenocorticism; urinary obstruction; if persistent ('silent atria') – due to muscular dystrophy or myocarditis; dilated cardiomyopathy
- Incomplete atrioventricular block: Normal variant (especially horses and resting dogs); increased vagal tone; administration of digitalis glycosides narcotics or xylazine; AV nodal disease; cardiomyopathy; myocarditis; doxorubicin cardiotoxicity
- Complete atrioventricular block: AV nodal or junctional disease including infarction, degeneration or replacement with connective tissue; neoplasia; severe drug toxicity (digitalis, xylazine, doxorubicin); aortic valve bacterial endocarditis; (?) Lyme disease
- Intraventricular (bundle branch and fascicular) conduction blocks: May be observed with almost any congenital or acquired heart disease including atrial and ventricular septal defects, pulmonary and aortic stenosis, and cardiomyopathy; smoke inhalation and other causes of acute cor pulmonale; digitalis intoxication; Chagas' disease; doxorubicin toxicity; hyperthyroidism

23.2 Clinical associations of common cardiac arrhythmias.

Dysrhythmia	Initial therapy	Chronic therapy	Comments
Sinus bradycardia; sinus arrest	Atropine Glycopyrrolate Dopamine Dobutamine Transvenous pacing	Pacemaker – permanent transvenous or epicardial pacing system; terbutaline or oral anticholinergic if pacing is unavailable	Rule out hypothyroidism Refer for a pacemaker which is the most effective therapy when due to sick sinus syndrome. Terbutaline may stimulate beta$_2$ receptors in SA node to discharge more effectively if pacing is unavailable.
Atrial premature complexes	Generally unnecessary unless paroxysmal atrial tachycardia; rule out hypokalaemia	Beta blockers Digoxin Diltiazem Quinidine Procainamide	Treatment of underlying condition is important; digoxin if heart failure; beta blockers if not. Quinidine or procainamide are occasionally effective but are second choices.
Atrial tachycardia	Verapamil or diltiazem (dog/cat); quinidine (horse)	Diltiazem, beta blocker, and/or digoxin (dog/cat) Quinidine Procainamide	If CHF then digoxin plus a beta blocker or diltiazem; isolated atrial arrhythmias may respond to a beta blocker +/- an antiarrhythmic drug; rule out re-entrant tachycardias that use the AV node – such arrhythmias should be referred for optimal management. Quinidine for horses.
Atrial flutter or atrial fibrillation	For attempted conversion to sinus rhythm: Quinidine or digoxin + quinidine (dog/horse); or verapamil or diltiazem (dog/cat); correct electrolyte disturbances (cattle)	For control of ventricular rate at rest and with exercise: digoxin plus a beta blocker or diltiazem (dog/cat) Recurrent AF in horses is treated per initial therapy unless there is heart failure, then use digoxin if indicated	Conversion to sinus rhythm may be attempted if no other signs of serious cardiac disease are evident – this is most commonly done in horses or in dogs with acute onset of AF. Options for failed conversion of AF in horses using q2h oral therapy are: • Oral quinidine, q6h, for 48–72 h or • Digitalization for 48–72 h followed by oral quinidine, q6h. Beware digoxin/quinidine drug interaction that approximately doubles serum digoxin concentration.
Ventricular extrasystoles Ventricular tachycardia	Lidocaine (dog); procainamide (dog,horse); quinidine (dog, horse); beta blocker (cat); propafenone (horse); potassium or magnesium chloride infusion	Procainamide, quinidine, mexiletine, or tocainide often with a beta blocker; sotolal for refractory cases (dog) Beta blocker (cat)	Determine need for therapy; first correct hypoxia, metabolic and electrolyte disturbances; consider Holter (tape recorder) ECG to assess need and effectiveness of therapy; consider consulting a cardiac specialist. Be aware of potential proarrhythmia effects of antiarrhythmic drugs.
High grade second degree or complete AV block	Atropine; if not effective administer dopamine; if no effect initiate or refer for transvenous pacing	Permanent transvenous or epicardial pacing	Refer to cardiac specialist for cardiac pacing.
Atrial standstill (hyperkalaemia)	Correct underlying disorder; intravenous saline; IV sodium bicarbonate solution. Calcium salts (calcium chloride or gluconate), atropine, adrenaline or regular insulin plus dextrose are occasionally indicated in severe cases	Prevent by treating the primary condition	Addison's disease and excessive doses of mitotane for Cushing's disease are important causes in dogs; in cats and in large animals obstruction or rupture of the urinary conduit are most important. These conditions also must be managed for effective therapy. Rare cases of persistent atrial standstill, unrelated to hyperkalemia, are managed by permanent ventricular pacing

23.3 Therapy of common cardiac arrhythmias. See Appendix A2 for drug formulary and doses.

All ECGs were recorded with simultaneous leads I and II at 10 mm/mV and 25 mm/sec unless otherwise stated.

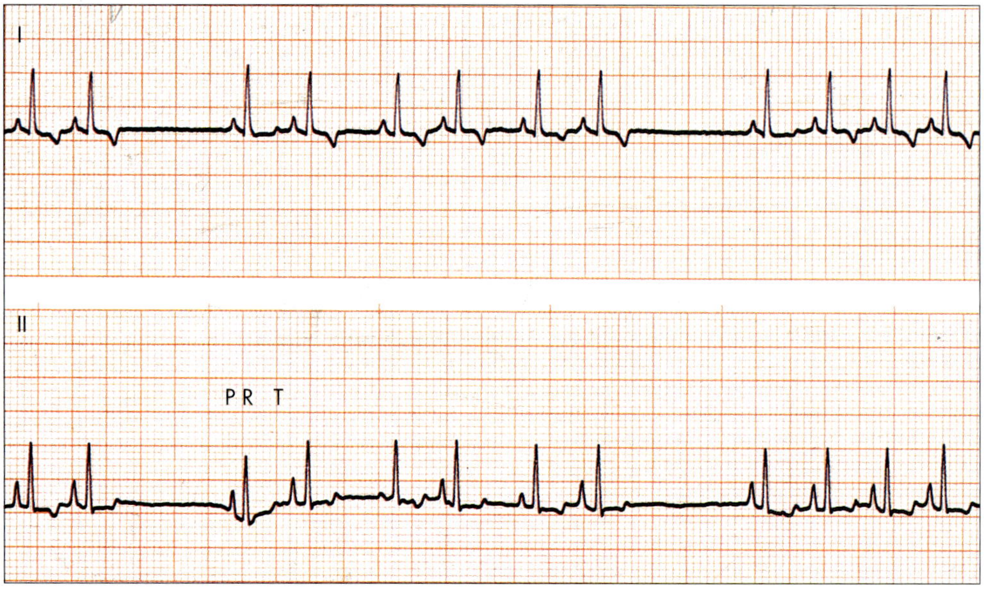

23.4 ECG from a Japanese chin with brachycephalic airway obstruction. There is marked sinus arrhythmia, and marginal P pulmonale (courtesy of Virginia Luis Fuentes).

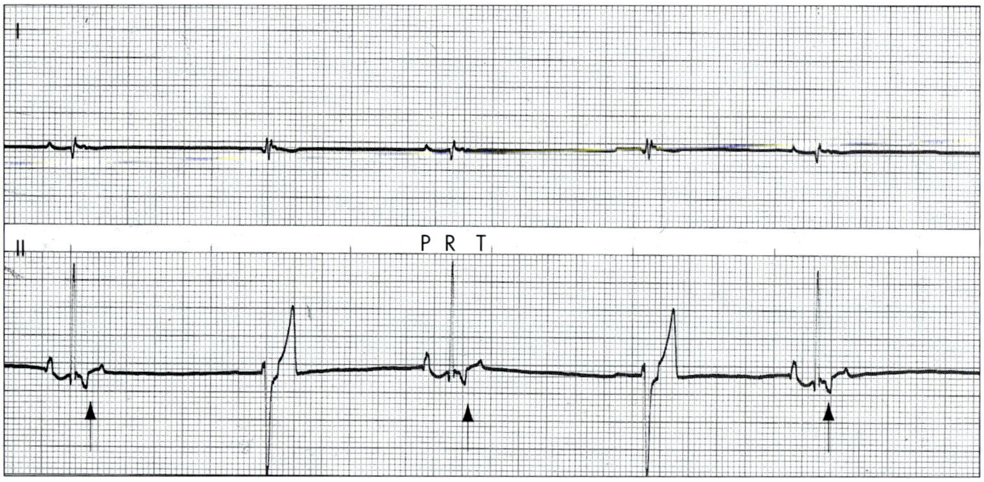

23.5 ECG from a golden retriever with sinus bradycardia and escape beats following beta blockade and digoxin as therapy for atrial tachycardia. Negative retrograde P waves (arrows) can still be seen in the S–T segment of the normally conducted beats.

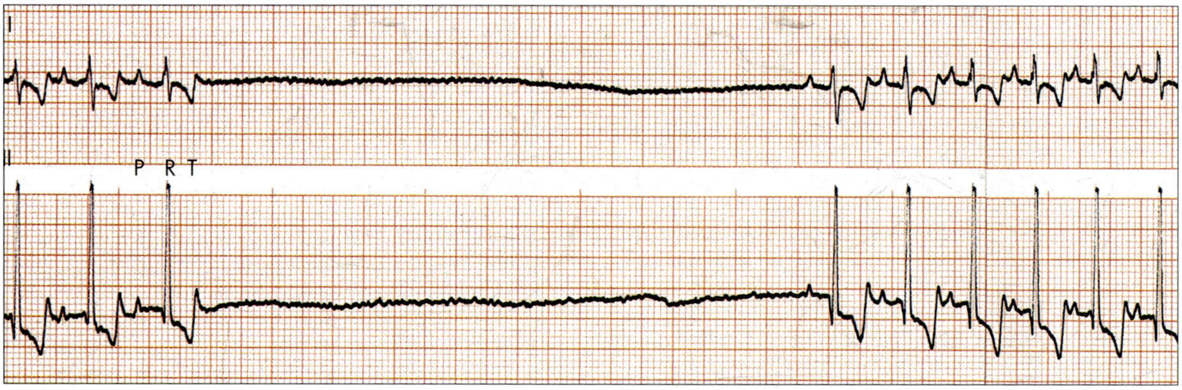

23.6 ECG from a springer spaniel with episodes of syncope. There is sinus arrest (a form of sick sinus syndrome) and variable first-degree AV block. This dog received a cardiac pacemaker.

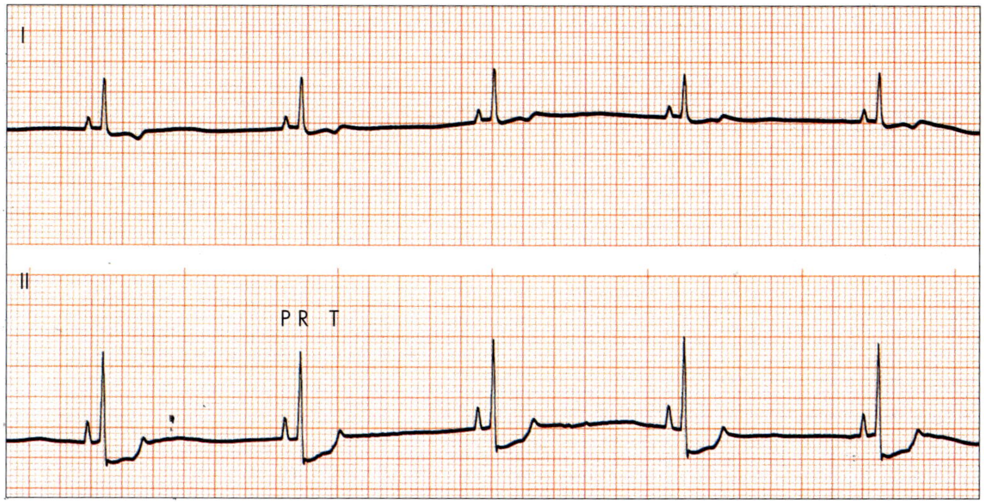

23.7 ECG from a 12-year-old West Highland white terrier with lethargy, sinus bradycardia and S–T segment depression. This dog subsequently received a pacemaker.

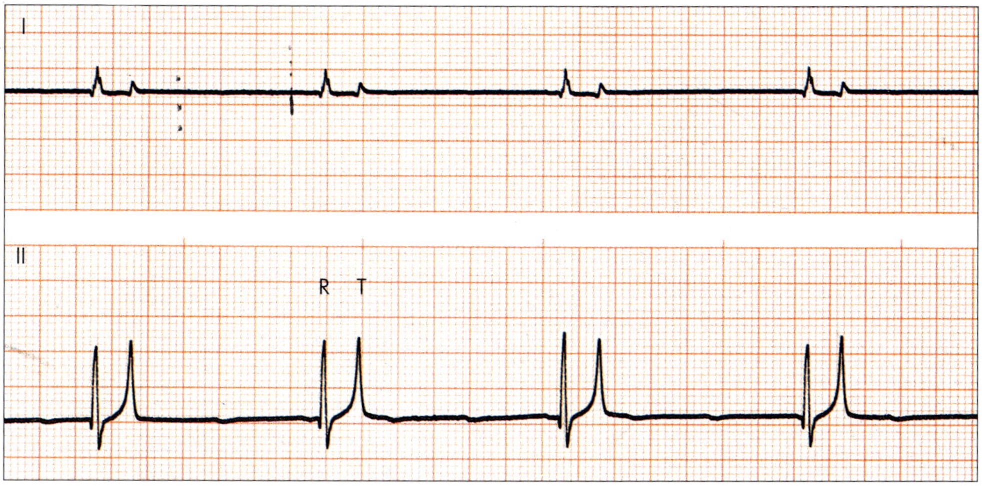

23.8 ECG from a standard poodle with hypoadrenocorticalism (Addison's disease), showing almost complete absence of P waves (nearly atrial standstill), bradycardia (45 bpm) and spiked T waves, all features typical of hyperkalaemia.

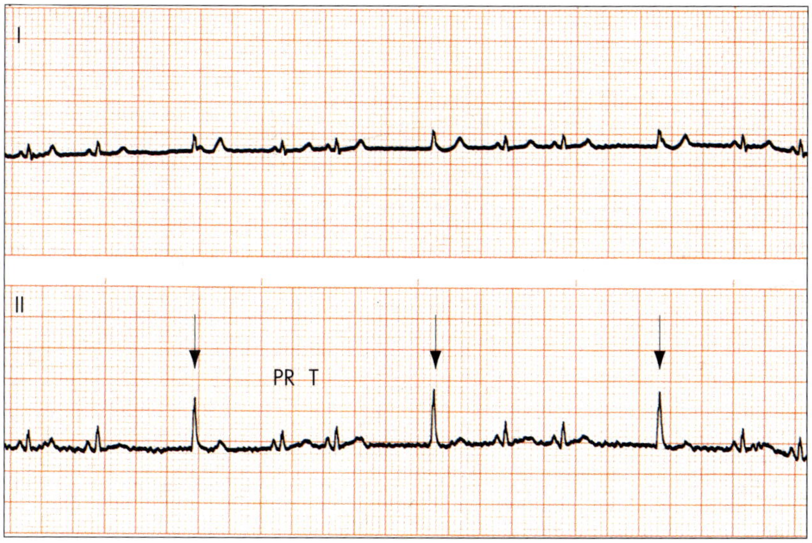

23.9 ECG from a cat with head trauma following a road traffic accident. There is sinus arrest with escape beats (arrows).

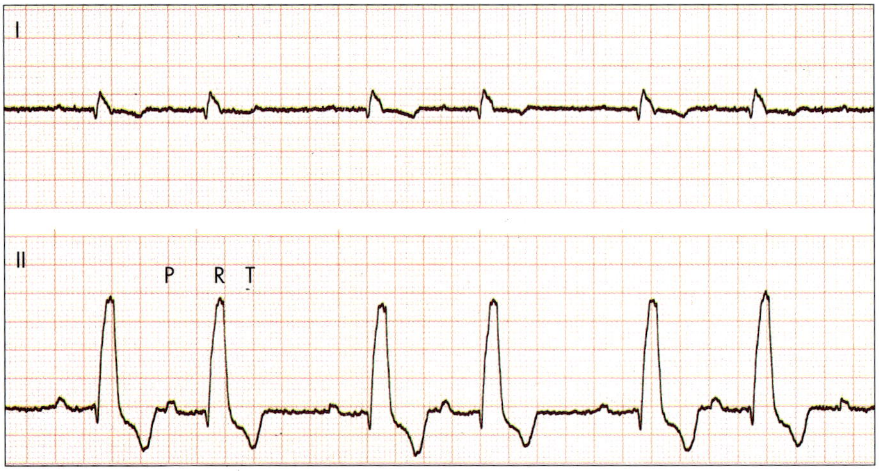

23.10 ECG recorded at 50 mm/sec and 0.5 cm/mV from a cocker spaniel with dilated cardiomyopathy, following therapy that included digoxin. There is first-degree AV block and left-bundle branch block (courtesy of Virginia Luis Fuentes).

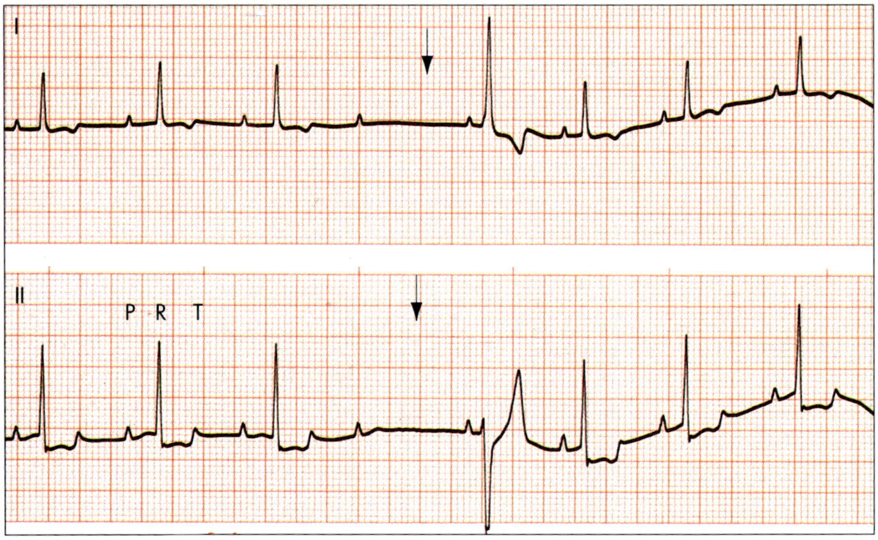

23.11 ECG from the West Highland terrier shown in **23.7**. There is now first-degree AV block with Wenckebach phenomenon and second-degree AV block (arrows).

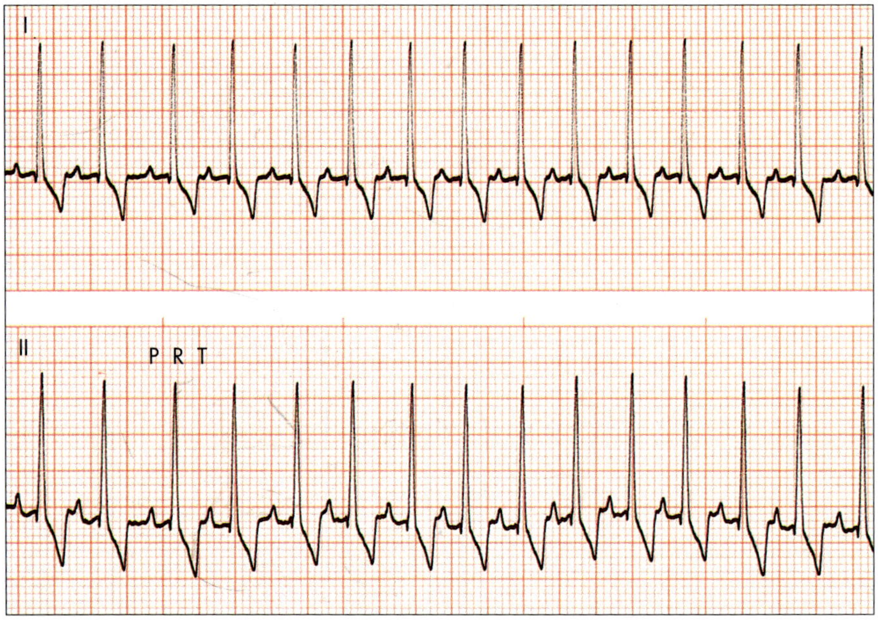

23.12 ECG from a cavalier King Charles spaniel with mitral regurgitation, following therapy with glycosides. There is still sinus tachycardia (180 bpm), but first-degree AV block suggests adequate digitalization.

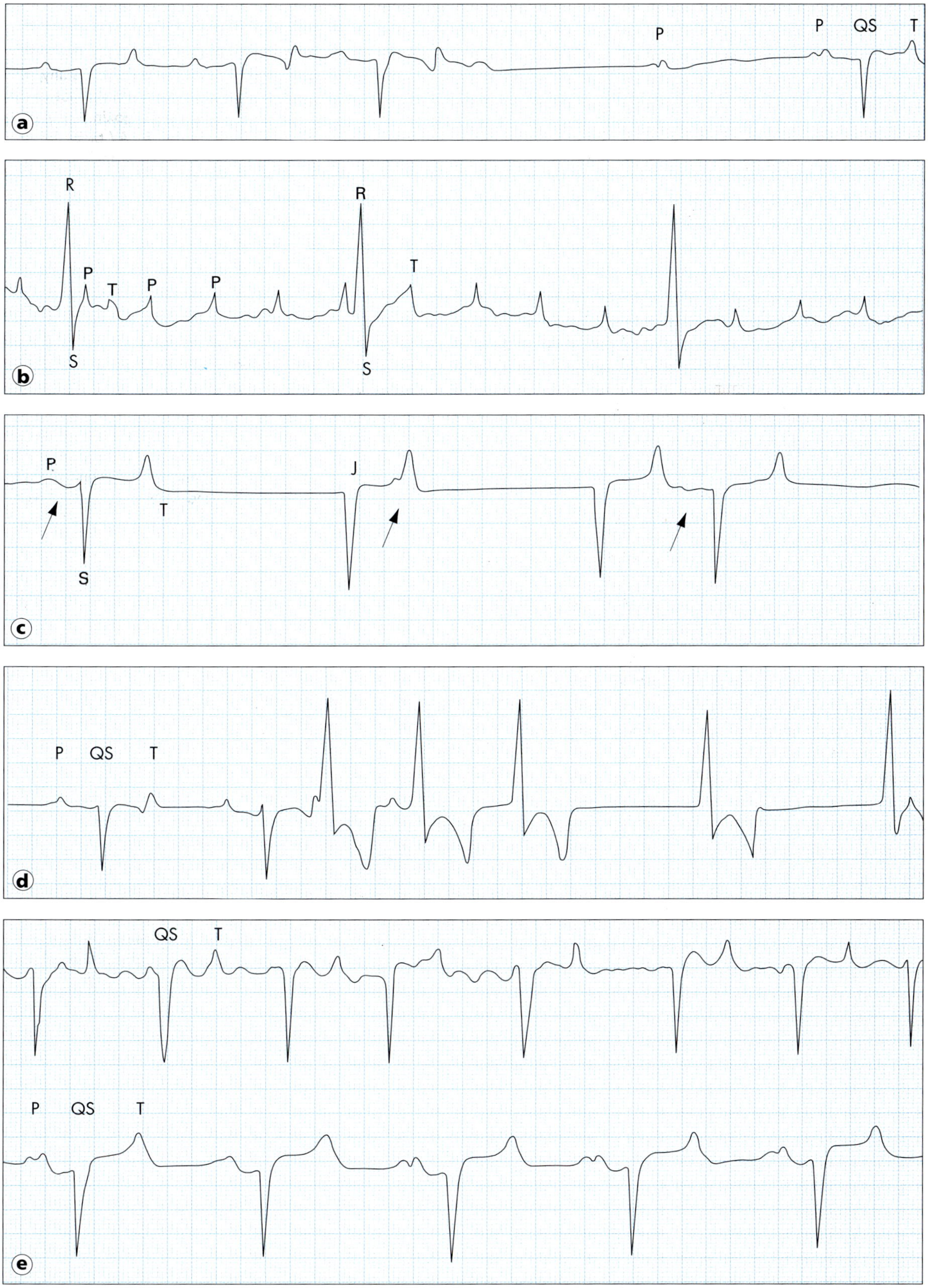
a
P
P
QS
T
b
R
S
P
T
P
P
R
S
T
c
P
S
T
J
d
P
QS
T
e
QS
T
P
QS
T

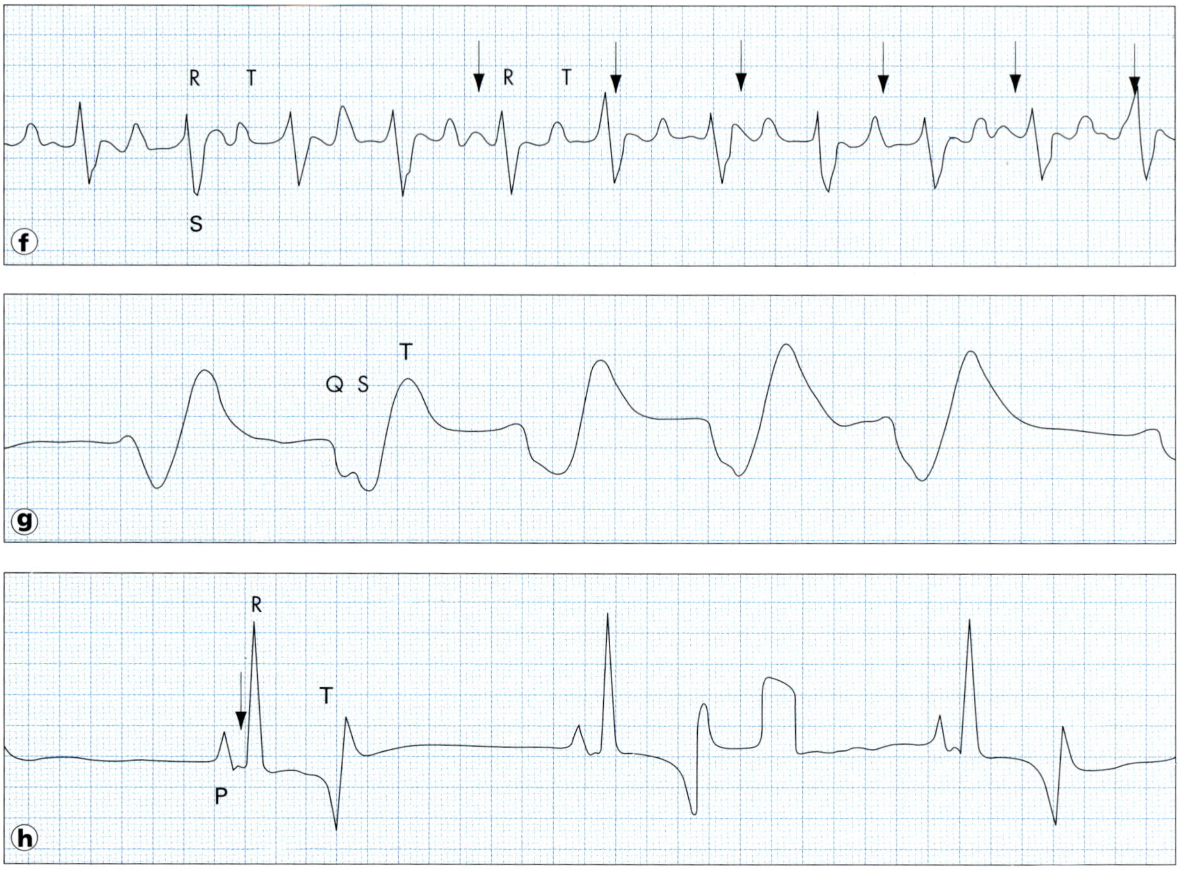

23.13 ECG traces recorded from various horses (at 25 mm/sec and using a base–apex lead unless otherwise stated): **(a)** Trace from a healthy horse with sinus arrhythmia and second-degree atrioventricular (AV) block. Waveforms are marked. **(b)** ECG from a horse with complete (third-degree) atrioventricular block. There are frequent unconducted P waves (some of which are marked) and ventricular escape beats. **(c)** ECG from an anaesthetized horse demonstrating sinus bradycardia and an idionodal (junctional) rhythm. P waves are indicated by arrows. The first junctional complex (J) is not preceded by a P wave, and it is followed by a brief period of atrioventricular dissociation. The last complex is a sinus 'capture' that is preceded by a P wave, conducted with a prolonged P–Q interval (first-degree AV block). **(d)** ECG recording from a horse with colic. Two sinus beats are followed by five ventricular ectopic complexes, discharging irregularly. **(e)** Two recordings from the same horse, before and after administration of quinidine sulphate. The top strip demonstrates coarse atrial fibrillation with an irregular ventricular response. QRS complexes (negative) are normal for this lead, and the T waves are positive. The second strip was recorded after conversion to sinus rhythm. **(f)** ECG demonstrating AV dissociation due to a nodal or high ventricular tachycardia. The QRS complexes (RS in form) are not associated with the P waves, which are physiologically blocked by the competing ventricular impulse. Note that the P waves (arrowheads) 'march' through the QRS complexes without disturbing the ventricular rhythm. **(g)** Sinoventricular rhythm in a foal with severe hyperkalaemia. P waves are absent and the QRS complexes and T waves are markedly widened (50 mm/sec). The foal had uroabdomen. **(h)** Ventricular pre-excitation is demonstrated in this ECG recorded in lead II at 50 mm/sec. A very brief interval (arrow) follows the P wave. The tiny positive deflection between the P and R waves represents an area of pre-excited ventricular depolarization (a 'delta' wave). The QRS complex is slightly widened. A 1 mV calibration signal is inscribed prior to the last complex.

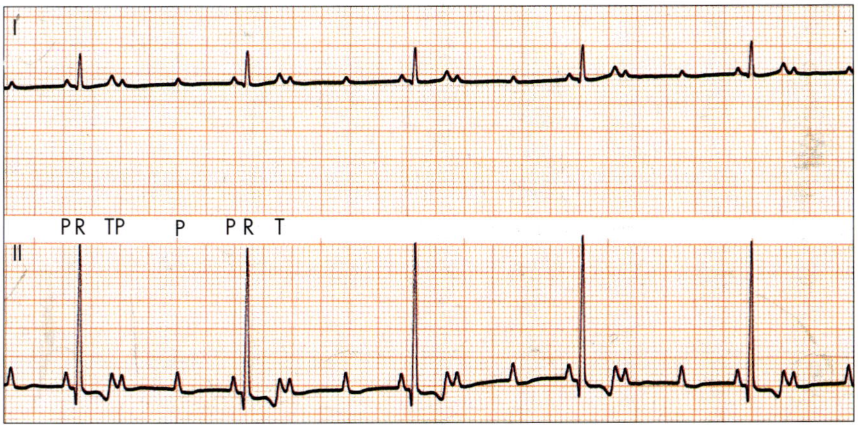

23.14 ECG from a Labrador retriever bitch with episodes of syncope. There is Mobitz type 2 second-degree AV block with 3:1 conduction (and no evidence of the Wenckebach phenomenon). An invasive tumour in the upper interventricular septum was subsequently demonstrated post mortem.

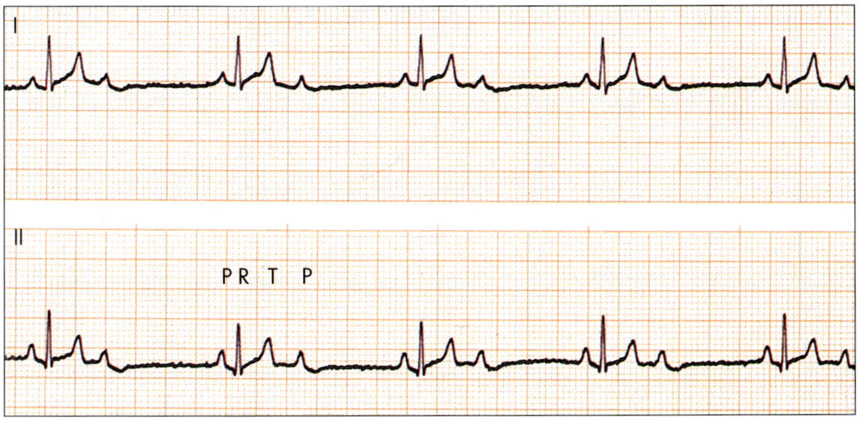

23.15 ECG from a Labrador retriever with advanced Mobitz type 2 AV block and a conduction ratio that varied between 2:1 (shown here) and 4:1. This dog subsequently received a pacemaker.

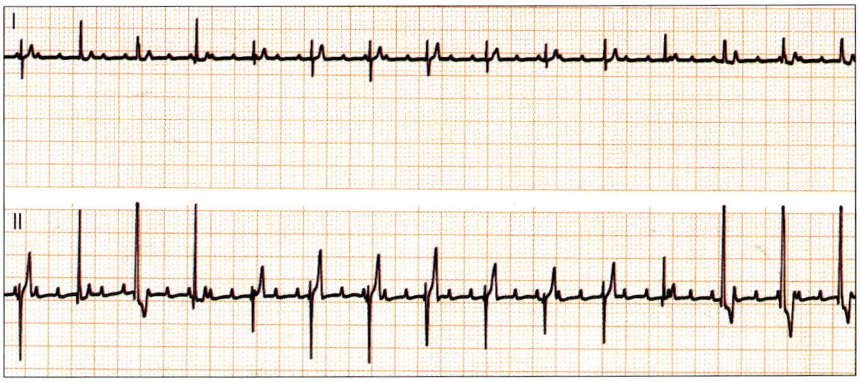

23.16 ECG recorded at 10 mm/sec and 0.5 cm/mV from another Labrador retriever with third-degree (complete) AV block and episodes of syncope, showing an escape rhythm of variable morphology. Most of the time escape beats discharged at the unusually high rate of 70 bpm.

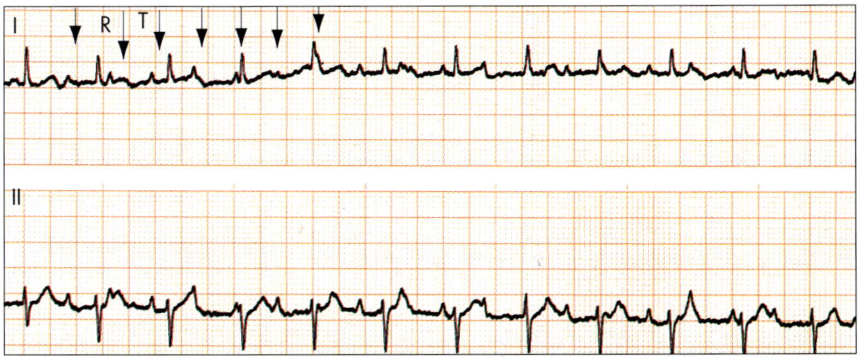

23.17 ECG from a 12-year-old cat with iatrogenic hypercalcaemia following resection of a thyroid adenoma. There is third-degree AV block, with escape ventricular complexes at about 110 bpm. P waves are indicated by arrows. The escape rhythm in cats is usually much more rapid than in dogs. There is considerable baseline artefact. (Courtesy of Mr Darren Foster.)

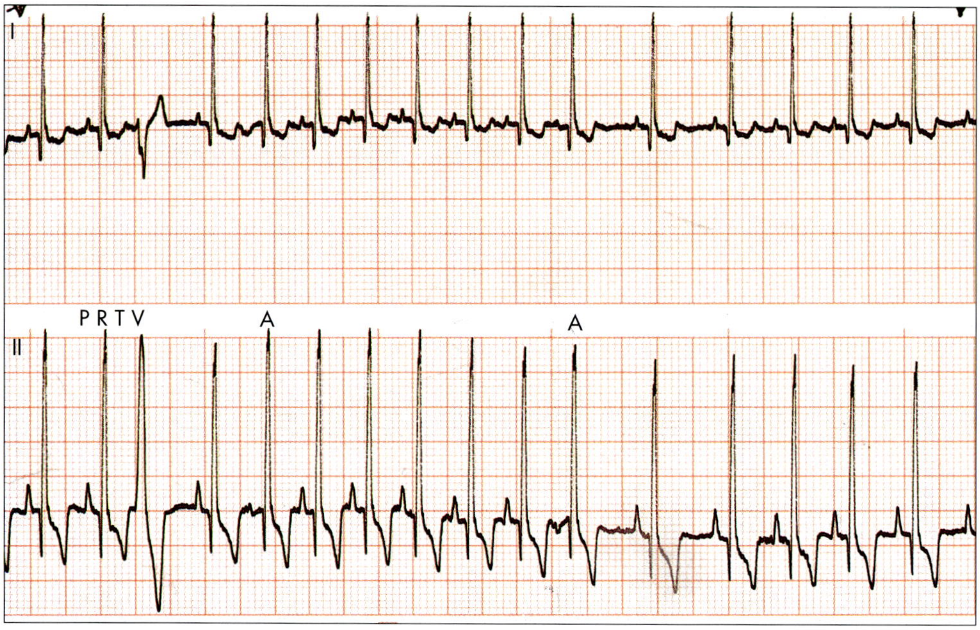

23.18 ECG from a boxer with subaortic stenosis. There are atrial (A) premature and ventricular (V) premature beats and S–T coving. Ventricular premature complexes (VPCs) are found commonly with the myocardial ischaemia associated with severe stenosis.

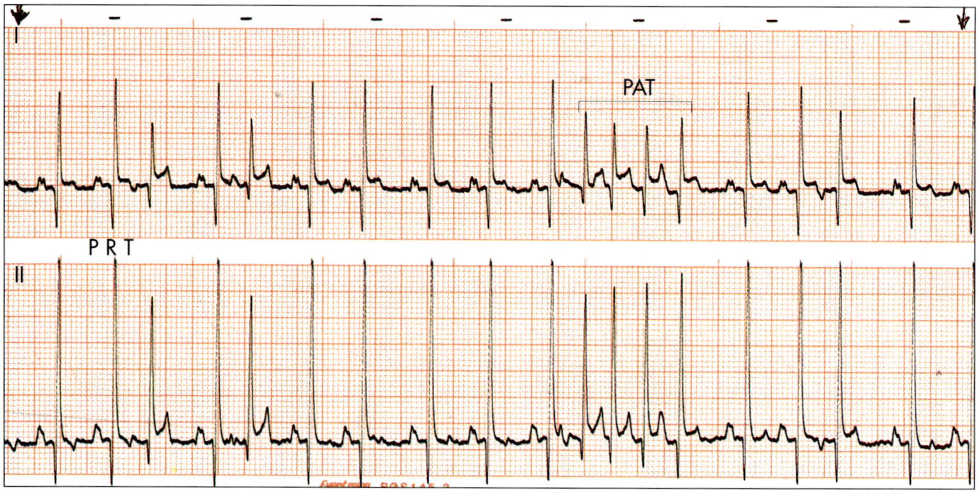

23.19 ECG from an aged cocker spaniel with mitral regurgitation. There is evidence of left-sided cardiac enlargement, with P mitrale, and a tall and wide QRS complex. There are atrial premature beats and paroxysms of atrial tachycardia (PAT), probably due to left atrial dilatation.

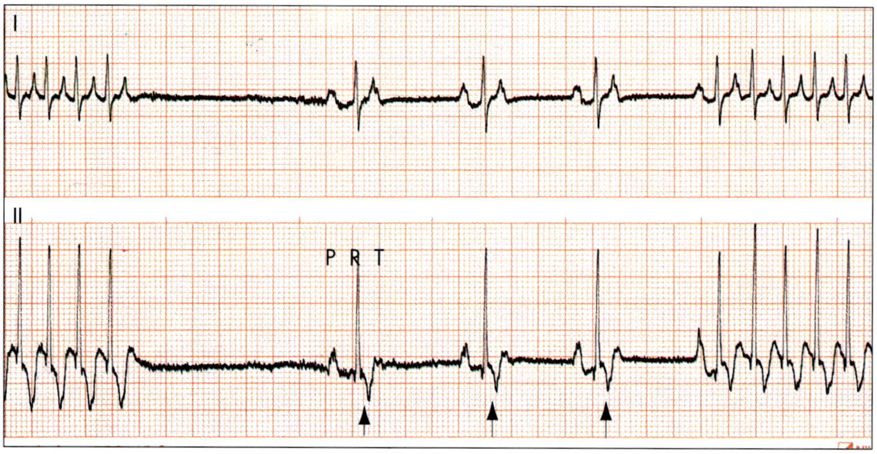

23.20 ECG from a young Labrador retriever with severe mitral regurgitation and probable re-entrant supraventricular tachycardia (SVT), undergoing carotid sinus massage. This causes temporary sinus arrest/bradycardia, with failure to conduct the negative atrial ectopic P waves seen in the S–T segment during the pause (arrow). The SVT recurs at the end of the trace

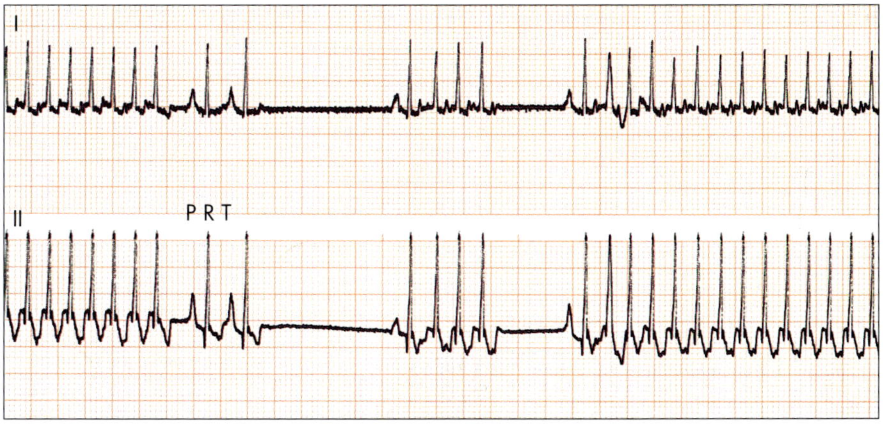

23.21 ECG from a cocker spaniel with dilated cardiomyopathy. There is supraventricular tachycardia (nearly 400 bpm) which is arrested by the intravenous administration of an ultra short-acting beta blocker, esmolol. The tachycardia was almost certainly associated with re-entry (with negative P waves in the S–T segments, but there is no re-entry P wave in the S–T segment of the first two sinus beats in the pause. P pulmonale is also seen for the first beats during the pause. This is commonly found at cessation of tachycardias or during bradycardias.

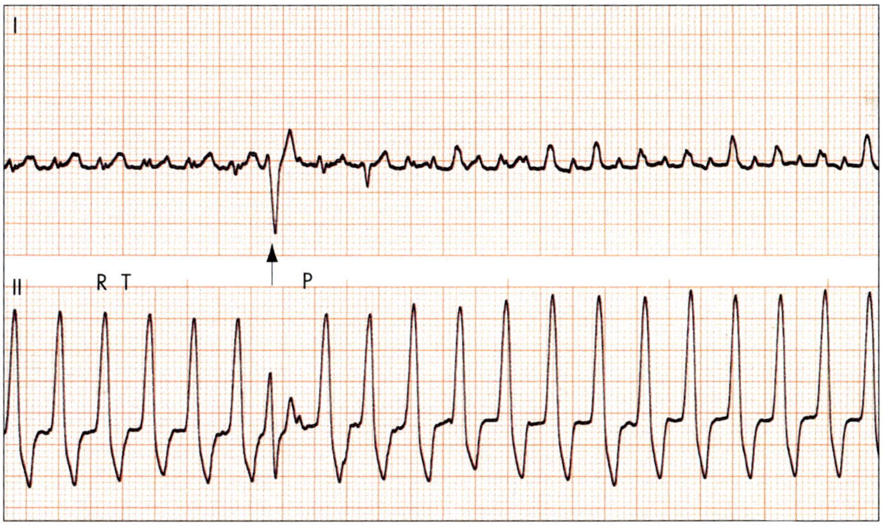

23.22 ECG from another cocker spaniel with dilated cardiomyopathy. There is sustained sinus tachycardia, with one separate ventricular premature complex (arrow). The tachycardia appears to be ventricular in origin on initial inspection. However, a P wave (with first-degree AV block) is evident after the premature beat, and subsequent ECGs revealed sinus tachycardia with left-bundle branch block, which can mimic ventricular tachycardia (courtesy Virginia Luis Fuentes).

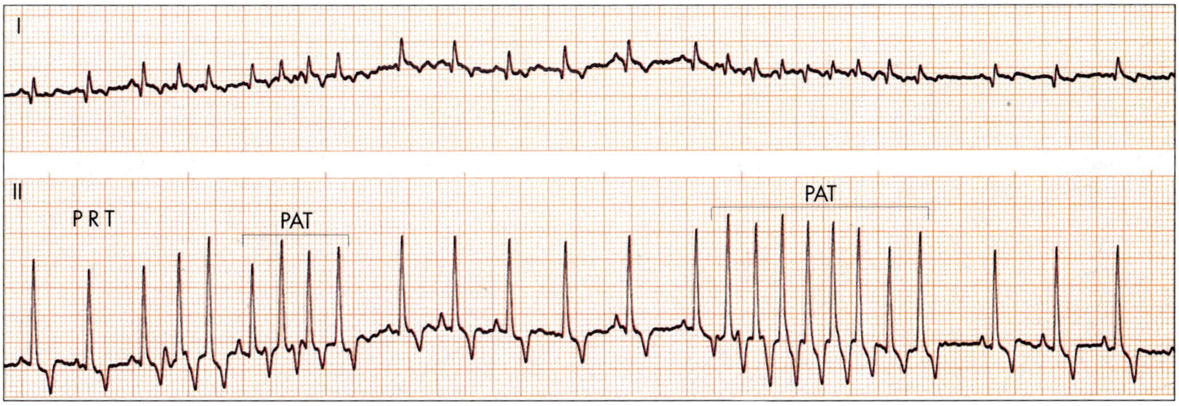

23.23 ECG from a 13-year-old Labrador retriever with hyperadrenocorticism. These paroxysms of atrial tachycardia (PAT) were an incidental finding, in a dog with sinus arrhythmia and wandering pacemaker.

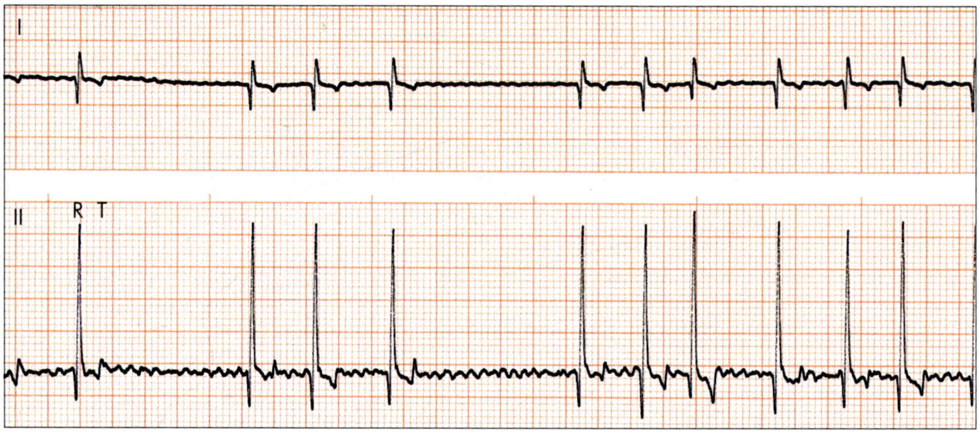

23.24 ECG from a Bouvier de Flandres with 'benign' atrial fibrillation (AF). AF is confirmed by irregular QRS complexes and absence of P waves. There are also prominent f waves to be seen at this slow heart rate (115 bpm).

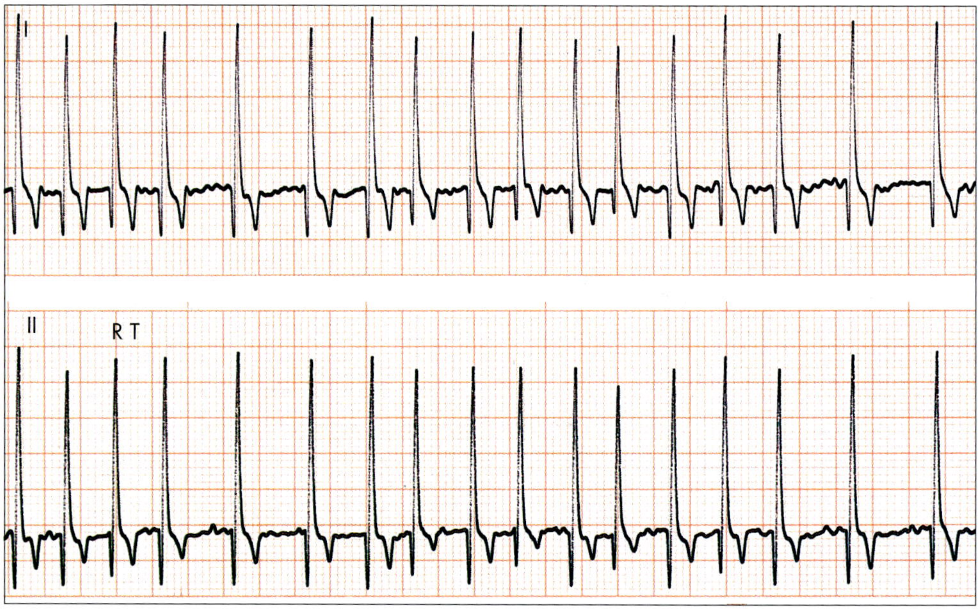

23.25 ECG from a cocker spaniel with dilated cardiomyopathy. There is atrial fibrillation with a fast ventricular rate (about 170 bpm). Marginally prolonged QRS complexes are consistent with left ventricular enlargement.

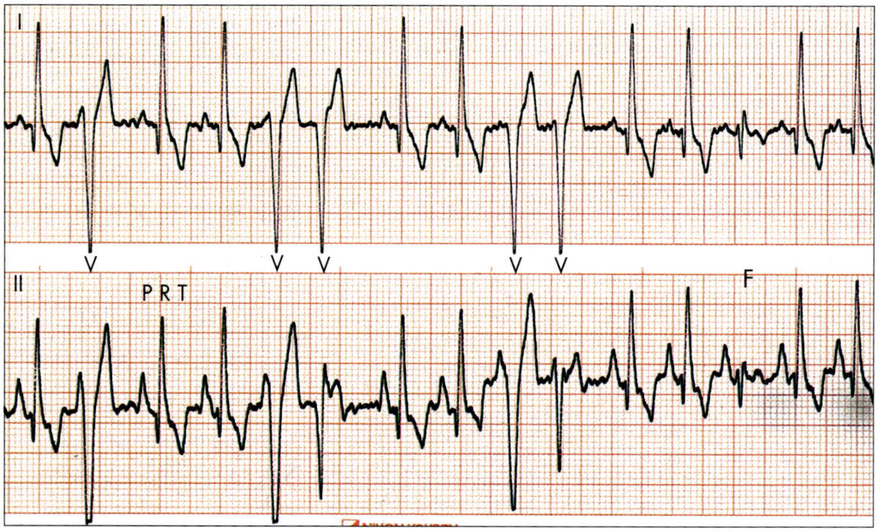

23.26 ECG from a Doberman pinscher with dilated cardiomyopathy. There is sinus tachycardia with multiple ventricular premature complexes (VPCs: V) and fusion beats (e.g. F). There is also evidence of atrial and left ventricular enlargement. Dobermans show atrial fibrillation much less often than dogs with cardiomyopathy from other large breeds, and VPCs are often found. This dog died within a few weeks. (Courtesy Virginia Luis Fuentes).

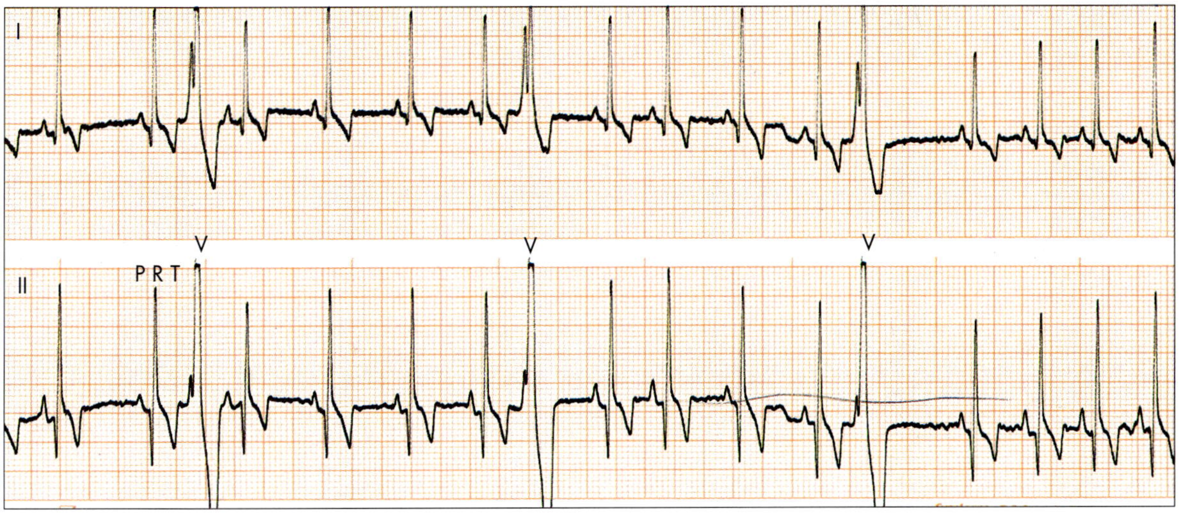

23.27 ECG from an 11-year-old Irish setter cross with chronic gastritis. There are frequent ventricular premature complexes (V), but these were an incidental finding, in a dog with sinus arrhythmia and wandering pacemaker.

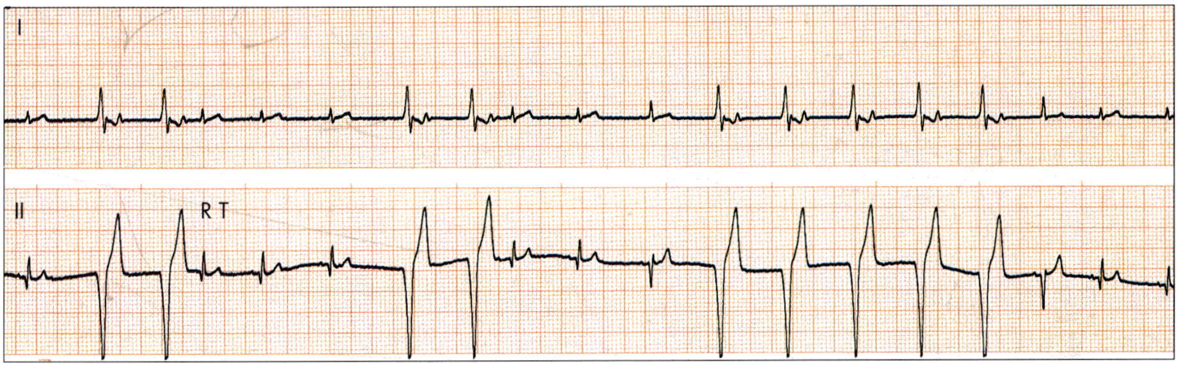

23.28 ECG recorded from a German shepherd dog during general anaesthesia for surgical investigation of a lumbosacral spondylopathy. There is sinus bradycardia with slow ventricular tachycardia. This bradycardia might be reversed by increased oxygenation or reduction in depth of anaesthesia, and it might respond to vagolytic drugs.

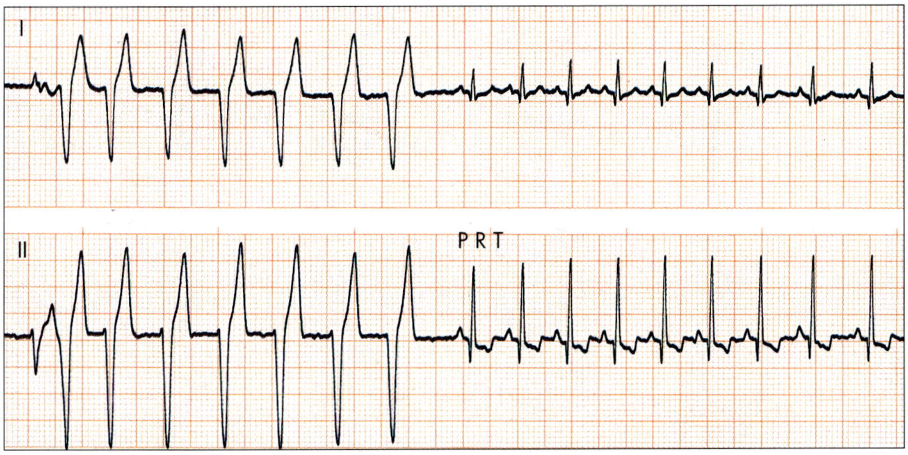

23.29 ECG from a Labrador retriever with a splenic haemangiosarcoma. There is paroxysmal ventricular tachycardia (VT). VT is commonly seen with abdominal disorders, especially those involving the spleen. At this slow rate of discharge, the value of therapy is debatable.

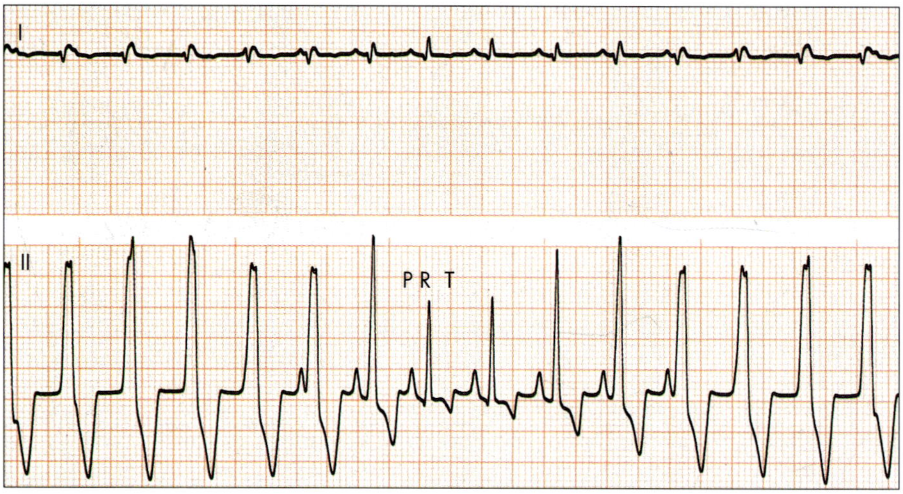

23.30 ECG recorded at 0.5 cm/mV from a cocker spaniel with dilated cardiomyopathy. There is variable atrioventricular dissociation due to slow ventricular tachycardia, with a period of normal sinus 'capture' of the ventricular rhythm. Elsewhere, P waves are seen to wander into and out of QRS complexes. Again, the value of therapy for this rhythm is debatable.

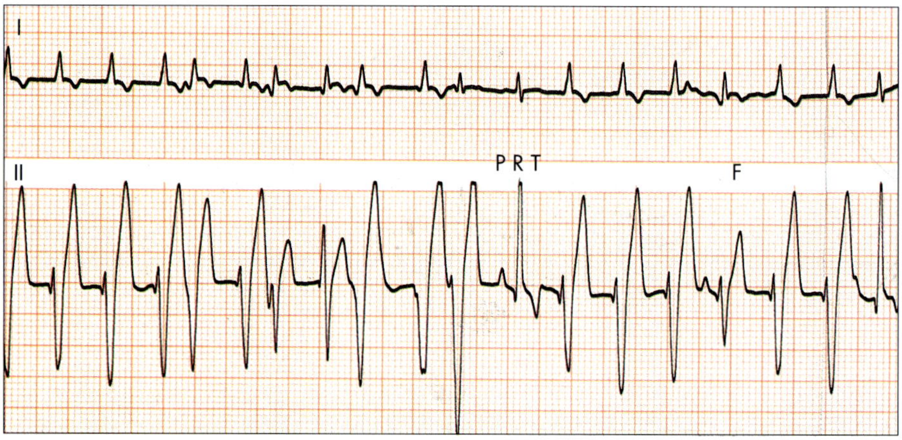

23.31 ECG from a 9-year-old golden retriever with pulmonary thrombosis following surgery to remove a splenic tumour. There is rapid ventricular tachycardia with polymorphic ventricular complexes, a fusion beat (F) and one 'capture' beat (marked). This dog died soon after this recording, despite aggressive therapy.

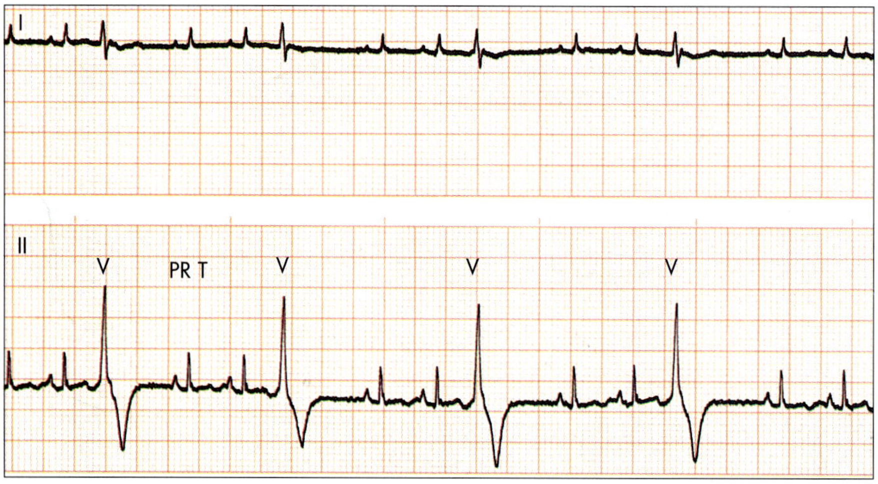

23.32 ECG from a cat with a splenic tumour. There are regular ventricular premature complexes (V).

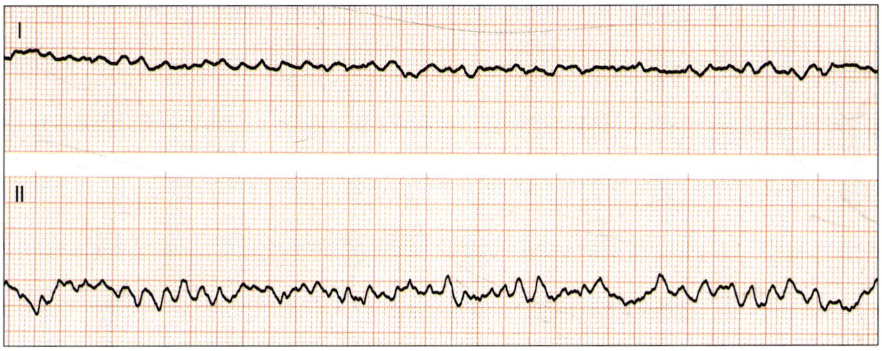

23.33 ECG from a golden retriever with cardiac arrest. due to ventricular fibrillation. However, this must be differentiated from artifacts such as electrode displacement or shivering. Defibrillation is the only effective therapy. (Courtesy Virginia Luis Fuentes.)

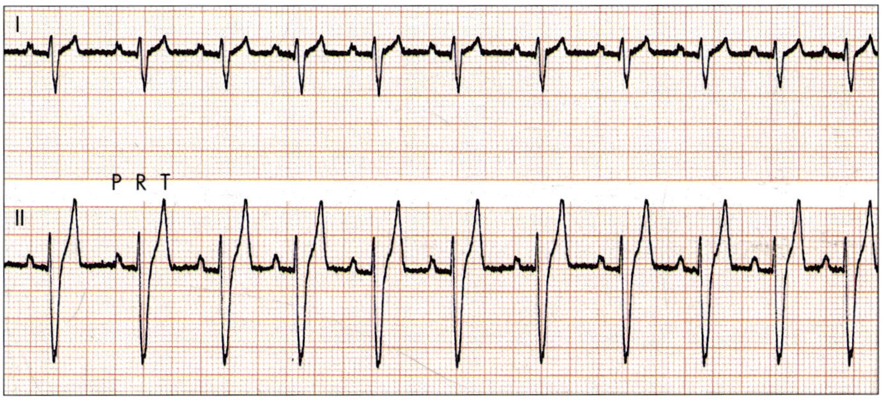

23.34 ECG recorded at 0.5 cm/mV from a symptomless aged greyhound, with right-bundle branch block of unknown aetiology. There is also sinus arrhythmia at a heart rate of about 100 bpm.

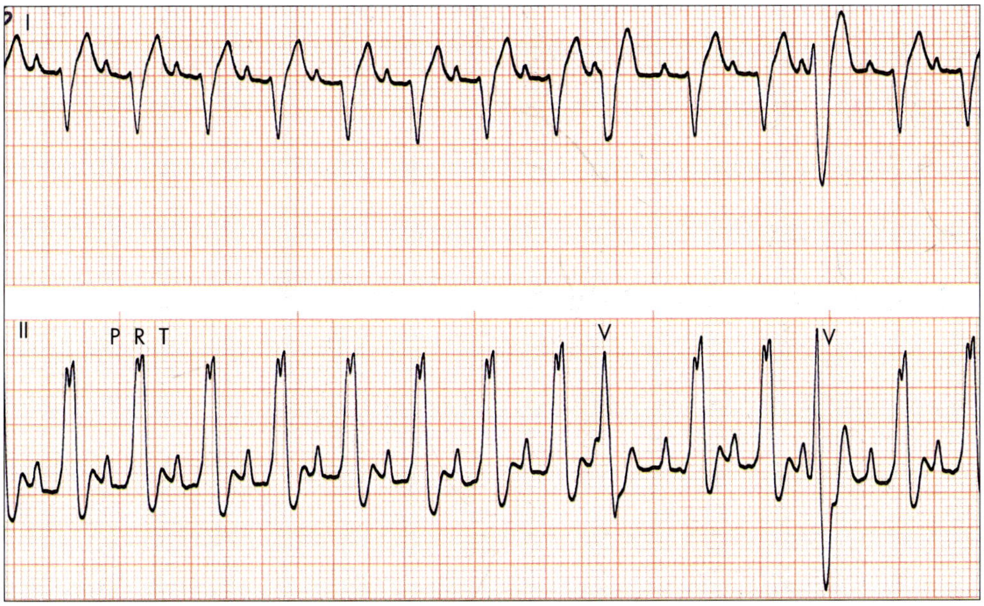

23.35 ECG from a cocker spaniel with dilated cardiomyopathy. There is an advanced intraventricular conduction disturbance with ventricular premature complexes (V). (Courtesy Virginia Luis Fuentes.)

Appendices

Applications for Cardiovascular Drugs			
Type of drug	**Drugs**	**Principal effects**	**Examples of use**
Cardiotonics	Digitalis glycosides (digoxin, digitoxin)	Positive inotropic drug, neurotropic drug (increases vagal tone and reduces sympathetic tone), slows heart rate	CHF due to dilated cardiomyopathy, chronic valvular disease, atrial fibrillation
	Dobutamine	Positive inotropic drug	Cardiogenic shock, severe CHF
	Amrinone	Positive inotropic drug/vasodilator	Cardiogenic shock, severe CHF
Diuretics	Furosemide (frusemide)	Diuretic	Pulmonary oedema, ascites, pleural effusion
	Hydrochlorothiazide & spironolactone	Combination diuretic, antagonizes aldosterone, retains potassium	Refractory ascites or pleural effusion due to CHF
Vasodilators	Hydralazine	Systemic arteriolar vasodilator, decreases left ventricular afterload, reduces mitral regurgitation	Mitral regurgitation, pulmonary oedema, concurrent systemic hypertension
	Nitroglycerine ointment	Systemic venodilator, pools blood in systemic veins	Pulmonary oedema, left-sided CHF
	Enalapril, Captopril, Lisinopril	Angiotensin converting enzyme inhibitors, vasodilators, decrease aldosterone	Chronic CHF due to cardiomyopathy or valvular heart disease
	Sodium nitroprusside	Direct arteriolar and venodilator	Emergency therapy of pulmonary oedema
Calcium-channel antagonists	Diltiazem Amlodipine besylate	Vasodialtor/antihypertensive. Decreases AV nodal conduction, improves ventricular relaxation, vasodilator	Atrial fibrillation, hypertrophic cardiomyopathy, hypertension
	Verapamil	Decreases AV nodal conduction	Acute i.v. therapy of supraventricular tachycardia
Beta blockers	Propranolol, atenolol, nadolol, metoprolol	Decreases heart rate, slows AV nodal conduction, decreases outflow obstruction	Hypertrophic cardiomyopathy, atrial fibrillation, antiarrhythmic therapy
Anti-arrhythmic drugs	Lidocaine (lignocaine), procainamide, quinidine, mexiletine, tocainide, amiodarone, sotalol	Perscribed primarily for control of ventricular tachydysrhythmias	Cardiac arrhythmias

A.1 Applications for Cardiovascular Drugs.

Dosages for Cardiovascular Drugs		
DRUG	**PREPARATION(S)**	**USUAL DOSAGE [*]**
AMIODARONE	Cordarone: 200 mg tablets	5–15 mg/kg, TID
AMLODIPINE	Norvasc 2.5 mg tablet	CAT – $^1/_4$ of 2.5 mg tablet daily
AMRINONE	Inocor: 5 mg/ml (20 ml vials)	1–3 mg/kg, IV followed by 30–100 µg/kg/min infusion
ATENOLOL	Tenormin: 25, 50 mg tablets	DOG – 6.25–25 mg q12h CAT – 6.25–12.5 mg daily
ATROPINE	0.4 mg/ml for injection	0.01–0.04 mg/kg. IV, IM, SQ
CAPTOPRIL	Capoten: 12.5, 25, 50 mg tablets	DOG, CAT – 0.5–2.0 (to 3.0) mg/kg q8h
DIGOXIN	Lanoxin, Cardoxin, 0.125, 0.25, 0.5 mg tablets; 0.05mg/ml and 0.15 mg/ml elixirs; 0.25 mg/ml Lanoxin for injection	Maintenance dose – DOG – 0.0055 – 0.011 mg/kg q12h; or 0.22 mg/sq metre body surface area q12h CAT – 0.0035 to 0.0055 mg/kg once or twice daily; Tablet (0.125 mg) – $^1/_4$ tablet daily or bid HORSE – 1.0 mg total IV bid; 2.0–3.5 mg/100 kg BW, once daily (in feed)
DILTIAZEM	Dilzem, Cardizem: 30, 60, 90, 120 mg tablets	DOG – 0.5–1.3 mg/kg q8h CAT – 0.5–2.0 mg/kg q8–12h
DOBUTAMINE	Dobutrex: 250 mg (20 ml) vial for injection	DOG – 2.5–20 µg constant rate IV infusion CAT – 2.5–10 µg/kg/min constant rate infusion
DOPAMINE	Intropin 200, 400 and 800 mg vials for injection	2–10 µg/kg/min, constant rate IV infusion
ENALAPRIL	Enacord; Cardiovet: 2.5, 5, 10, 20 mg tablets	DOG, CAT – 0.25–0.5 mg/kg once or twice daily
EPINEPHRINE	Adrenaline, 1:10,000 (0.1 mg/ml) & 1:1000 (1 mg/ml)	IV dose – 20 µg/kg
ESMOLOL	Brevibloc: 100 mg/ml – 10 ml vial	DOG, CAT – 25–150 µg/kg/min following a loading dose of 75–100 µg/kg administered over 3 minutes
FUROSEMIDE (FRUSEMIDE)	Lasix: 20, 40, 80 mg tablets; 1% syrup (10 mg/ml); 50 mg/ml ampoules	DOG – 2–6 mg/kg repeated q8–12h as needed (IV, IM, SQ, oral) CAT, HORSE – 1–4 mg/kg repeated q12h as needed (IV, IM, SQ, oral)
HYDRALAZINE	Apresoline: 10, 25, 50 mg tablets	DOG – 1–3 mg/kg q12h (initial dose 0.5 mg/kg, titrate to effect or to at least 1 mg/kg q12h)
HYDROCHLORO-THIAZIDE/ SPIRONOLACTON E	Hydrodiuril, Vitidrex: 25, 50 mg tablets; Aldactazide: 25 mg HCT combined with 25 mg spironolactone	DOG, CAT – 2–4 mg/kg once or twice daily (of either thiazide or combined product)
ISOSORBIDE DINITRATE	Sorbitrate oral tabs, Isordil: 5, 10 mg tablets	DOG – 2.5 to 5 mg bid

A.2 Cardiovascular drugs. *N.B. This list is a guide only. Preparations vary from country to country.

Cardiovascular Drugs		
DRUG	**PREPARATION(S)**	**USUAL DOSAGE [*]**
LIDOCAINE (LIGNOCAINE)	Xylocaine, Lidocaine USP: 2% (20 mg/ml) for injection (without epinephrine)	DOG – 2 mg/kg IV up to 8 mg/kg over 10 min; 25–75 (occasionally up to 100) μg /kg/min constant rate IV infusion CAT and HORSE – 0.25–0.75 mg/kg IV over 3–5-min
LISINOPRIL	Prinivil: 2.5, 5, 10, 20 mg tablets	DOG – 0.25–0.5 mg/kg daily
MEXILETINE	Mexitil: 150, 200, 250 mg capsules	DOG – 5–8 mg/kg q8–12h
MORPHINE SULPHATE	15 mg/ml (5–15 mg/ml ampoules)	DOG – 0.1–0.25 mg/kg, IV, IM
NADOLOL	Corgard: 20, 40, 80, 120 mg tablets	DOG, CAT – 0.25–0.5 mg/kg q12h
NITROGLYCERINE OINTMENT (2%)	Nitrol, Nitro-bid, Nitrostat Percutol: one inch ≡ 15 mg; Minitran transderm patches 2.5, 5, 10, 15 mg/24 h	DOG – 4–12 mg (up to 15 mg) topically q12h CAT – 2–4 mg topically q12h (doses approximate)
PROCAINAMIDE	Pronestyl (-SR); Procan SR: capsules & tablets (SR): 250, 375, 500 mg	DOG – 2mg/kg IV to a maximum of 20 mg/kg over 30-min; 25–40 μg/kg/min IV infusion; 8–20 mg/kg, IM q4-6h or orally q6–8h CAT – 3–8 mg/kg, IM or orally q6–8h
PROPRANOLOL	Inderal LA, 1 mg ampoule for injection; 10, 20, 40, 60, 80 mg tablets; Inderal LA capsules – 60, 80, 120, 160 mg	DOG – 0.2–1.0 mg/kg orally q8h CAT – 2.5–5.0 mg orally tid; IV dose: 20–60 μg/kg over 5–10 min
TOCAINIDE	Tonocard: 400, 600 mg tablets	DOG – 10–20 mg/kg q8h
QUINIDINE	Quinidine gluconate (80 mg/ml for injection), Quinidex (sulphate – sustained release) and Quinora (sulphate) 300 mg tablets [= 250 mg Q-base], Quinaglute (gluconate) 324 mg [= 202 mg Q-base]	DOG – 6–20 mg/kg IM, q6h; 6–20 mg/kg orally q6–8h (Note: 'base-equivalent' of quinidine varies with the quinidine salt) HORSE – 0.5–1.0 mg/kg IV; 2 gm/100 kg bodyweight q2–6h to effect COW – 40 mg/kg in 4L sterile water; 1 L/h to effect
SODIUM BICARBONATE	Sodium bicarbonate: 8.4% (= 1 mEq/ml of $NaHCO_3$)	0.5–1 mEq/kg IV or as guided by blood gas analysis
SOTALOL	Betapace: 80, 160, 240 mg tablets	DOG – 0.5–1.0 mg/kg bid
SPIRONO-LACTONE	Aldactone: 25, 50, 100 mg tablets	DOG – 2–4 mg/kg orally daily
THEOPHYLLINE and related salts	Corvental–D, Theo-dur, Slo-phyllin; Choledyl (oxtriphyllin); aminophyllin(e): 100, 200 [300, 400] mg tablets; Aminophylline 250 mg/10 ml vials	DOG – 8–10 mg/kg orally q8h; 6–10 mg/kg IV slowly CAT – 6–10 mg/kg orally q12h
VERAPAMIL	Cordilox Isoptin 5, 10 mg ampules for injection; Isoptin, Calan 40, 80, 120 mg tablets	DOG – 0.05 mg/kg, IV every 10–30 min to a maximum cumulative dose of 0.15 mg/kg; oral dose is uncertain CAT – as per dog

Congenital Heart Disease in Animals – Summary of Essential Facts

Defect and effect	Lesions – observed at necropsy or by echo- or angiography	History	Pulse	Auscultation	Thoracic radiographs	ECG	Doppler studies	Cardiac catheterization findings
PDA (volume overload; left-to-right shunt)	Persistent ductus arteriosus (between descending Ao & PA) Left heart dilatation & hypertrophy	Canine > feline Possible left-sided CHF Most common heart defect in dogs	↑	Continuous murmur detected over the left craniodorsal base (i.e. over the main PA)	↑ PA, LA, LV Dilated descending Ao. Pulmonary overcirculation	LA ↑ LV ↑	High-velocity, continuous flow in PA; ↑ transmitral and transaortic RBC velocities	Oxygen step-up in the PA; ↑ LVEDP from volume overload of the LV
VSD (volume overload; left-to-right shunt)	Defect is usually subaortic and beneath the TV (high on ventricular septum); defect size determines clinical significance	All species affected; the most common cardiac defect of large animals and cats; possible left-sided CHF	N	Holosystolic murmur over the right sternal border; also systolic murmur of relative pulmonic stenosis over left cranial dorsal cardiac base	↑ PA, LA, LV +/– RV ↑ Pulmonary overcirculation	Vari-able	High-velocity systolic flow across VSD into RV; ↑ velocities across mitral & pulmonic valves	Oxygen step-up in the RV; ↑ LVEDP from volume overload of LV; variable RV pressures
ASD (volume overload; left-to-right shunt)	Ostium secundum (in fossa ovale) or ostium primum lesion (lower atrial septum) RV eccentric hypertrophy	Ruminants & cats > horses or dogs; possible right-sided CHF; (cyanosis if concurrent obstructive TV or pulmonic valve)	N	Systolic ejection murmur of relative PS detected over left craniodorsal base; no murmur from shunt across the ASD owing to low velocity of shunted blood	↑ RA, RV, PA +/– LA ↑ Pulmonary overcirculation	RA ↑ RV ↑	Low-velocity shunt flow across the ASD; high-velocity flow across the tricuspid and pulmonic valves	Oxygen step-up at level of right atrium (compared to haemoglobin saturation in vena cava); ↑ RVEDP due to volume overload
Pulmonic stenosis (pressure overload of RV)	Malformed, often hypoplastic pulmonic valve Concentric RVH	Lesion most common in dogs; signs: Sudden death Syncope Right-sided CHF	N	Ejection murmur of PS detected over pulmonic valve and left craniodorsal cardiac base	↑ RV +/– RA Dilated PA (post-stenotic dilation) Pulmonary undercirculation	RV ↑	High-velocity systolic flow across the stenotic valve	Systolic pressure gradient RV to PA; giant a-wave in RA pressure trace; elevated RVEDP
Aortic stenosis (pressure overload of LV)	Congenital subaortic fibrous obstruction Concentric LVH	Very common in dogs; signs: Syncope Sudden death Left-sided CHF	↓	Ejection murmur near aortic valve; often radiates loudly over the right cardiac base (ascending aorta)	↑ LV Dilated ascending aorta (post-stenotic flow disturbances)	LV ↑ Often VPCs	High-velocity systolic flow across stenosis	Systolic pressure gradient LV to aorta; elevated LVEDP
Tetralogy of Fallot (right-to-left shunt)	Unrestrictive VSD + PS + RV hypertrophy +'over-riding aorta'	Dogs, cats, horses, cattle Cyanosis	N	Ejection murmur of PS; VSD not heard due to equal RV and LV pressures	↑ RV ↓ Pulmonary circulation	RV ↑	Low-velocity systolic flow from RV to LV; high-velocity flow across PS	Systolic pressure gradient across RV to PA; equilibration of RV and LV presssure
Mitral & tricuspid valve malformations	Variety of lesions of valve & support apparatus causing an incompetence +/– valve stenosis	Dogs, cats, less often large animals	N	Valvular regurgitation murmurs over affected valve areas (left apex or tricuspid area)	Similar to acquired mitral or tricuspid regurgitation = atrial + ventricular dilatation	LV ↑ (MR) or RV ↑ (TR)	High velocity systolic flow from ventricle to atrium across AV valve; if stenotic valve: increased diastolic inflow velocity	Elevated ventricular EDP from volume overload; giant C–V waves in atrial pressure curves; if stenosis: diastolic gradient from atrium to ventricle detected

A.3 Congenital heart disease in animals – summary of essential facts.

References and Further Reading

General References

Birchard SJ and Sherding RG (Eds): *Saunder's Manual of Small Animal Practice.* Philadelphia, W.B. Saunders, 1994. 396–606.

Bonagura JD (Ed): Symposium on cardiology. *Vet Clin N Am (Equine Pract)* 1985; **1**:265–435.

Bonagura JD (Ed): *Cardiology.* Churchill Livingstone, 1987.

Bonagura JD (ed): *Kirk's Current Veterinary Therapy XII.* Philadelphia, W.B. Saunders, 1995. 771–927.

Bonagura JD: Cardiovascular Diseases; 1995. in *The Cat: Diseases and Clinical Management* 1995. Ed: Sherding RG. W.B. Saunders, Philadelphia. 819–946.

Bonagura JD, Muir WW: The Cardiovascular System; in *Equine Anesthesia.* 1991. Eds: Muir WW and Hubbell JAE. Mosby Year Book, St Louis. 39–104.

Braunwald E (Ed) : *Heart Disease: A Textbook of Cardiovascular Medicine.* Philadelphia, W.B. Saunders, 1992.

Edwards NJ: *Bolton's Handbook of Canine and Feline Electrocardiography.* Philadelphia, W.B. Saunders, 1987.

Ettinger SJ and Feldman EC: *Textbook of Veterinary Internal Medicine.* Philadelphia, W.B. Saunders, 1995. 844–1068.

Fox PR (Ed): *Canine and Feline Cardiology.* New York, Churchill Livingstone, 1988.

Kirk RW and Bonagura JD (Eds): *Kirk's Current Veterinary Therapy XI.* Philadelphia, W.B. Saunders, 1992. 646–816.

Liu SK: Acquired cardiac lesions leading to congestive heart failure in the cat. *Am J Vet Res* 1970; **31**: 2071–88.

Miller MS and Tilley LP: *Manual of Canine and Feline Cardiology.* Philadelphia, W.B. Saunders, 1995.

Opie LH: *The heart: Physiology and Metabolism.* New York, Raven Press, 1991.

Opie LH: *Drugs for the Heart.* 4th edition. Philadelphia, W.B. Saunders. 1995.

Cardiovascular Pathology

(See also reference list at the end of Chapter 2)

Else RW, Holmes JR: Cardiac pathology in the horse. I: Gross pathology. *Equine Vet J* 1972; **4**:1–8.

Liu SK: Pathology of feline heart disease. *Vet Clin N Am (Small Anim Pract)* 1977; **7**:323–39.

Marcus LC, Ross JN: Microscopic lesions in the hearts of aged horses and mules. *Vet Pathol* 1967; **4**:162–85.

Van Mierop LSH: Pathology and pathogenesis of the common cardiac malformations. *Cardiol Clin* 1970; **2**:28–59.

Whitney JC: Cardiovascular pathology. *J Small Anim Pract* 1967; **8**:459–65.

Heart Failure

Bonagura JD: Congestive-heart-failure in the horse. *Proceedings of the Eleventh Annual Veterinary Medical Forum,* American College of Veterinary Internal Medicine, Lakewood, Colorado 1993; 614–8.

Clinical Examination and Diagnostic Studies of the Cardiovascular System

Auscultation and clinical examination

Bonagura JD: Equine heart disease. An overview. *Vet Clin N Am (Equine Pract)* 1985; **1**:267–74.

Fregin GF: Medical evaluation of the cardiovascular system. *Vet Clin N Am (Equine Pract)* 1992; **8**:329–46.

Gerring EL: Auscultation of the equine heart. *Equine Vet Educ* 1990; **2**:22–3.

Harpster NK: Clinical examination of the feline cardiovascular system. *Vet Clin N Am* 1977; **7**:241–256.

Patteson MW, Cripps PJ: A survey of cardiac auscultatory findings in horses. *Equine Vet J* 1993; **25**:409–15.

Reef VB: Clinical approach to poor performance in horses. *Proceedings of the Seventh Annual Veterinary Medical Forum, American College of Veterinary Internal Medicine, Lakewood, Colorado* 1989;566–9.

Reef VB: The significance of cardiac auscultatory findings in horses – insight into the age-old dilemma. *Equine Vet J* 1993; **25**: 393–4.

Cardiac Radiography

Buchanan JW, Bucheler J: Vertebral scale system to measure canine heart size in radiographs. *J Amer Vet Med Assn* 1995; **206**:194–9.

Stickle RL, Anderson LK: Diagnosis of common congenital heart anomalies in the dog using survey and nonselective contrast radiography. *Vet Radiology* 1987; **28**:6–12.

Suter PF, Lord PF: Cardiac diseases; in *Thoracic Radiography of the Dog and Cat.* 1984. Ed: Suter PF. Published by the author (Peter F. Suter), Wettswil, Switzerland. 351–516.

Cardiac Catheterization and Angiocardiography

Bonagura JD, Meyers CW, Pensinger RR: Angiocardiography. *Vet Clin N Am (Small Anim Pract)* 1982; **12**:239–58.

Buchanan JW, Patterson DF: Selective angiocardiography in dogs with congenital cardiovascular disease. *J Am Vet Radiol Soc* 1965; **6**:21.

Electrocardiography

Bonagura JD, Miller MS: Electrocardiography; in *Equine Sports Medicine.* 1985. Ed: Jones WE. Lea and Febiger, Philadelphia. 89–106.

Fregin GF: The equine electrocardiogram with standardized body and limb positions. *Cornell Vet* 1982; **72**:304–24.

Goodwin JK, Lombard CW: The electrocardiographic and radiographic features of common congenital heart defects. *Vet Med* 1990; **85**:48–62.

Hilwig RW: Cardiac arrhythmias in the horse. *J Am Vet Med Assoc* 1977; **170**:153–63.

Echocardiography

Bonagura JD, O'Grady MR, Herring DS: Echocardiography: I - Principles of interpretation;II - Congenital heart disease; III - Acquired heart disease; *Vet Clin N Am (Small Anim Pract)* 1985; **15**:1177–1224.

Brown DJ, Knight DH, King RR: Use of pulsed-wave Doppler echocardiography to determine aortic and pulmonary velocity and flow variables in clinically normal dogs. *Am J Vet Res* 1991; **52**:543–50.

Darke PGG: Doppler echocardiography. *J Small Anim Pract* 1992; **33**:104–12.

Fox PR, Bond BR, Peterson ME: Echocardiographic reference values in healthy cats sedated with ketamine hydrochloride. *Am J Vet Res* 1985, **46**:1479–84.

Long KJ, Bonagura JD, Darke PG: Standardised imaging technique for guided M-mode and Doppler echocardiography in the horse. *Equine Vet J* 1992; **24**:226–35.

Moise NS: Doppler echocardiographic evaluation of congenital cardiac disease. *J Vet Intern Med* 1989; **3**:195–207.

O'Grady MR, Bonagura JD, Powers JD, *et al*: Quantitative cross-sectional echocardiography in the normal dog. *Vet Radiology* 1986; **27**:34–49.

Thomas WP: Two-dimensional, real-time echocardiography in the dog. *Vet Radiology* 1984; **25**:50–64.

Thomas WP, Gaber CE, Jacobs GJ, *et al*: Recommendations for standards in transthoracic two-dimensional echocardiography in the dog and cat. Echocardiography Committee of the Specialty of Cardiology, American College of Veterinary Internal Medicine. *J Vet Intern Med* 1993; **7**:247–52.

Yuill CDM, O'Grady MR: Doppler-derived velocity of blood flow across the cardiac valves in the normal dog. *Canad J Vet Res* 1991, **55**:185–192.

Congenital Heart Disease

Patterson DF: Hereditary congenital heart defects in dogs. *J Small Anim Pract* 1989; **30**:153–65.

Septal Defects

Bolton GR, Ettinger SJ, Liu SK: Tetralogy of Fallot in three cats. *J Am Vet Med Assoc* 1972; **160**:1622–31.

Lombard CW, Scarratt WK, Buergelt CD: Ventricular septal defects in the horse. *J Am Vet Med Assoc* 1983; **183**:562–65.

Reef VB: Cardiovascular disease in the equine neonate. *Vet Clin N Am (Equine Pract)* 1985; **1**:117–29.

Ringwald RJ, Bonagura JD: Tetralogy of Fallot in the dog: clinical findings in 13 cases. *J Am Anim Hosp Assoc* 1988; **24**:33–43.

Patent Ductus Arteriosus

Birchard SJ, Bonagura JD, Fingland RB: Results of ligation of patent ductus arteriosus in dogs: 201 cases (1969-1988). *J Am Vet Med Assoc* 1990; **196**:2011–13.

Cohen JS, Tilley LP, Liu SK, *et al*: Patent ductus arteriosus in five cats. *J Am Anim Hosp Assoc* 1975; **11**:95–101.

Eyster GE, Eupler JT, Cords GB, *et al*: Patent ductus arteriosus in the dog: characteristics of occurrence and results of surgery in one hundred consecutive cases. *J Am Vet Med Assoc* 1976; **168**:435–8.

Patterson DF, Pyle RL, Buchanan JW, *et al*: Hereditary patient ductus arteriosus and its sequelae in the dog. *Circulation Res* 1971; **29**:1–13.

Pyle RL, Park RD, Alexander, A.F. *et al*: Patent ductus arteriosus with pulmonary hypertension in the dog. 1981, *J Am Vet Med Assoc.* **178**:565–71.

Congenital Valvular Heart Disease

Fingland RB, Bonagura JD, Myer CW: Pulmonic stenosis in the dog: 29 cases (1975–1984). *J Am Vet Med Assoc* 1986; **189**:218–26.

Hamlin RL, Smetzer DL, Smith CR: Congenital mitral insufficiency in the dog. *J Am Vet Med Assoc* 1965; **146**:1088–1100.

Lehmkuhl LB, Ware WA, Bonagura JD: Mitral stenosis in 15 dogs. *J Vet Intern Med* 1994; **8**:2-17. **35**:169–72.

Liu SK, Tilley LP: Dysplasia of the tricuspid valve in the dog and cat. *J Am Vet Med Assoc* 1976; **169**:625–9.

Roth L: Bacterial aortic valvular endocarditis associated with subaortic stenosis. *J Small Anim Pract* 1994; **35**:169–72.

Stepien RL, Bonagura JD: Aortic stenosis clinical findings in six cats. *J Small Anim Pract* 1991; **32**:341–50.

Valvular Heart Disease – Acquired

Bishop SP, Cole CR, Smetzer DL: Functional and morphologic pathology of equine aortic insufficiency. *Vet Pathol* 1966; **3**:137–58.

Buchanan JW: Chronic Valvular Disease (Endocardiosis) in dogs. *Adv Vet Sci Compar Med* 1979; **21**:75–106.

Holmes JR, Miller PJ: Three cases of ruptured mitral valve chordae in the horse. *Equine Vet J* 1984; **16**:125–35.

Miller PJ, Holmes JR: Observations on seven cases of mitral insufficiency in the horse. *Equine Vet J* 1985; **17**:181–90.

Infective Endocarditis

Buergelt CD, Cooley AJ, Hines SA, *et al*: Endocarditis in six horses. *Vet Pathol* 1985; **22**:333–7.

Elwood CM, Cobb MA, Stepien RL: Clinical and echocardiographic findings in 10 dogs with vegetative bacterial-endocarditis. *J Small Anim Pract* 1993; **34**:420–27.

Roussel AJ, Kasari TR: Bacterial endocarditis in large animals. Part II. Incidence, causes, clinical signs, and pathologic findings. *Compend Cont Educ Pract Vet* 1989; **11**:769–74.

Sisson D, Thomas WP: Endocarditis of the aortic valve in the dog. *J Am Vet Med Assoc* 1984; **184**:570–7.

Myocardial Diseases

Atkins CE, Gallo AM, Kurzman ID, *et al*: Risk factors, clinical signs, and survival in cats with a clinical diagnosis of idiopathic hypertrophic cardiomyopathy: 74 cases (1985–1989). *J Am Vet Med Assoc* 1992; **201**:613–18.

King JM, Roth L, Haschek WM: Myocardial necrosis secondary to neural lesions in domestic animals. *J Am Vet Med Assoc* 1982; **180**:144–8.

Liu SK, Maron BJ, Tilley LP: Hypertrophic cardiomyopathy in the dog. *Am J Path* 1979; **94**: 497–507.

Liu S, Peterson ME, Fox PR: Hypertrophic cardiomyopathy and hyperthyroidism in the cat. *J Am Vet Med Assoc* 1984; **185**:52–7.

Lombard CW: Echocardiographic and clinical signs of canine dilated cardiomyopathy. *J Small Anim Pract* 1984; **25**:59–70.

Monnet E, Orton EC, Salman M, *et al*: Idiopathic dilated cardiomyopathy in dogs – survival and prognostic indicators. *J Vet Intern Med* 1995; **9**:12–17.

Pion PD, Kittleson MD, Thomas WP, *et al*: Clinical findings in cats with dilated cardiomyopathy and relationship of findings to taurine deficiency. *J Am Vet Med Assoc* 1992; **201**:267–74.

Pericardial Diseases

Berg RJ, Wingfield W: Pericardial effusion in the dog: a review of 42 cases. *J Am Anim Hosp Associ* 1984; **20**:721–30.

Bernard W, Reef V, Clark ES, *et al*: Pericarditis in horses: Six cases (1982-1986). *J Am Vet Med Assoc* 1990; **196**:468–71.

Cobb MA, Brownlie SE: Intrapericardial neoplasia in 14 dogs. *J Small Anim Pract* 1992; **33**:309–16.

McGuirk SM: Treatment of cardiovascular disease in cattle. [Review]. *Vet Clin N Am (Food Anim Pract)* 1991; **7**:729–46.

Thomas WP, Reed JR, Bauer TG, *et al*: Constrictive pericardial disease in the dog. *J Am Vet Med Assoc* 1984; **184**:546–53.

Thomas WP, Sisson D, Bauer TG, *et al*: Detection of cardiac masses in dogs by two-dimensional echocardiography. *Vet Radiology* 1984; **25**:65–72.

Cor Pulmonale

Angel KL, Tyler JW: Pulmonary hypertension and cardiac insufficiency in three cows with primary lung disease. *J Vet Intern Med* 1992; **6**:214–19.

Henry CJ, Dillon R: Heartworm disease in dogs. *J Amer Vet Med Assn* 1994; **204**:1148–51.

Vascular Disorders

Helphrey ML: Vascular ring anomalies in the dog. *Vet Clin N Am (Sm Anim Pract)* 1979; **9**:207–18.

Hosgood G: Arteriovenous fistulas: pathophysiology, diagnosis, and treatment. *Compend Cont Educ Pract Vet* 1989; **11**:625–36.

Kelly DF, Gaskell CJ, Lee MA: Arteriosclerosis of extramural coronary arteries in Labradors with congestive heart failure. *J Small Anim Pract* 1992; **33**:437–42.

Cardiac Arrhythmias

Holmes JR, Henigan M, Williams RB, et al: Paroxysmal atrial fibrillation in racehorses. *Equine Vet J* 1986; **18**:37–42.

McGuirk SM, Muir WW: Diagnosis and treatment of cardiac arrhythmias. *Vet Clin N Am (Equine Pract)* 1985; **1**: 353–70.

Muir WW: Antiarrhythmic drugs. Treatment of cardiac arrhythmias. *Vet Clin N Am (Small Anim Pract)* 1991; **21**:957–87.

Reef VB, Reimer JM, Spencer PA: Treatment of atrial fibrillation in horses – new perspectives. *J Vet Intern Med* 1995; **9**:57–67.

Reimer JM, Reef VB, Sweeney RW: Ventricular arrhythmias in horses: 21 cases (1984-1989). *J Am Vet Med Assoc* 1992; **201**: 1237–43.

Index